MW01064514

Clinical Guide to Antineoplastic Therapy

A Chemotherapy Handbook

Edited by
Mary Magee Gullatte, RN, MN, ANP, AOCN®, FAAMA

To Wesley & Shirley

Mary Gullatte RN 3/17/2004

Oncology Nursing Society
Pittsburgh, PA

ONS Publishing Division
Publisher: Leonard Mafrica, MBA, CAE
Technical Publications Editor: Barbara Sigler, RN, MNEd
Senior Staff Editor: Lisa M. George, BA
Copy Editor: Krista Ramsey
Creative Services Assistant: Dany Sjoen

Clinical Guide to Antineoplastic Therapy: A Chemotherapy Handbook

Copyright © 2001 by the Oncology Nursing Society

All rights reserved. No part of the material protected by this copyright may be repro-
duced or utilized in any form, electronic or mechanical, including photocopying, recording, or by an information storage and retrieval system, without written permission from the copyright owner. For information, write to the Oncology Nursing
Society, 501 Holiday Drive, Pittsburgh, PA 15220-2749.

Library of Congress Control Number: 2001098481

ISBN 1-890504-25-4

Publisher's Note
This book is published by the Oncology Nursing Society (ONS). ONS neither repre-
sents nor guarantees that the practices described herein will, if followed, ensure safe
and effective patient care. The recommendations contained in this book reflect ONS's
judgment regarding the state of general knowledge and practice in the field as of the
date of publication. The recommendations may not be appropriate for use in all
circumstances. Those who use this book should make their own determinations regarding specific safe and appropriate patient-care practices, taking into account the
personnel, equipment, and practices available at the hospital or other facility at which
they are located. The editors and publisher cannot be held responsible for any liability incurred as a consequence from the use or application of any of the contents of this
book. Figures and tables are used as examples only. They are not meant to be all-
inclusive, nor do they represent endorsement of any particular institution by ONS.
Mention of specific products and opinions related to those products do not indicate
or imply endorsement by ONS.

ONS publications are originally published in English. Permission has been granted by
the ONS Board of Directors for foreign translation. (Individual tables and figures
that are reprinted or adapted require additional permission from the original source.)
However, because translations from English may not always be accurate and precise,
ONS disclaims any responsibility for inaccurate translations. Readers relying on precise information should check the original English version.

Printed in the United States of America

Oncology Nursing Society

A special thanks to God, from whom I have received many special blessings. I thank my father and mother, Bilbo and Hazel Magee, for instilling in me a strong work ethic, integrity, a sense of self esteem, and a "you can" attitude. To my immediate family, husband, Rodney, Sr., and children, Rodney, Jr., and Ronda, thanks for always being there for me and allowing me to pursue my personal and professional aspirations. You are my source of joy, love, and support always. To my brothers and sisters, Selma, Billy, Lester, Amanda, Winnie, Wallace, Hope, Donna, and Sue Ann, who have helped me to grow as a sister and friend. To Javonne S. Reese, whose friendship, clerical assistance, and support have been invaluable. To Veda Burns, Reverend Kenneth and Cassandra Marcus, thanks for your spiritual support. I also dedicate this book to the many patients with cancer and their families whose lives I have touched and who have equally touched my life.

To all of you, thanks and God bless you.

CONTRIBUTORS

Joyce Alexander, RN, MSN, AOCN®
Clinical Nurse Specialist, Oncology/
  Bone Marrow Transplant
Halifax Medical Center
Daytona Beach, Florida
Chapter 7. Symptom Management

Delcina Brown, MN, RN, CS, AOCN®
Adult Nurse Practitioner
Oncology Clinical Nurse Specialist
Georgia Cancer Specialists
Atlanta, Georgia
*Chapter 1. Cellular Mechanisms of Chemo-
  therapy*

Mary Jensen Camp, PharmD, BCPS,
  BCOP
Regional Clinical Affairs Manager
Ortho Biotech Products, L.P.
Atlanta, Georgia
Chapter 5. Antineoplastic Agents

Anjeanette Christensen, BA, JD
Law Clerk
The Law Offices of Scott R. Erwin,
  Attorney at Law
DeKalb, Illinois
*Chapter 6. Legal Issues in Chemotherapy
  Administration*

Veronica A. Clarke-Tasker, PhD, RN,
  MBA
Assistant Professor
Howard University College of Pharmacy,
  Nursing and Allied Health Sciences
Division of Nursing
Washington, DC
*Chapter 10. Public and Professional Cancer
  Resources*

Barbara Johnson Farmer, MSN, MSA,
  RN, FNP
Doctoral Fellow
University of Wisconsin-Milwaukee
*Chapter 9. Psychosocial Support of the
  Patient Receiving Chemotherapy*

Marilyn Frank-Stromborg, EdD, JD,
  ANP, FAAN
Chair and Presidential Research
  Professor
School of Nursing
Northern Illinois University
DeKalb, Illinois
*Chapter 6. Legal Issues in Chemotherapy
  Administration*

Janese S. Gaddis, RN, MSN, OCN®
Primary Oncology Nurse
Oncology Ambulatory Clinic
Grady Health System
Atlanta, Georgia
*Chapter 2. Pharmacologic Principles of
  Chemotherapy*

James W. Gilmore, PharmD
Oncology Program Manager
Atlanta Medical Center
Atlanta, Georgia
Chapter 5. Antineoplastic Agents

Mary Magee Gullatte, RN, MN, ANP,
  AOCN®, FAAMA
Director of Nursing–Oncology Services
Winship Cancer Institute, Emory
  University Hospital, and Crawford
  Long Hospital
Atlanta, Georgia
Adjunct Clinical Faculty
Nell Hodgson Woodruff School of
  Nursing
Emory University
Atlanta, Georgia
Adult Nurse Practitioner, Primary Care
  Practice of Imani Vannoy, MD, PC
Marietta, Georgia
*Chapter 2. Pharmacologic Principles of
  Chemotherapy; Chapter 3. Principles and
  Standards of Chemotherapy Administra-
  tion; Chapter 5. Antineoplastic Agents;
  Chapter 8. Clinical Trials*

Annette Humble, MN, RN, CS, AOCN®
Director of Advanced Practice Nursing
Georgia Cancer Specialists
Clinical Adjunct Faculty
Nell Hodgson Woodruff School of Nursing
Emory University
Atlanta, Georgia
Chapter 1. Cellular Mechanisms of Chemotherapy

Donald A. Hutcherson, RPh
Clinical Pharmacist, Hematology/Bone Marrow Transplant
Emory University Hospital
Atlanta, Georgia
Chapter 5. Antineoplastic Agents

Judith Ann Kostka, RN, MS, MBA
Nurse Manager, Oncology Services
Cape Cod Healthcare
Hyannis, Massachusetts
Chapter 8. Clinical Trials

Jennifer S. Webster, MN, RN, CS, AOCN®
Oncology Clinical Nurse Specialist
Adult Nurse Practitioner
Georgia Cancer Specialists
Atlanta, Georgia
Chapter 4. Vascular Access Devices

CONTENTS

Evolving knowledge of cancer genetics and molecular mechanisms of cellular behavior are creating a new paradigm for the treatment of cancer. On a daily basis, scientific discoveries continue to enhance our understanding of the pathophysiology of the cancer process and are facilitating the development of antineoplastic therapies based on specific molecular characteristics of the disease. In addition to standard therapies, targeted interventions increasingly are becoming available for individuals who manifest distinct characteristics of certain types of cancer. Chemotherapy will continue to play a major role in the armamentarium of cancer treatment. New agents, new combinations of agents, and novel delivery strategies will challenge the way patients are currently managed in the clinical setting. In concert with this, supportive care interventions for this population will continue to be optimized.

The effective delivery of cancer chemotherapy requires very specific knowledge and the expertise of a multidisciplinary team. Physicians, oncology nurses, social workers, and pharmacists in particular are integral to the delivery of this service. An ongoing commitment to maintaining current state of the knowledge on the topic is essential to effective practice. Mary Gullatte's *Clinical Guide to Antineoplastic Therapy: A Chemotherapy Handbook* provides an excellent reference for practitioners. Working with a team of multidisciplinary authors with defined expertise in the field, Gullatte has fashioned an extraordinary clinical resource for cancer professionals. The handbook begins with a sound discussion of the theoretical underpinnings and pharmacologic principles of chemotherapy administration. An excellent discussion of the nuances and complexities of drug administration, including a thorough review of vascular access device issues, follows. Standards of practice for chemotherapy administration also are presented. Chapter 5 consists of a collection of drug monographs that outline clinically pertinent information on each of the antineoplastic agents. The easy-to-use format makes this section of the book an extremely practical resource for busy clinicians.

Providing effective supportive interventions to patients receiving chemotherapy is associated with improved outcomes. The development of symptoms from both the disease and treatment is common in this population. As professionals directly involved in chemotherapy administration, oncology nurses are well positioned to assess and manage symptoms. In Chapter 7, readers will find a thoughtful review of the management of symptoms typically associated with chemotherapy administration. In addition, Chapter 9 offers specific information on psychosocial support, providing insight into the complex psychosocial issues that often accompany a cancer diagnosis and the treatment experience. A discussion of caregiver issues and survivorship concerns are unique aspects of this chapter and contribute to its comprehensiveness. Chapter 10 provides excellent resource and referral information, which are particularly relevant in today's healthcare context.

Continued evolution of the knowledge base on cancer treatment and supportive care relies on patient participation in clinical trials, yet national statistics indicate that only a small percentage of patients enroll in studies. All cancer-care professionals have a responsibility to be knowledgeable about the process of clinical cancer investigation so that they can provide accurate and reliable information to patients. Ongoing research programs are leading to discoveries that will pave the way for more effective therapies and future improvements in cancer care. Chapter 8 provides a review of clinical trials and includes information that should be in the repertoire of all cancer professionals. Comprehensive discussions of the informed consent process and additional legal considerations are presented in Chapter 6.

Knowledgeable professionals are essential to the delivery of quality cancer care. An ongoing commitment to ensuring that their knowledge is current is a hallmark of cancer professionals. *Clinical Guide to Antineoplastic Therapy: A Chemotherapy Handbook* is an excellent source of current information for the practicing clinician. Comprehensive in scope and practical in format, the book is destined to become an essential resource and should be required reading for all oncology professionals involved in the preparation and delivery of cancer chemotherapy.

Regina S. Cunningham, MA, RN, AOCN®
Chief Nursing Officer
Director of Ambulatory Services
The Cancer Institute of New Jersey
New Brunswick, New Jersey

As we embrace the new millennium, cancer continues to be the second leading cause of death from disease in the United States. With the tremendous advances in screening, early detection, and treatment in the 20th century, especially in the last decade, the American Cancer Society reported in 2000 an overall decrease in cancer mortality. Advances in pharmacotherapeutic research has placed in the armamentarium of the oncology care team an arsenal of new therapies to prevent and control many of the historical dose-limiting side effects of cancer chemotherapy. With these advances came new challenges and hope for patients with cancer, caregivers, and medical providers.

It is of critical importance that the professional responsible for administering chemotherapy be knowledgeable, competent, and skilled. *Clinical Guide to Antineoplastic Therapy: A Chemotherapy Handbook* is divided into three sections. The first two chapters review the pharmacology of chemotherapy, including cellular mechanisms and growth of cancer cells. Chapters Three through Six cover chemotherapy administration, including more than 70 antineoplastic drug monographs, and a unique section on legal implications of chemotherapy administration. The remaining chapters include information on symptom management, clinical trials, and psychosocial support issues and conclude with a listing of public and professional cancer resources.

Cancer survival statistics indicate that cancer mortality can be reduced by early detection and treatment of most cancers. This reference is intended to be a practical handbook for physicians, nurses, nurse practitioners, physician assistants, and pharmacists involved in the treatment of patients with cancer receiving antineoplastic agents. The information provided on each drug is based on the current use and dosage approved by the manufacturer and U.S. Food and Drug Administration. The practitioner is encouraged to follow prescribed and approved protocols when dosing and administering chemotherapy and to consult other primary literature on chemotherapeutic agents as appropriate. No liability will be assumed for the use of any dosing and scheduling tables in this publication and the absence of typographical errors is not guaranteed.

ACKNOWLEDGMENTS

The editor wishes to express thanks to special individuals and mentors who have had a positive impact on helping to shape her professional growth and practice and for encouraging her to pursue personal and professional goals with persistence and determination.

Nurses: Mary Beth McDowell, Mary F. Woody, Mary Huch, Annette Tardy Morgan, Charlotte McHenry, Laura Porter Kimble, Marla Salmon, Brenda Brown, Robbin Moore, T.K. and Amy Lee, Carrie Gullatte, Sarah Carter, Clara Jenkins, Jessie Anderson, and the late Marsha Kelly.

Oncology nurses: Edith Folsom Honeycutt, Nelza Levine, Rose McGee, Jane Clark, Sandra Millon Underwood, Janice Phillips, Pearl Moore, Cynthia Crank, Ryan Iwamoto, Kevin Sowers, Sharon Krumm, Melba Hill Paschel, Marjorie Kagawa-Singer, Roberta Strohl, Deborah McGuire, Ann Belcher, Susan Baird, Carol Sheridan, Shirley Otto, Marlene Cohen, Brenda Nevidjon, Susan Beck, and all of those nurses with whom I have worked and who have coached and mentored me over the decades.

Physicians: James Bennett, James Fisher, Imani Vannoy, Douglas Murray, Daniel Nixon, Warren Sommerlot, David Lawson, Harold Freeman, Charles Huguley, Ravi Sarma, Leonard Heffner, Elliot Winton, William Wood, Louis Sullivan, Tina Jones, Robert Hermann, Toncred Styblo, James Keller, and Edmond Waller.

I also wish to express sincere gratitude to my employers at Emory University Hospital and Crawford Long Hospital, Alice Vautier, chief nursing officer; John D. Henry, Sr., chief executive officer; and Jonathan Simons, medical director of the Winship Cancer Institute, for their support of my professional growth.

The editor wishes to express deep appreciation to all the contributing authors, consultants, and reviewers of this master work. Everyone was gracious, accommodating, committed, and prompt in the preparation of the manuscripts.

Special thanks to the following reviewers of chapter manuscripts:

Anne E. Belcher, PhD, RN, AOCN®, FAAN
Professor and director of the Undergraduate Program
Department of Nursing
College of Health Professions
Thomas Jefferson University
Philadelphia, Pennsylvania

Colleen Bittinger, RN IV, BSN
Nurse clinician
BMT/Leukemia
Emory University Hospital
Atlanta, Georgia

Georgie Cusack, RN, MSN, AOCN®
Clinical nurse specialist
Clinical Center
National Institutes of Health
Bethesda, Maryland

Michael Fanucchi, MD
Associate professor
Winship Cancer Institute
Emory University School of Medicine
Atlanta, Georgia

W. Gale Gaines, RN IV
Nurse clinician
Hematology/Oncology
Emory University Hospital
Atlanta, Georgia

Lloyd G.Geddes, Jr., MD
Associate professor
Section of Hematology Oncology
Morehouse School of Medicine
Medical director
DeKalb Cancer Treatment Center
Atlanta, Georgia

Ruth Canty Ghotz, RN, MS, AOCN®
Oncology clinical nurse specialist
Hematology/Oncology
Cincinnati Veterans Administration
   Center
Cincinnati, Ohio

David R. Kohler, PharmD
Oncology clinical pharmacy specialist
National Institutes of Health
Bethesda, Maryland

Sharon L. Krumm, PhD, RN
Administrator and director of nursing
The Johns Hopkins Oncology Center
Baltimore, Maryland

David H. Lawson, MD
Associate professor
Winship Cancer Institute
Emory University School of Medicine
Atlanta, Georgia

Helen Mouzon, RN IV
Nurse clinician
Medical Oncology
Crawford Long Hospital
Atlanta, Georgia

Peter Ripley, MD
Principle investigator and medical
director
   Clinical Studies
Cape Cod, Massachusetts

Barbara Rogers, CRNP, MN, AOCN®
Adult oncology nurse practitioner
Fox Chase Cancer Center
Philadelphia, Pennsylvania

Paula Saunders, MSW
Oncology social worker
BMT/Leukemia
Department of Social Services
Emory University Hospital
Atlanta, Georgia

Special thanks to Barbara Sigler and the staff of the ONS Publishing Division for their work on this publication.

CHAPTER 1

Cellular Mechanisms of Chemotherapy

Delcina Brown, MN, RN, CS, AOCN®
Annette Humble, MN, RN, CS, AOCN®

Overview

Cancer continues to be a significant economic and emotional burden on the community in terms of significant expenditure of financial resources, time, unquantifiable human suffering, and loss of life. As individuals and healthcare providers, we want to provide the best care to increase patient survival and quality of life. Understanding the etiology of cancer shows us that prevention must be a goal in populations at risk. Research on the treatment of cancer helps to further define the relationship between risk and cause, growth, response, and resistance. The problem of cancer, in terms of normal and malignant cell growth, the role of the immune system, the action of chemotherapy and tumor response, and goals of treatment, is described in this chapter.

Normal and Malignant Cell Growth

Cancer is an abnormal growth of cells beyond their intended size, site, and functional capabilities. The initiation of this process occurs when carcinogenic agents damage the deoxyribonucleic acid (DNA) of the cell. This is followed by promotion of cell proliferation and progression and change in its morphology, which potentiates the cell's malignant behavior.

To explain this process, it is helpful to understand the cell's normal function. The growth of all cells occurs in a cell cycle that includes mitosis, G_1, S phase, G_2, and G_0 (i.e., the resting phase) (see Figure 1-1). Mitosis is the process of cell division that allows cells to replicate and begins in a single parent cell with a diploid number of chromosomes (equal to 23 pairs). This results in two daughter cells, each with a complete set of chromosomes. Plant alkaloids and taxanes are effective in this period. The cell cycle begins with the interphase, or the

Figure 1-1. The Cell Cycle

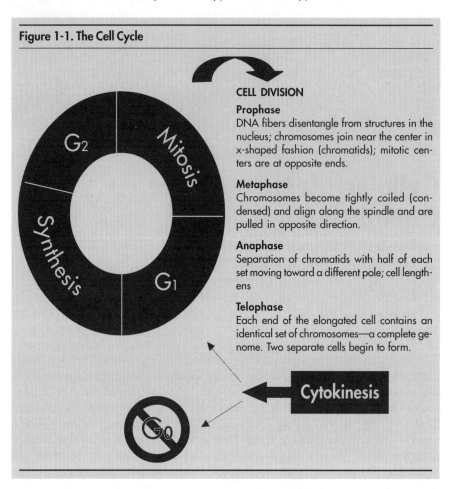

CELL DIVISION

Prophase
DNA fibers disentangle from structures in the nucleus; chromosomes join near the center in x-shaped fashion (chromatids); mitotic centers are at opposite ends.

Metaphase
Chromosomes become tightly coiled (condensed) and align along the spindle and are pulled in opposite direction.

Anaphase
Separation of chromatids with half of each set moving toward a different pole; cell lengthens

Telophase
Each end of the elongated cell contains an identical set of chromosomes—a complete genome. Two separate cells begin to form.

postmitotic G_1 period, in which the chromosomes are uncondensed. In the first part of this growth phase, the DNA directs the synthesis of ribonucleic acid (RNA) and proteins. In late G_1, the crucial restriction point determines the rate of cellular proliferation (Lee & Dang, 1995). Both steroids and asparaginase are effective in this phase. The S phase follows, in which chromosomes actually replicate in preparation for mitosis and each daughter cell consists of a complete set of chromosomes (23 pairs each). Drugs effective in this period are procarbazine and antimetabolites (e.g., methotrexate, fluorouracil, hydroxyurea). The premitotic G_2 phase follows the S phase. This is the second growth phase in which there is RNA and protein synthesis for mitosis. Examples of drugs effective in this period are etoposide, topotecan, and bleomycin (Association of Community Cancer Centers, 2000). Mitosis includes prophase, metaphase, anaphase, and telophase, together producing cytokinesis. Simply put, in prophase, the chromosomes condense into distinct entities and the nuclear membrane breaks down. The chromosomes attach and line up before separating and spindle fibers draw them in opposite directions. The fibers' attractive properties are known as the mitotic spindle (i.e., metaphase).

When the daughter chromatids are drawn to separate locations, anaphase results. Next, they develop new nuclear membranes to form telophase. Finally, all the cellular components, excluding the nucleus, divide, resulting in cytokinesis. Cytokinesis produces two daughter cells that have identical chromosomes to the parent cell. Drugs effective in this period are bleomycin and plant alkaloids. The cycle begins again with interphase (i.e., resting period, G_0). In G_0, cells are programmed for specific functions. It is important to note that they also are refractory to chemotherapy (Groenwald, Frogge, Goodman, & Yarbro, 1998).

Immunology: Host Defense

The body has several lines of natural defenses. The goals of the body's defense systems are to protect the body against invading microorganisms, to remove normal cells at the end of the life cycle, and to recognize and destroy foreign and abnormal cells, such as cancer and virally infected cells. One of the body's defense systems is the immune system, which is divided into innate immunity and adaptive immunity (Rieger, 1999). Both branches of the immune system are important in fighting malignant cell growth within the body. Innate immunity is the primary line of defense in the body. It is nonspecific and has no memory and, therefore, does not require antigen and antibody production; the origin of the foreign cell is irrelevant. Innate immunity consists of physical barriers (skin), mechanical barriers (ciliary action of the respiratory system), chemical barriers (tears), and certain white blood cells (WBCs [neutrophils, monocytes, and macrophages]). It also includes a large granular lymphocyte branch known as natural killer (NK) cells. NK cells are large cytotoxic T cells that bind to malignant and virally infected cells to release cytotoxic agents and cause apoptosis (cell death) and cell lysis (Murphy, 2000) (see Table 1-1).

Table 1-1. Immune System Cells and Their Functions

Immune System Cells	Function
Innate immunity	
Neutrophils	Present phagocytosis in acute infection.
Basophils	Release histamine at local infection.
Eosinophils	Present in allergic reaction.
Monocytes	Phagocytosis present in chronic infection.
Natural killer cells	Provide immunity against viruses and tumors.
Adaptive immunity	
Lymphocytes	
B lymphocytes	Bind to antigen via membrane-bound immunoglobulin.
Plasma cells	Produce immunoglobulin; most mature form of B cell.
Memory cells	Maintain memory effect.
T lymphocytes	Bind to antigen via membrane-bound receptors.
T helper cells	Initiate immune response, assist in production of antibody.
T cytotoxic cells	Kill cells via lysis.
T suppressor cells	Decrease immune response to T and B cells.
T memory cells	Maintain memory effect.

Adaptive immunity is the second line of defense within the body. The acquired branch consists of the humoral immunity, cellular immunity, and cytokines. These components work together with specificity and memory. This immune system includes lymphocytes, T cells (cell-mediated immunity), B cells and immunoglobulins (humoral immunity), and lymphokines and monokines (cytokines) to develop antibodies against foreign and abnormal cells. Cytokines are proteins within the blood that stimulate acquired immune responses and promote communication within the cell lines. The T lymphocyte functions as a cytotoxic antisense sensitive cell, such as a macrophage or dendritic cell, against malignant cells. The macrophage presents a malignant cell to the T lymphocyte. After the T lymphocyte is exposed to the malignant cell antigen, it produces T lymphocytes and B cells that are specific to the antigen. These activated T cells have an antigen receptor. The T lymphocyte then targets the malignant cell and binds to the antigen on the malignant cell surface. The T lymphocyte and B cells develop a memory response after a subsequent exposure. Helper T lymphocytes activate the production of cytotoxic and helper T cells. Suppressor T cells stop the function of the cytotoxic and helper T cells (Kastan, 1997; Volker, 1998). When the immune system fails to remove all abnormal and malignant cells, the cells are allowed to proliferate. Dendritic cell therapy has recently demonstrated evidence supporting the value of the immune system through the use of patient-individualized cancer vaccines and antisense proteins in lymphoma. In Timmerman et al.'s (1999) study, fresh tumor was removed from each patient and was used to create a specific antibody (called "Id" for idiotype), which was then incubated with peripheral dendritic cells. Of the 26 patients treated, 17 remained progression free of their lymphoma for a median of 25 months. Antisense also is an amazing new protein (known as BCL-2 antisense RNA in lymphoma) that allows for upregulation and overexpression of BCL-2 that induces chemotherapy resistance in lymphomas. Patients exposed to antisense experienced a reduction in the BCL-2 protein, inhibition of cellular proliferation, and stimulation of apoptosis. These noted agents are only available in clinical trials at present, but many new biologic therapies are currently utilized. Table 1-2 provides an overview of agents on the market as of the time of this publication.

Cellular Transformation to Malignancy

The transformation from normal to malignant cell has several characteristics. These include change in appearance (size and shape), function, and growth. These changes occur through alterations in molecular and genetic function of the cell's surface, internal structures, and rate of growth (mitosis) and cell death (apoptosis), which result in uncontrolled growth. In addition, the body's ability to recognize the cells through the immune system is altered. The surface of the cell contains molecules and receptors that communicate contact inhibition, which is the signaling that notifies the cells to stop reproduction. This regulatory property stops cell growth once a given directive is achieved. For example, if the skin is cut, the cells receive a message to accelerate growth to repair the function of protection to the body. As cells replicate, the wound continually becomes visibly smaller

Table 1-2. Major Biological Agents in Clinical Use

Category	Agent	Example	Use
Cytokines	Interferon	Interferon-alpha	Hairy cell leukemia, Kaposi's sarcoma, hepatitis B and C, melanoma, follicular lymphoma
		Interferon gamma	Chronic granulomatous disease
		Interferon beta	Multiple sclerosis
	Interleukins	Interleukin-2 (IL-2) (aldesleukin)	Melanoma, renal cell cancer
		Interleukin-11 (Neumega®a)	Thrombocytopenia
	Hematopoietic growth factors	Granulocyte-colony-stimulating factor (CSF)	Neutropenia
		Granulocyte-macrophage-CSF	Anemia Thrombocytopenia
		Erythropoietin	
		Interleukin 11	
	Tumor necrosis factor		
Monoclonal antibodies		Rituximab (Rituxan®b)	Low-grade, CD20+ non-Hodgkin's lymphoma
		Trastuzumab (Herceptin®c)	Metastatic breast cancer with overexpression of HER2
			Treatment of rejection in organ transplants
Differentiation agents		Muromonab-CD3 (Orthoclone®d)	
Cellular therapies	Retinoids	All-trans retinoic acid	Induction for acute promyelocytic leukemia
	Lymphokine-activated killer cells (LAKs)	LAK + IL-2	Metastatic melanoma, renal cell cancer
	Tumor-infiltrating lymphocytes		Melanoma, renal cell cancer
Immunostimulants	Bacillus Calmette-Guérin		Carcinoma in situ of the bladder
	Levamisole		

(Continued on next page)

Table 1-2. Major Biological Agents in Clinical Use *(Continued)*

Category	Agent	Example	Use
Immunostimulants (cont.)	Vaccines	Active specific immuno-therapy	Melanoma trials
Gene therapy Fusion proteins		Denileukin difitox (ONTAK™[e])	Recurrent cutaneous T cell lymphoma; binds to IL-2 for direct cytocidal action, inhibits protein synthesis

[a] Genetics Institute, Cambridge, MA
[b] IDEC Pharmaceuticals Corporation, San Diego, CA
[c] Genentech Inc., South San Francisco, CA
[d] Ortho Biotech Inc., Raritan, NJ
[e] Ligand Pharmaceuticals Inc., San Diego, CA

Note. Based on information from Rieger, 1999.

until it heals. Cancer cells lose contact inhibition ability and continue to grow despite overcrowding or loss of anchorage. Malignant cells lose this ability and can become stimulated by mutated genes to develop clonal selection, which allows mutation and survival of malignant cells. These genes, known as oncogenes, attach to the receptors on the membrane of the cell to stimulate uncontrolled growth. This inability to control growth is called loss of restriction in cell cycle. These cells also require less growth factor. In contrast, the opposing gene is known as an anti-oncogene or cancer suppressor gene, which blocks the action of the oncogene (Fidler, 1997).

Histology of Cancer

Defining the origin of a cancer involves determining the histology. This nomenclature refers to differentiation of the tissue from which the tumor derived. Any cell in the body has the potential for becoming malignant, and many tumors retain some of their cellular characteristics. From inception of life begins the development of three germ layers that become cells, tissue, and organs. The first layer, the ectoderm, differentiates into skin and the nervous system. The second layer, the mesoderm, differentiates into connective tissue and several structures: bones, blood, cartilage, fat, muscle, fibrous tissue, and lymph vessels. Finally, the endoderm becomes the digestive and respiratory tract and lining of the urinary tract (Lee & Dang, 1995).

The characteristic that allows malignant cell recognition is called the histogenetic classification system. The origin of the tumor is retained in the base name along with a suffix, such as sarcoma or carcinoma. The base name is *oma,* which is Greek for "tumor." As an example, an epithelial tumor that arises from glandular tissue would be known as an adenoma if benign but as an adenocarcinoma if malignant.

Cancer Physiology

Whereas benign tumors have characteristics of abnormal cell division, cancerous tumors appear to be dissimilar from the cell of origin, with edges that move outward irregularly, a very rapid growth rate, the ability to invade surrounding tissue, systemic effects, metastases to distant sites, and recurrence (Fidler, 1997).

Metastasis refers to the intricate process that allows spread to distant sites in the body and involves five phases: invasion, cell detachment, dissemination, arrest and establishment, and proliferation. Invasion occurs when malignant cells grow outside of their original location, invading adjacent cells by breaking through the cell basement membrane and between endothelial cells into capillaries to obtain nutrition and blood supply. Initially, neoplastic cells proliferate by utilizing nutrients supplied by diffusion in the microenvironment of the organ. Through excretion of vessel growth (neovascularization) molecules and suppression of inhibitory agents, the neoplastic cell establishes a capillary network to support growth. Cell detachment is separation from the primary neoplasm. Neoplastic cells can downregulate the cohesion of normal cells, which allows increased mobility and aids in detachment. The most common site of invasion is via thin walled capillaries and lymphatic channels that have little ability to resist penetration (Morton, Ollila, Hseuh, Essner, & Gupta, 1999). Dissemination occurs when cells detach and move to other areas of the body. This takes place when malignant emboli shed from the tumor into the vessels and become trapped by lymph nodes. These neoplastic cells aggregate to survive the host defenses. A main site of lymphatic and vascular communication is the thoracic duct, which empties into the venous circulation and the portal venous system, terminating in the liver. Arrest, establishment, and proliferation occur when tumor cells break through vessels to find interstitial spaces that are conducive to growth. To survive, neoplastic cells must continue this phenomena of extravasation, evasion of host defenses, and angiogenesis to ensure growth. With this process, the malignancy now has the environmental niche in which to grow (Pritchard, 1999).

Goals of Chemotherapy

The goals of chemotherapy include cure, control, and palliation. Prevention is a goal recently added to this list. The term *cure* refers to the absence of cancer over an observed length of time. Statistics usually are based on five years of disease-free survival. Aggressive combination regimens frequently are used when cure is the goal. Agents selected for combination regimens have individual activity, have dose-limiting toxicities that differ in combination, have proven effectiveness, and may be synergistic in action. For example, in the treatment of breast cancer, the primary treatment may be mastectomy, followed by combination chemotherapy as the adjuvant treatment. Control and palliation of disease also can be accomplished with the use of chemotherapy. Control allows the prolonging of a patient's life through relatively stabilizing the disease, although this may not mean that signs and symptoms related to a tumor are relieved. Palliation refers to the lessening of morbidity with the cancer process. For example, a patient may have a tumor that obstructs the digestive tract and prevents enjoying food and causes significant distress related to nausea and vomiting. Palliation occurs when chemotherapy decreases the tumor burden and size, allowing the patient to eat and digest food naturally (Groenwald et al., 1998). Both control and palliation are viable goals for patients who may never be cured of cancer.

Cell Phase Specificity

Chemotherapeutic drugs can be placed into two main categories that relate to cell-cycle specificity: phase nonspecific and phase specific (see Figure 1-2). Phase nonspecific drugs are further classified as cycle nonspecific or cycle specific phase nonspecific and have a linear response curve. A linear response curve means that the more drug given, the greater the injury and cell kill. Cycle nonspecific drugs, such as steroids and some antitumor antibiotics, kill nondi-

Figure 1-2. Examples of Cell-Cycle Specific and Cell-Cycle Nonspecific Drugs

Cell-Cycle (Phase) Specific Drugs	Cell-Cycle (Phase) Nonspecific Drugs
G_1 phase Asparaginase Prednisone Ifosfamide	Alkylating agents Busulfan Chlorambucil Cisplatin Cyclophosphamide Mechlorethamine Melphalan Temozolamide Carboplatin Ifosfamide
S phase (antimetabolites) Fluorouracil Carboplatin Cytarabine Hydroxyurea Mercaptopurine Methotrexate Thioguanine Fluorouracil and leucovoran	Antibiotics Dactinomycin Daunorubicin Epirubicin Mitomycin Mitoxantrone Piroxantrone Valrubicin
G_2 phase Bleomycin Etoposide Teniposide Amsacrine Ifosfamide	Nitrosoureas Carmustine Streptozocin Lomustine Semustine
M phase (vinca alkaloids) Vincristine Vinblastine Vinorelbine tartrate Vindesine	Miscellaneous agents Dacarbazine Procarbazine

Note. Based on information from Groenwald et al., 1998; Miaskowski, 1997; Rieger, 1999; Skeel, 1995.

viding cells. Cycle specific phase nonspecific drugs, such as alkylating agents, injure cells at any point in the cell cycle but only if they proceed through the generation cycle. Phase specific drugs are further categorized as cycle specific phase specific and can cause cell injury only if present during a specific phase in the cell cycle. Because of this restriction, these drugs have limited ability despite increased dose. An example is fluorouracil, which is cell-cycle S-phase specific. However, if the drug is administered over a period of time and the concentration is maintained, the cell kill is greater (Miaskowski, 1997).

Tumor Response Criteria

The outcome criteria for chemotherapy are measured as objective and subjective responses to treatment. Objective responses usually are measured radiologically. A complete response (CR) is the complete disappearance of all identifiable tumor volume that lasts at least one month. A partial response (PR) is a 50% or greater decrease in tumor volume that lasts at least one month with no increase during therapy.

A minimal response (MR) is less than a 50% decrease in measurable tumor volume that lasts at least one month with no growth during therapy. Progression (P) of disease is defined as a 25% increase in tumor volume either in the same lesions or the growth of new lesions. Stable (S) disease is tumor volume that is unchanged. A subjective response is reported as improvement (I) of symptoms. These symptoms may include a decrease in pain, improved appetite with weight gain, increased sense of well being and strength, and decreased fatigue.

Factors Affecting Chemotherapy Response

As noted previously, the goal of therapy is to prevent the cancer from overtaking and killing the host. Halting the process of multiplication, invasion, and metastasis can occur in several ways, including inhibition of macromolecular synthesis and function, cytoplasmic organization, and cell membrane function (Skeel, 1995). Interference with macromolecular synthesis and function refers to interference of the synthesis of DNA or RNA in the nucleus to trigger cell death. The cytoplasm surrounds the nucleus and consists of fluid called cytosol and organelles suspended in it. The majority of cellular metabolism takes place within the cytosol, which includes the production of energy and the biosynthesis of nutrients. The cell membrane is a flexible layer that selectively controls passage of chemicals into and out of the cell, thus maintaining homeostasis. Response to chemotherapy can be altered by tumor burden and growth fraction, the use of single agent versus combination therapy, dose, and development of resistance to chemotherapeutic agents (Schiffer, 1999).

The tumor burden or number of tumor cells present in a tumor affects its response to chemotherapy. Tumors have a growth fraction, which is the number of cells actively dividing in a specific period. The growth fraction and tumor size are inversely proportional to the chemotherapeutic response (Lee & Dang, 1995). When the tumor is small, the growth fraction is fast, and an increased number of cells take up the drug. Thus, the number of cells killed is greater with exposure to antineoplastic agents. As the tumor grows, the growth fraction slows and the response to chemotherapy is less. The greater the tumor burden and slower the growth fraction, the greater the potential for chemotherapy resistance (Kastan, 1997).

Another reason for chemotherapy resistance is tumor heterogeneity. Genetic differences among the individual cells occurs by accidental mutations during the cell life cycle. These differences result in different growth rates, invasiveness and metastatic potential, hormone responsiveness, and susceptibility to chemotherapeutic agents. These mutations can result in resistance to chemotherapeutic drugs (Volker, 1998).

One method of overcoming drug resistance is the use of multidrug regimens that work in different phases of the cell cycle. Reasons for using combination therapy include the prevention of resistant clones, cytotoxicity to resting and dividing cells, enhancement of drug activity (synergism), sanctuary access by change in drug solubility or tissue affinity, and rescue of the host from the toxic effects of another drug (Skeel, 1995).

Dosage and timing of drug delivery can be modified to affect chemotherapy response rates. Delivery of cell-cycle specific chemotherapeutic agents (in intermittent doses), to cells that have a shorter duration in the cell life cycle, yields a lesser number of cells killed, whereas cell-cycle specific agents given via continuous infusion protocol result in a greater number of cells killed. There is a clear connection between the amount of the chemotherapeutic agent and the cell death rate. The higher the dose, the greater the number of cells killed. Toxicity is the dose-limiting factor, as it may lead to increased morbidity and mortality. Dose is determined in clinical trials with the goal of high cell death and limitation of toxicity. Dose intensity also is important to tumor response. Dose intensity is the total prescribed amount of chemotherapy delivered in a specific amount of time. Inadequate dosing can compromise the therapeutic benefit of the chemotherapy. Dose reductions and decreased dose rate have been associated with compromised patient outcome, whereas those maintained in compliant regimens respond better (Groenwald et al., 1998).

Another method of overcoming drug resistance is the use of chemosensitizers. Calcium channel blockers, such as verapamil, as well as B vitamins (i.e., leucovoran), and even warfarin, have been used to sensitize or modulate chemotherapy responses. A nonpharmacologic method of chemosensitization is radiation therapy.

Summary

Treatment planning for a patient with cancer involves interdisciplinary decision making. This process should be based on the understanding of the immune system, which safeguards the body, the origination and growth patterns of malignant cells, morbidity and mortality expected of a malignancy and treatment, cure rates, and patient wishes. Future directions of cancer therapy will most likely focus on the chromosomal level. In the past decade, many new agents transformed the efficacy and tolerability of treatment. Research in the next decade will focus on development of tools to identify those at risk, prevention of genetic abnormalities, and the development of chemotherapeutic agents that are only toxic to tumor cells. The future truly holds the legacy of a multimechanistic approach to this problem.

References

Association of Community Cancer Centers. (2000). *USP DI oncology drug information* (3rd ed.). Rockville, MD: Author.

Fidler, I.J. (1997). Molecular biology of cancer: Invasion and metastasis. In V.T. DeVita, Jr., S. Hellman, & S.A. Rosenberg (Eds.), *Cancer: Principles and practice of oncology* (5th ed.) (pp. 135–151). Philadelphia: Lippincott-Raven.

Groenwald, S.L., Frogge, M.H., Goodman, M., & Yarbro, C.H. (1998). *Comprehensive cancer nursing review.* Boston: Jones and Bartlett.

Kastan, M.B. (1997). Molecular biology of cancer: The cell cycle. In V.T. DeVita, Jr., S. Hellman, & S.A. Rosenberg (Eds.), *Cancer: Principles and practice of oncology* (5th ed.) (pp. 121–133). Philadelphia: Lippincott-Raven.

Lee, W.M., & Dang, C.V. (1995). Control of cell growth, differentiation, and death. In R. Hoffman (Ed.), *Hematology* (2nd ed.) (pp. 69–73). New York: Churchill Livingstone.

Miaskowski, C. (1997). *Oncology nursing: An essential guide for patient care.* Philadelphia: W.B. Saunders.

Morton, D.L., Ollila, D.W., Hsueh, E.C., Essner, R., & Gupta, R.K. (1999). Cytoreductive surgery and adjuvant immunotherapy: A new management paradigm for metastatic melanoma. *CA: A Cancer Journal for Clinicians, 49,* 101–116.

Murphy, B. (2000, January). *Control of transcription and cell cycle.* Program and abstracts of the 4th Annual Winter American Society of Transplantation Meeting, Fajardo, Puerto Rico.

Pritchard, K. (1999, December). *Biology and preclinical studies of metastasis.* Program and abstracts of the 22nd Annual San Antonio Breast Cancer Symposium, San Antonio, TX.

Rieger, P.T. (1999). *Clinical handbook for biotherapy.* Boston: Jones and Bartlett.

Schiffer, C.A. (1999, December). *Modulating drug resistance.* Program and abstracts of the 41st American Society of Hematology Annual Meeting, New Orleans, LA.

Skeel, R.T. (1995). Biologic and pharmacologic basis of cancer chemotherapy. In R.T. Skeel & N.A. Lanchant (Eds.), *Handbook of cancer chemotherapy* (4th ed.) (pp. 3–17). New York: Little, Brown & Co.

Timmerman, J.M., Davis, T.A., Hsu, H.J., Caspar, C., Benike, C., Liles, T.M., Czerwinski, D., Taidi, B., Van Beckhoven, A., Fazio, M., Engleman, E., Levy, R., & Hanna, M. (1999). Idiotype-pulsed dendritic cell vaccination for B-cell lymphoma: Clinical and immunological responses in 26 patients (Abstract 1714). Program and abstracts of the 41st American Society of Hematology Annual Meeting. *Blood, 94,* 386A.

Volker, D.L. (1998). Carcinogenesis. In J.K. Itano & K.N. Taoka (Eds.), *Core curriculum for oncology nursing* (3rd ed.) (pp. 357–382). Philadelphia: W.B. Saunders.

CHAPTER 2

Pharmacologic Principles of Chemotherapy

Janese S. Gaddis, RN, MSN, OCN®
Mary Magee Gullatte, RN, MN, ANP, AOCN®, FAAMA

Overview

Prior to the invention of the microscope, cancer was not detected until there were obvious physical manifestations. The development of complex biotechnology has enabled scientists to acquire knowledge about cancer cells' uncontrolled trigger mechanisms and deadly growth. With the aid of molecular biology and genetics, scientists have made great advances in the discovery and relationship of genes and chromosomes to the development of cancer (National Cancer Institute [NCI], 1998). Researchers' efforts continually lead to improvements in cancer treatments and supportive therapies, which include hematopoietic growth factors, antiemetic agents, and cytoprotective agents (Wood, 1998). With the recent mapping of the human genome, more targeted therapies for prevention, detection, and treatment of human cancers are expected to be available in the near future.

An effective chemotherapy treatment regimen requires a comprehensive understanding of the principles of pharmacodynamics and tumor biology; knowledge of the natural history of the cancer being treated; the goal of treatment; and patient-family expectations of treatment. Some chemotherapy agents have cytotoxic effects on cancer cells through interaction with deoxyribonucleic acid (DNA), ribonucleic acid (RNA), or protein synthesis. Drug action initially requires adequate drug delivery to the target site; to produce cell kill, the cell has to absorb the chemotherapeutic agent (Eckardt, Eckardt, Villalona-Calero, Drengler, & Von Hoff, 1995; McGovern, 1994). Drug delivery depends on a number of features: blood flow to the tumor, dose absorption, administration route, renal function, rate of delivery, schedule, and drug diffusion characteristics. Delivery also may be influenced by the extent of plasma protein binding, under normal and abnormal states, absorption, and first-pass metabolism in the liver (Schackney,

1995). Also to be considered is the presence and functional integrity of anatomic and physiologic barriers to drug exposure as a function of disease.

Pharmacokinetics is the study of drug absorption, distribution, metabolism, and excretion. Pharmacodynamics has been described as "what the drug does to the body," whereas pharmacokinetics describes "what the body does to the drug" (Kobayashi, Jordell, & Ratain, 1993; NCI, 1998; Rust & Jameson, 1998). A phenomenon that occurs in cancer antineoplastic therapy is drug interaction. This occurs when the effect of one drug is modified by the prior or concurrent administration of another pharmacologically active substance. These interactions may be antagonistic, synergistic, or unexpected responses (Findley, 1992). Pharmacokinetic interactions needed for optimal treatment response include changes in absorption, distribution, metabolism, and elimination of the anticancer drug (Lokiec, 1996).

Attempts are continually being made to improve treatment response. Strategies include high-dose chemotherapy, prolonged or continuous infusion regimens, use of agents that impair or reverse multidrug resistance, and biochemical modulation. Biochemical modulation entails an attempt to favorably alter the interaction of conventional agents with their targets. Knowledge of both drug metabolism and mechanism of chemotherapeutic resistance are required to develop appropriate strategies (Kobayasi et al., 1993; Toshihko et al., 1999). According to DeVita (1997), a major obstacle in the use of chemotherapy regimens is the presence of mutations in cells that lead to resistance. When developing cancer chemotherapy combination regimens, two factors are taken into consideration: combining drugs with complimentary mechanisms of action to enhance synergistic cytotoxicity and elimination of subpopulations of tumor cells with distinct patterns of drug sensitivity (Sznol & Longo, 1993; Wood, 1998). Current cancer treatment choices are constantly expanding. Treatment may include, singularly or in combination, chemotherapy, surgery, radiation therapy, biologic response modifiers, and immunotherapy (Kaufman & Chabner, 1996).

Drug Resistance

Eckardt et al. (1995) described chemotherapy resistance as a major concern that occurs in a significant number of patients; resistance may occur as a stable change within the cell or be inducible within the cell after administration of the chemotherapeutic agent (see Table 2-1). Mechanisms that may lead to chemotherapy resistance include glutathione transferase and DNA repair. Chemosensitizers have been utilized to reverse the process of resistance (e.g., calcium channel blockers, lysosomotropic agents, noncytotoxic drug analogues, other miscellaneous agents such as cyclosporine). Drug resistance may be natural (occurring from select innate resistance from natural cell lines) or acquired (occurring from drug-induced adaptation or mutation of cancer cells) (Chan et al., 1994; NCI, 1998). In an effort to combat this process and increase therapeutic effect, combination chemotherapy regimens can be used. These regimens would include drugs with different mechanisms of action and different toxicities given at full dose. Some drug combinations can produce antagonistic effects. By administering these agents in sequence or cycles, toxicities can be avoided while delaying drug resistance. Combination

Table 2-1. Antineoplastic Drug Classification

Class	Subclass	Mechanism of Action	Toxicity Profile	Examples of Agents
Alkylating agents Cell-cycle, phase non-specific		Produce break in DNA molecule and cross linking of strands; interfere with DNA replication and transcription; exerts activity on hematopoietic stem cells	Delayed and prolonged myelosuppression, amenorrhea, oligospermia, or azoospermia; in men, permanent infertility; secondary cancer	
	Bischloroethylamines (nitrogen mustard)	Produce highly reactive carbonium ions that react with the electron-rich areas of susceptible molecules	Myelosuppression, alopecia, nausea and vomiting, diarrhea, and mucositis	Chlorambucil, cyclophosphamide, ifosfamide, estramustine, mecholorethamine, melphalan
	Ethylenimine	Capable of the same kinds of reactions as nitrogen mustard		Thiotepa
	Alkyl sulfonates	Interact more with thiol groups than with nucleic acid		Busulfan
	Triazine	Acts as an alkylator after 5-aminoimidazole carboxamide is cleaved from active diazomethan		Dacarbazine
	Nitrosoureas	Undergo rapid spontaneous activation in aqueous solutions to form alkylation and carbamoylation products; non-cross-resistance with other alkylating agents; highly lipid soluble	Prolonged and delayed myelosuppression	Carmustine, lomustine, streptozocin

(Continued on next page)

Table 2-1. Antineoplastic Drug Classification (Continued)

Class	Subclass	Mechanism of Action	Toxicity Profile	Examples of Agents
Alkylating agents Cell-cycle, phase non-specific (cont.)	Heavy metals	Inhibit DNA synthesis through formation of intrastrand cross-links in DNA; react with DNA by chelation or by binding to the cell	Renal toxicity, ototoxicity, myelosuppression, neurotoxicity	Cisplatin, carboplatin, oxaliplatin
Antimetabolites Cell-cycle, phase specific		S-phase; interferes with DNA and RNA function; structurally similar to intracellular substances because of cell incorporation into essential sites of cellular metabolism and inability to divide; most active in tumors with high growth fraction and rapidly cycling cell population	Myelosuppression, stomatitis, diarrhea, other gastrointestinal (GI) sequelae	
	Folic acid analog	Antifolate; inhibits dihydrofolate reductase, thereby inhibiting DNA synthesis	Myelosuppression (thrombocytopenia, leukopenia), skin erythema, rash, hyperpigmentation, renal and hepatic dysfunction, pulmonary toxicity	Methotrexate, timetrexate
	Pyrimidine analog	Inhibits DNA polymerase, thus DNA synthesis; interferes with RNA function	Diarrhea, mucositis, rash, hyperpigmentation, hand and foot syndrome	Azacytidine, cytarabine, floxuridine, fluorouracil
	Purine analog	Inhibits purine synthesis, thereby inhibiting DNA and RNA synthesis	Myelosuppression, anorexia, nausea and vomiting, hepatic toxicity, peripheral neuropathy, neurotoxicity	Mercaptopurine, thioguanine, pentostatin, fludarubine

(Continued on next page)

Table 2-1. Antineoplastic Drug Classification (Continued)

Class	Subclass	Mechanism of Action	Toxicity Profile	Examples of Agents
Antitumor antibiotics, Cell-cycle specific		Bind with DNA to inhibit synthesis of DNA and RNA	Pulmonary toxicity, fever, chills, pain at the site of administration, myelosuppression, skin and GI toxicities, mucositis, hepatic and renal dysfunction, blood clotting disorders	
	Anthracyclines	Intercalation of DNA, topoisomerase II, DNA inhibition	Myelosuppression, cardiotoxicity (cumulative cardiac toxicity), alopecia, severe tissue necrosis if extravasation occurs	Daunorubicin, doxorubicin, idarubicin, epirubicin, valrubicin
	Chromomycin	Cell-cycle specific and phase nonspecific	Allergic reactions, nausea and vomiting, diarrhea, cumulative myelosuppression, alopecia, hepatotoxicity; vesicant	Dactinomycin, plicamycin
	Miscellaneous	Inhibition of DNA	Pulmonary toxicity, cutaneous hyperkeratosis	Mitomycin, bleomycin
Plant alkaloids Cell-cycle specific		Mitotic inhibitors; prevent cell division	Myelosuppression, neurotoxicity, GI toxicity, allergic reactions, distal neuropathy	

(Continued on next page)

Table 2-1. Antineoplastic Drug Classification (Continued)

Class	Subclass	Mechanism of Action	Toxicity Profile	Examples of Agents
Plant alkaloids Cell-cycle specific (cont.)	Vinca alkaloids	Bind to microtubule proteins, arrest mitosis during metaphase; active in S and M phases	Neurotoxicity, constipation, urinary retention, jaw pain, syndrome of inappropriate antidiuretic hormone, tissue necrosis if extravasation occurs	Vincristine, vinblastine, vindesine, vinorelbine
	Taxanes	Enhance microtubule assembly; inhibit tubulin depolymerization	Peripheral neuropathy, myelosuppression, anaphylaxis, alopecia, arthralgia, myalgia	Paclitaxel, docetaxel
	Podophyllotoxins	Inhibit DNA synthesis in S and G phases to prevent mitosis; cause single breaks in DNA	Hypotension, myelosuppression, nausea and vomiting, mucositis, alopecia, hypersensitivity reaction, fever, bronchospasms	Etoposide, teniposide
Hormones/hormone antagonists		Manipulate hormonally active tissue, thus inhibiting cell growth		
	Glucocorticoids	Lysis of lymphoid cells; may recruit malignant cells out of G_0 phase, making them vulnerable to damage caused by the cell-cycle specific agent	Electrolyte imbalance, GI disorders, osteoporosis, changes in secondary sex characteristics, increased susceptibility to infection, mood swings, increased appetite, fluid retention	Cortisone, hydrocortisone, dexamethasone, methylprednisolone, prednisone

(Continued on next page)

Table 2-1. Antineoplastic Drug Classification (Continued)

Class	Subclass	Mechanism of Action	Toxicity Profile	Examples of Agents
Hormones/hormone antagonists (cont.)	Androgens	Estrogen antagonists; suppress pituitary function	Fluid and sodium retention, obstructive jaundice, voice change, libido change, emotional change	Testosterone propionate, fluoxymesterone, testolactone, methyltestosterone, testosterone enanthate
	Estrogens	Suppress testosterone through hypothalamus in males and alter breast cancer cell response to prolactin in females	Thrombophlebitis, gynecomastia, fluid retention, bloating	Diethylstilbestrol, ethinyl estradiol, estramustine, chlorotrianisene, conjugated estrogens
	Progestin	Inhibits pituitary gonadotropin secretion	Weight changes, hot flashes, thrombophlebitis, menstrual problems	Progestin, megestrol acetate, medroxyprogesterone acetate
	Antiestrogens	Nonsteroidal; bind to estrogen receptors, form an abnormal complex that migrates to the cell nucleus and inhibits DNA synthesis	Increased risk for gynecologic malignancy, hot flashes, nausea and vomiting, menstrual abnormalities, bone pain, thrombotic disorders	Tamoxifen, toremifene, raloxifene
	GnRH agonists	Prevent the pulsed release of endogenous GnRH from the hypothalamus, stimulating the release of follicle stimulating hormone (FSH) and luteinizing hormone (LH)	Headache, insomnia, impotence, hot flashes, thrombophlebitis, vaginal dryness, decreased libido, nausea, vomiting, bone pain, myalgia, injection site irritation, cardiac arrhythmias, peripheral edema	Leuprolide acetate, goserelin, goserelin bicalutamide, nilutamide, flutamide

(Continued on next page)

Table 2-1. Antineoplastic Drug Classification (Continued)

Class	Subclass	Mechanism of Action	Toxicity Profile	Examples of Agents
Hormones/hormone antagonists (cont.)	Antiandrogens	Inhibit androgen uptake or inhibit nuclear binding of androgen in target tissues; inhibit pituitary gonadotropin, achieving a chemical orchiectomy	Hot flashes, impotency and decreased libido, tumor flare, nausea and vomiting	Bicalutamide, nilutamide, flutamide
Topoisomerase I inhibitors		Cause an irreversible double-strand DNA break that arrests cell division and results in cell death, RNA synthesis in cell division	Myelosuppression, headache, paresthesia, alopecia, nausea and vomiting, diarrhea, constipation, stomach pain, stomatitis	Topotecan, irinotecan
Biologic response modifiers		Stimulate division and differentiation of hematopoietic stem cells in the bone marrow	Fatigue, headache, pyrexia, urticaria, polycythemia	Epoetin alfa, filgrastim, sargramostim, oprelvekin, interferon alfa, aldesleukin, rituximab, levamisole, tumor necrosis factor

Note. Based on information from Agarwala,1994; Burke et al.,1995; Chabner & Collins, 1990; Clarke et al., 1991; Colvin & Chabner, 1990; Gullatte & Graves, 1990; Holland & Frei, 2000; Jordan, 1994; May & Morgan, 1994; McEvoy, 1998; Preston & Wilfinger, 1993.

regimens should include drugs that are effective singularly against the specific cancer, do not pose the same type of toxicities, do not have the same time of onset of the same toxicity, and, with synchronization, singularly potentiate the effects of the other drugs in the regimen (Guy & Ingram, 1996). Another strategy to reduce and/or delay toxicity and decrease drug resistance is the use of intermittent therapy. This may be more effective, less immunosuppressive, and less toxic than a low-dose continuous regimen. Because normal cells are better able to self-repair than most cancer cells, normal cells may recover during a drug-free period. This approach is used to produce maximum tumor cell kill while allowing regeneration of faster-growing normal tissue. Dose intensification may be used, which involves using a chemotherapeutic agent over a specific period of time for maximal cell kill (Cobb, 1998; Miller, Ratain, & Schilsky, 1996). Logarithmic changes in the tumor cell burden can be expected during the course of antineoplastic therapy.

Treatment Goals

The goals of cancer therapy include cure, control, and/or palliation. The potential for cure correlates with the tumor size, location, histology, and cytology. Primary treatment options may include surgery, radiation therapy, chemotherapy, immunotherapy, biologic response modifiers, or multimodality therapy. For purposes of this book, we will focus on chemotherapy. Control and palliation encompass remission or disease-free interval and survival time, prevention of recurrence, and relief of signs and symptoms of the cancer (Kaufman & Chabner, 1996; Lenhard, Lawrence, & McKenna 1995). With the advent of supportive therapies, palliative therapy can better achieve delays in disease progression, prolong overall survival, minimize disease complications and treatment toxicities, and maximize quality of life (Sots & Allegia, 1996). Chemotherapy may be administered as neoadjuvant, adjuvant, or primary treatment. Adjuvant therapies aid primary therapy, are used to improve therapeutic outcomes and prognosis, and often follow primary interventions. Adjuvant therapy is initiated for patients at high risk for recurrence. It has been established that, in high-risk subsets, systemic adjuvant therapy significantly lowers tumor recurrence through the early elimination of metastatic microfoci of disease. Neoadjuvant therapy involves administration of chemotherapy to reduce tumor load prior to surgery or radiation therapy. This therapy often improves the probability of total surgical resection, reduces the morbidity of surgery or radiation, and eradicates micrometastatic disease.

Cell-Cycle Response of Chemotherapy

The sequence of normal and malignant cell growth is reflected in the cell cycle, which aids in identifying potential therapeutic agents that act on cells during certain cycles of mitosis. Cell growth and replication involve five active phases (Baserga, 1981; Bingham, 1978).

1. G_0 resting phase: Cells can remain in this phase for various lengths of time; this phase does not include replication.

2. G_1: RNA and protein synthesis to prepare for DNA synthesis.
3. S: DNA synthesis, genetic code for information regarding growth, repair, and cell reproduction. Cells differ in time period spent here.
4. G_2: Second growth period, in which further protein and RNA synthesis occur and cell prepares for mitosis. Chromosomes prepare for division.
5. M: Actual cell division occurs. Involves prophase, metaphase, anaphase, and telophase.

The cellular response to chemotherapy is reviewed in Chapter 1 of this book. The pharmacologic influence of antineoplastic agents is exerted on enzymes or substrates acted upon by enzyme systems involved in DNA, RNA, and protein synthesis. Additionally, antineoplastic agents act on biochemical pathways that are common to normal cells as well as cancer cells. Thus, the antineoplastic agents are classified as cytotoxic rather than tumoricidal, accounting for the toxicities experienced by the host on rapidly proliferating tissues, such as the bone marrow, gastrointestinal (GI) epithelium, skin, hair follicles, gonads, and embryonic structures (McEvoy, 1998).

Classification of Antineoplastic Agents

The terms *cancer chemotherapy drugs* and *cytotoxic compounds* generally are used interchangeably. Antineoplastic agents usually are grouped into numerous classes based on cellular activity and pharmacologic properties of the drugs, specific to the neoplasm to be treated. These agents may be classified according to the basis of their mechanism of action, derivation, and chemical structure: alkylating agents, heavy metals, antimetabolites, antibiotics, plant alkaloids, hormones, miscellaneous agents, and investigational agents (Burke, Wilkes, & Ingwersen, 1995). Although agents may be assigned to a specific group, their properties may overlap with other classes. Antineoplastic drugs also may be classified based on their relationship to cell life cycle activity. This classification is not absolute, as some agents act by multiple mechanisms, and the precise mechanism is unknown in others (McEvoy, 1998; Yasko, 1998).

Alkylating Agents

The first alkylating agents originated in military efforts to launch a chemical and biological offensive during World Wars I and II (Gilman, Rall, Nies, & Palmer, 1990). Alkylating agents are uni- and multifunctional compounds that have the ability to substitute alkyl groups for hydrogen ions, which then react with molecular ions of the body such as phosphate, amino, hydroxyl, sulfhydryl, carboxyl, and imidazole groups (May & Morgan, 1994). These molecular reactions produce abnormalities in DNA, RNA, and proteins by interfering with replication, transcription, and disruption of nucleic acid, thus preventing normal cell function (Chabner & Collins, 1990).

Alkylating agents do not rely on the cell cycle to be effective; hence, they are classed as cell-cycle nonspecific. However, these agents inhibit overall protein synthesis as well as RNA and DNA function. Another classic characteristic of alkylating agents is their ability to produce DNA cross-links. Alkylating agents are divided into six classes based on their chemical structure and covalent bonding mechanisms: bischloroethylamines (nitrogen mustards, ifosfamide, chlorambucil); aziridines (thiotepa, mitomycin C, and diaziquone [AZQ]); alkyl alkane sulfonates (busulfan); nitrosoureas (streptozocin, carmustine [BCNU], lomustine [CCNU]); nonclassic agents (triazenes, hydrazines [dacarbazine, procarbazine]); and platin (heavy metal) compounds (cisplatin, carboplatin) (May & Morgan, 1994). Although cisplatin and carboplatin often are categorized as alkylating agents because they form adducts with proteins, DNA, and RNA, there is not an actual alkylating portion to the active molecule. They are, instead, heavy metal or platinating agents. Alkylating agents have mutagenic, teratogenic, and carcinogenic effects. It is postulated that tumor cell resistance to alkylating agents is mediated by tripeptide glutathione conjugation or DNA repair processes within the target cell (Colvin, 2000; McGovern, 1994).

Toxicity of Alkylating Agents

A major target of alkylating agents is the hematopoietic system, causing leukopenia, thrombocytopenia, and anemia. Hematologic toxicity often is dose-dependent and cumulative. Hematologic nadirs for oral alkylating agents may occur in three to six weeks, whereas toxicities from agents administered by the intravenous route may appear within one to two weeks and linger for one to two weeks post-treatment depending on dose and schedule (Gilman et al., 1990; McGovern, 1994). The severity of GI toxicities, such as nausea, vomiting, diarrhea, mucositis, and stomatitis, also are dose- and drug-dependent. Symptom management and treatment of hematologic and GI side effects of alkylating agents are outlined in Chapter 7. Some alkylating agents possess vesicant properties and should be administered with extreme caution when given intravenously. Extravasation into the soft tissues may cause severe local tissue damage (e.g., burning at the injection site, sloughing, necrosis). Other toxicities may include ototoxicity, nephrotoxicity, peripheral and central neuropathy, hemorrhagic cystitis, alopecia, hyperuricemia, hepatotoxicity, nephrotoxicity, and pulmonary, cardiac, and gonadal toxicity, as well as secondary malignancies.

Antimetabolites

Antimetabolic agents have been used in cancer treatment since the late 1940s. These agents are analogs of naturally occurring metabolites in the human body. The antineoplastic effect of the antimetabolites occurs during the S phase of the cell cycle. This class of agents is cell-cycle dependent, affecting DNA, RNA, and protein synthesis. Antimetabolites are most effective against cancer cells that have a high growth fraction (i.e., are rapidly dividing). Another mechanism of action of the antimetabolites is the ability to inhibit purine and pyrimidine nucleotide synthesis, thereby exerting an effect on enzymes needed for

DNA and RNA synthesis, resulting in cell death or apoptosis. Biochemical modulation is designed to enhance the cytotoxic effectiveness of antimetabolites and overcome cellular resistance to the drug. An example of this effective strategy is the combination of fluorouracil and leucovorin calcium in the treatment of colorectal cancers (Delap, 1994; Kamen, Cole, & Bertino, 2000).

Antimetabolite Toxicity

Treatment with antimetabolic agents results in suppression of cell growth in mitotically active tissues (e.g., GI mucosa, hematopoietic system). Purines are abundant in the normal bone marrow and are essential to marrow growth and function. Therefore, a purine antimetabolite such as thioguanine is toxic to the normal bone marrow yet quite effective in treating hematologic malignancies (Delap, 1994). There are three classes of antimetabolic agents: folate antagonists (methotrexate [MTX]); purine antagonists (thioguanine, mecaptopurine, pentostatin, fludarabine phosphate); and pyrimidine antagonists (fluorouracil, floxuridine, cytarabine).

Folate analogs: Depending on dose and schedule, the folate antagonist MTX has a myelosuppressive nadir of one to two weeks. GI effects of MTX include stomatitis, mucositis, and diarrhea (Delap, 1994; McGovern, 1994). A leucovorin rescue often is employed when administering high-dose MTX. Leucovorin calcium (a reduced form of folic acid) is administered to protect the normal cells from the antagonistic action of MTX, thereby reducing serious toxicities to normal cells. This is accomplished because of the conversion of folic acid to leucovorin and does not affect the action of leucovorin itself (Govoni & Hayes, 1988). The initial half-life of the folate antagonists is 2–3 hours with a terminal half-life of 8–10 hours. The initial and/or terminal half-life may vary based on dose administered and hepatic and renal function.

Purine analogs: The purine antagonists (mecaptopurine and thioguanine) are analogs of the naturally occurring purines hypoxanthine and guanine. There appears to be no significant differences in the efficacy or indications of thioguanine compared with mercaptopurine (Delap, 1994). The toxicities associated with the purine analogs include myelosuppression, nephrotoxicity, immunosuppression, and neurotoxicity. These toxicities vary based on the drug and the dose; however, myelosuppression is common to all of the purine antimetabolites.

Pyrimidine analogs: The pyrimidine antimetabolites are thymidylate synthase inhibitors, blocking DNA synthesis. The antineoplastic agent, fluorouracil, is one of several pyrimidine analogs. The half-life of these antimetabolites ranges from 3–20 minutes, depending on the agent. The myelosuppressive nadir of fluorouracil is one to two weeks. While, generally, the antimetabolites are cell cycle phase specific and exert their effect on cells with a rapid growth curve, some of the pyrimidines have demonstrated activity in all phases (Delap, 1994). Toxicities associated with the pyrimidine analogs expectedly include myelosuppression, mucositis, diarrhea, nausea, vomiting, and chemical hepatitis (associated with intraarterial floxuridine).

Antitumor Antibiotics

Antitumor antibiotics are a heterogenous group of antineoplastic agents. Many of these agents are topoisomerase II inhibitors. The topoisomerases are one of several groups of enzymes that regulate the topologic, or twisting and winding, state of a DNA double-strand molecule around itself (Delap, 1994). Topoisomerase enzymes are vital to DNA and RNA transcription and replication. This class of drugs has vesicant properties and should be administered with extreme caution. Antitumor antibiotic agents are clinically valuable because of their antitumor activity across a broad spectrum of cancers. The anthracyclines are derived from bacterial cultures. Examples of these antibiotic agents include dactinomycin *Streptomyces parvulus,* doxorubicin *Streptomyces peutius,* and daunorubicin *Streptomyces coeruleorubidus.* While dactinomycin was the first approved antitumor antibiotic of natural origin, doxorubicin is considered the most active anthracycline agent against a broad spectrum of diseases (Delap). Bleomycin *Streptomyces verticillis* has activity in several phases of the cell cycle including S, G_2, and M phases. Bleomycin is very toxic to the skin and lungs and can produce cumulative and irreversible interstitial fibrosis and death (Delap; Kamen et al., 2000). Anthracyclines are reactive to metal ions such as aluminum. As a result of the organometallic chemistry of these agents, prolonged contact with aluminum needles and surfaces should be minimized or avoided (Chabner & Collins, 1990; Williamson, Luce, & Hausmann, 1983). Toxicities associated with antitumor antibiotic agents can be life-threatening. Because of the iron-binding effect of these agents, which results in oxidative cell damage, cardiac tissue is most vulnerable to their effects. Recommendations for the total lifetime cumulative dose of doxorubicin is 400 mg/m^2. It is important to establish exclusion criteria for patients considered for treatment with anthracyclines. A cardioprotective agent may be used prior to administration of anthracyclines and should be considered for doses greater than 300 mg/m^2. Other antitumor antibiotics include mitomycin (also classed as a bioreductive alkylator) and plicamycin. For most of these antitumor antibiotic agents, the dose-limiting factor is the effect on the hematopoietic system (myelosuppression). GI toxicities are manifested by nausea, vomiting, and stomatitis. Dermatologic effects include alopecia, extravasation, tissue necrosis, and radiation recall phenomenon.

Biologic Agents

Biologic agents (biotherapy) are used to promote tumor regression, stimulate the immune system, and promote hematopoiesis (Creekmore, Walter, & Longo, 1991). The use of biologic response modifiers (BRMs) dates back to the early years of treating leukemia with the immunomodulator agent bacillus Calmette-Guérin (BCG). Science and technology have progressed light years beyond these early agents and limited knowledge of the value of cell mediated immunity in the treatment of disease. Continuing research is needed to maximize the benefit of the BRMs and immune modulators (e.g., interferon, interleukin) in disease management. Through the use of cytokines or colony-stimulating factors (i.e., filgrastim, sargramostim, erythropoietin, or oprelvekin), which control hematopoiesis, the oncology team has reversed and shortened the myelosuppressive dose-limiting toxicities of many antineoplastic therapies. In many cases, these agents have allowed patients to continue their treatment cycle without interruption. The oncology team now has access to hematopoietic growth factors for granulocytes, erythrocytes, and platelets. Other biologic agents include octreotide, a soma-tostatin analog, and retinoids. Some toxicities associated with these biologic agents (drug-, dose-, and duration-dependent) include nausea, vomiting, diar-rhea, fever, chills, myalgia, and arthralgia; exacerbation of hypertension; pruri-tus; dry skin; hair loss; dysuria; mental status changes; and myelosuppression. Detailed and specific toxicities and management are addressed in other chapters in this handbook.

Hormones

Hormone agonists and hormone antagonists are employed in the treatment of hormone-derived or hormone-sensitive tumors. These include those cancers arising in organs or tissues that rely on hormones for growth and development, such as breast, ovary, endometrium, and prostate. To maintain the growth of breast and prostate tumors, a supply of estrogen and androgen, respectively, is needed. The therapeutic strategy in the treatment of these cancers is to reduce or block the source of the hormone or the receptor site where the hormone is active. As an example, an alternative approach to gonadectomy or estrogen therapy in treating prostate cancer is to use the luteinizing hormone-releasing hormone superagonists to desensitize the pituitary gland and prevent release of gonadotrophins (Jordan, 1994). Likewise, an antiestrogen (tamoxifen) is used to treat postmenopausal women with breast cancer. The results of the National Surgical Adjuvant Breast Project breast cancer prevention trials have shown a reduction in the incidence of breast cancer in women at risk for the disease when treated prophylactically with the antiestrogen tamoxifen (Fisher et al., 1998; Gail et al., 1999). In women, estrogen is key to preventing osteoporosis and maintaining a healthy coronary system. An advantage to the use of tamoxifen is its estrogen-like effect on the bones and heart. This is important in postmeno-pausal women who are prescribed tamoxifen at a time when the naturally occur-ring circulating estrogen levels are diminishing or nearly absent. In contrast, the long-term use of estrogen-like tamoxifen increases the risk of thromboembolic disorders and endometrial cancer (Jordan).

Other hormonal agents include aminoglutethimide, diethylstilbestrol (a syn-thetic estrogen), fluoxymesterone (synthetic androgen), flutamide, goserelin ac-etate, leuprolide acetate, megestrol acetate, toremifene, raloxifene, anastrozole, fadrozole, and letrozole. These hormonal agents are administered orally or as a depot intramuscular injection. Drug distribution, absorption, half-life, and elimi-nation are reviewed in Chapter 5 under each specific agent. General toxicities of the hormonal agents include changes in weight, mood, skin, and heart, as well as nausea, vomiting, anorexia, hirsutism, and male pattern baldness.

Plant Alkaloids

The use of plants in medicinal therapy dates as far back as the beginning of time itself. The oldest recorded plant alkaloid used as a chemotherapeutic agent is colchicine, which had an observed effect in interfering with mitosis (Agarwala, 1994). Later plant alkaloids included vincristine and vinblastine and their semi-synthetic derivatives vinorelbine and vinzolidine (which are derived from the periwinkle plant). The latest plant alkaloids are the taxanes paclitaxel (derived from the Western yew tree) and docetaxel. Other derivatives include the podophyllotoxins, teniposide and etoposide. The plant alkaloids are cell-cycle phase specific and are primarily metabolized by the liver. Dose reductions may be necessary in patients with hepatic dysfunction. Absorption of the oral etoposide is not affected by food. General toxicities of the plant alkaloids include myelosuppression, neuropathy, allergic reactions, hypotension, alopecia, cardiac arrhythmias, constipation, myalgia, mucositis, nausea, and vomiting. The vinca alkaloids are vesicants, and caution should be taken to avoid extravasation.

References

Agarwala, S.S. (1994). Plant derived agents. In J.M. Kirkwood, M.T. Lotze, & J.M. Yasko (Eds.), *Current cancer therapeutics* (pp. 74–81). Philadelphia: Current Medicine.

Baserga, R. (1981). The cell cycle. *New England Journal of Medicine, 304,* 453–459.

Bingham, C.A. (1978). The cell cycle and cancer chemotherapy. *American Journal of Nursing, 78,* 1201–1205.

Burke, M., Wilkes, G., & Ingwersen, K. (1995). *Cancer chemotherapy. A nursing process approach* (pp. 30–35). Boston: Jones and Bartlett.

Chabner, B., & Collins, J. (Eds.). (1990). *Cancer chemotherapy: Principles and practice.* Philadelphia: J.B. Lippincott.

Chan, H.S.L., DeBoer, G., Thorner, P.S., Haddad, G., Gallie, B.L., & Ling, V. (1994). Multidrug resistance: Clinical opportunities in diagnosis and circumvention. *Hematology/Oncology Clinics of North America, 8,* 383–410.

Clarke, S.J., Jackman, A.L., & Harrap, K.R. (1991). Antimetabolites in cancer chemotherapy. *Advances in Experimental Medicine and Biology, 309A,* 7–13.

Cobb, S. (1998). Multimodality and new therapies. In J.M. Yasko (Ed.), *Nursing management of symptoms associated with chemotherapy* (pp. 27–34). West Conshohocken, PA: Meniscus Health Care Communications.

Colvin, D.M. (2000). Alkylating agents and platinum antitumor compounds. In J.F. Holland & E. Frei (Eds.), *Cancer medicine* (5th ed.) (pp. 648–669). London: B.C. Decker, Inc.

Colvin, D.M., & Chabner, B.A. (1990). Alkylating agents. In B.A. Chabner & J.M. Collins (Eds.), *Cancer chemotherapy: Principles and practice* (pp. 276–313). Philadelphia: Lippincott.

Creekmore, S., Walter, U., & Longo, D. (1991). Principles of the clinical evaluation of biologic agents. In V.T. DeVita, S. Hellman, & S.A. Rosenberg (Eds.), *The biologic therapy of cancer* (pp. 67–86). Philadelphia: Lippincott.

Delap, R.J. (1994). Antimetabolic agents. In J.M. Kirkwood, M.T. Lotze, & J.M. Yasko (Eds.), *Current cancer therapeutics* (pp. 32–47). Philadelphia: Current Medicine.

DeVita, V.T. (1997). Principles of cancer management: Chemotherapy. In V.T. DeVita, S. Hellman, & S.A. Rosenberg (Eds.), *Cancer: Principles and practice of oncology* (5th ed.) (pp. 333–334). Philadelphia: Lippincott-Raven.

Eckardt, J., Eckardt, G., Villalona-Calero, M., Drengler, R., & Von Hoff, D. (1995). New anticancer agents in clinical development. *Oncology, 9,* 1326.

Findley, R.S. (1992). Drug interaction in the oncology patient. *Seminars in Oncology, 8,* 95–101.

Fisher, B., Costantino, J.P., Wickerham, D.L., Redmond, C.K., Kavanah, M., Cronin, W.M., Vogel, V., Robidoux, A., Dimitrov, N., Atkins, J., Daly, M., Wieand, S., Tan-Chiu, E., Ford, L., & Wolmark, N. (1998). Tamoxifen for prevention of breast cancer: Report of the National Surgical Adjuvant Breast and Bowel Project P-1 Study. *Journal of the National Cancer Institute, 90,* 1371–1388.

Gail, M.H., Costantino, J.P., Bryant, J., Croyle, R., Freedman, L., Helzlsouer, K., & Vogel, V. (1999). Weighing the risks and benefits of tamoxifen treatment for preventing breast cancer. *Journal of the National Cancer Institute, 91,* 1829–1846.

Gilman, A., Rall, T., Nies, A., & Palmer, T. (Eds.). (1990). *Goodman and Gillman's the pharmacological basis of therapeutics* (8th ed.) (pp. 1202–1276). New York: Pergamon Press.

Govoni, L., & Hayes, J. (Eds.). (1988). *Drugs and nursing implications.* Norwalk, CT: Appleton & Lange.

Gullatte, M.M., & Graves, T. (1990). Advances in antineoplastic therapy. *Oncology Nursing Forum, 17,* 867–875.

Guy, J., & Ingram, B. (1996). Medical oncology–The agents. In R. McCorkle, M. Grant, M. Frank-Stromborg, & S. Baird (Eds.), *Cancer nursing: A comprehensive textbook* (pp. 359–394). Philadelphia: W.B. Saunders.

Holland, J.F., & Frei, E. (Eds.). (2000). *Cancer medicine* (5th ed.). London: B.C. Decker, Inc.

Jordan, V.C. (1994). Hormonal agents. In J.M. Kirkwood, M.T. Lotze, & J.M. Yasko (Eds.), *Current cancer therapeutics* (pp. 65–73). Philadelphia, PA: Current Medicine.

Kamen, B.A., Cole, P.D., & Bertino, J.R. (2000). Folate antagonists. In J.F. Holland & E. Frei (Eds.), *Cancer medicine* (5th ed.) (pp. 612–624) London: B.C. Decker, Inc.

Kaufman, D., & Chabner, B. (1996). Clinical strategies for cancer treatment: The role of drugs. In B. Chamber & D. Longo (Eds.), *Cancer chemotherapy and biotherapy: Principles and practice* (pp. 1–15). Philadelphia: Lippincott.

Kobayashi, K., Jordell, D., & Ratain, M. (1993). Pharmacodynamics–Pharmacokinetic relationships and therapeutic drug monitoring. *Cancer Survival, 17,* 51–78.

Lenhard, R., Jr., Lawrence, W., Jr., & McKenna, R. (1995). General approaches to the patient. In G. Murphy, W. Lawrence, & R. Lenhard (Eds.), *Clinical oncology* (pp. 64–74). Washington, DC: Health Organization Publishers.

Lokiec, F. (1996). Drug interaction in cancer chemotherapy. In R. Schilesky, G. Milano, & M. Ratain (Eds.), *Principles of antineoplastic drug development and pharmacology* (pp. 189–201). New York: Marcel Dekker, Inc.

May, D.M., & Morgan, B. (1994). Alkylating agents. In J.M. Kirkwood, M.T. Lotze, & J.M. Yasko (Eds.), *Current cancer therapeutics* (pp. 1–18). Philadelphia: Current Medicine.

McEvoy, G. (Ed.). (1998). *AHFS 98 drug information*. Bethesda, MD: American Society of Health-System Pharmacists.

McGovern, J.P. (1994). Pharmacologic principles. In R.T. Dorr & D.D. von Hoff (Eds.), *Cancer chemotherapy handbook* (2nd ed.) (pp. 15–34). Norwalk, CT: Appleton & Lange.

Miller, A., Ratain, M., & Schilsky, R. (1996). Principles of pharmacology. In M.C. Perry (Ed.), *The chemotherapy source book*. Baltimore: Williams & Wilkins.

National Cancer Institute. (1998). *Closing in on cancer: Solving a 5000-year-old mystery*. (NIH Publication No. 98–2955). Bethesda, MD: U.S. Department of Health and Human Services National Institutes of Health.

Preston, F.A., & Wilfinger, C. (1993). *Memory bank for chemotherapy*. (2nd ed.). Boston: Jones and Bartlett.

Rust, D., & Jameson, G. (1998). The novel lipid delivery system of amphotericin B: Drug profile and relevance to clinical practice. *Oncology Nursing Forum, 25,* 35–48.

Schackney, S. (1995). Cell kinetics and cancer chemotherapy. In P. Calabresi, S.A. Schein, & S.A. Rosenberg (Eds.), *Medical oncology: Basic principles and clinical management of cancer* (pp. 41–60). New York: McMillan.

Sots, G., & Allegia, C. (1996). Biochemical modulation of cancer chemotherapy. In R. Schilsky, G. Milano, & M. Tatain (Eds.), *Principles of antineoplastic drug development and pharmacology* (pp. 174–176). New York: Marcel Dekker.

Sznol, M., & Longo, D.L. (1993). Chemotherapy drug interactions with biological agents. *Seminars in Oncology, 20,* 80–93.

Toshihko, K., Lubert, R., Steele, V., Kelloff, G., Kaskey, R., Rao, C., & Reddy, B. (1999). Chemoprevention effects of curicum, a naturally occurring anti-inflammatory agent during the promotion/progression stages of colon cancer [Abstract]. *Cancer Research, 59,* 597.

Williamson, M.J., Luce, J.K., & Hausmann, W.K. (1983). Doxorubicin hydrochloride-aluminum interaction [Letter to the editor]. *American Journal of Hospital Pharmacy, 40,* 214.

Wood, L. (1998). New therapies, new nursing challenges. In B.A. Sigler (Ed.), *ONS symposia highlights: 1998 Annual Congress* (p. 25). Pittsburgh: Medical Association Communications and the Oncology Nursing Society.

Yasko, J. (1998). *Nursing management of symptoms associated with chemotherapy* (pp. 235–265). West Conshohocken, PA: Meniscus Health Care Communications.

CHAPTER 3

Principles and Standards of Chemotherapy Administration

Mary Magee Gullatte, RN, MN, ANP, AOCN®, FAAMA

Introduction

The administration of chemotherapy requires a knowledgeable and competent oncology professional. Although chemotherapy administration has become widely performed over the last half century, it remains a therapy that requires specialized knowledge, skill, and expertise. Issues of concern include safe handling, preparation, administration, and disposal. This chapter will address specific issues of administration, including vesicant and extravasation management, routes of administration, and patient and family education.

Industry and oncology specialty organizations have written or supported documented standards and recommendations for safe handling of cytotoxic agents. These guidelines and recommendations have been formulated or published by The Occupational Safety and Health Administration (OSHA), the American Society of Health-System Pharmacists (ASHP), the Oncology Nursing Society (ONS), the Joint Commission on Accreditation of Healthcare Organizations (JCAHO), the National Institutes of Health (NIH) Clinical Center Nursing Department, and the Centers for Disease Control (CDC).

Cytotoxic and antineoplastic compounds are known to have carcinogenic, mutagenic, and teratogenic potential (Shapiro, Gotfried, & Lishner, 1990). Special safety precautions are required when handling antineoplastic agents to protect workers from and minimize exposure to these agents. Figure 3-1 outlines the safe handling recommendations and guidelines from ASHP, government regulatory agencies, and ONS. Adhering to these safety precautions will minimize the exposure risk for healthcare workers responsible for administration of cytotoxic agents. It is imperative that the healthcare professional responsible for administering cytotoxic agents have knowledge and skill in principles of medication administration and intravenous therapy. Adherence to the

Figure 3-1. Antineoplastic Safe Handling Guidelines

Preparation

Review agency policy and procedure.
Verify patient, drug, dose, route, and time.
Prepare route/site per guidelines or policy.
Review pertinent laboratory values.
Review patient history.
Conduct physical assessment.
Review chemotherapy order.
Calculate and verify dose.
Gather supplies for preparation of dose:
  • Gloves (0.007–0.009-inch-thick, powder-free latex)
  • Disposable gown (long sleeves and cuffed to the wrist)
  • Safety goggles
  • N95 respirator mask
Use biological safety cabinet (BSC) (Class II or III) to mix and prepare cytotoxic drugs (CD).
Place absorbent, plastic-backed pad on work surface.
Have spill kit available.
Use disposal paraphernalia (e.g., chemotherapy waste bucket).
Ensure that emergency drugs are available based on agents and patient history of hypersensitivity reaction.
Have extravasation medications appropriate to the agent on hand.
Have patient consents signed as appropriate.
Label all syringes and IV bags or bottles.
  • Name
  • Drug
  • Dose
  • Route
Priming: The American Society of Health-System Pharmacists recommendation is threefold: (a) prime within the BSC; (b) when preparing at the site of administration, prime IV line with non-CD-containing fluid or a backflow closed system; and (c) purge air from single-dose syringes under BSC or as above.
Transport CD in a leak-proof, impervious container.

Administration

Explain process to patient.
Verify drug and dose with second provider.
Wash hands before donning gloves.
Don personal protective equipment (PPE [e.g., gloves, gown, goggles, mask]).
Check PPE for nicks or tears; if present, change PPE.
Administer premedications (e.g., antiemetics).
Hydrate per protocol.
Verify patient, drug, dose, route, and time at patient's side.
Wipe container with sterile alcohol gauze.
Apply sterile gauze at injection ports to prevent spraying when connecting and disconnecting.
Verify patency of venous access by aspirating for blood return.
Use fresh IV site for vesicants.
Flush before and after administration of CD with compatible fluid.
Monitor tubing and IV site for leaks.
Use only Luer-Lok® connections.
Monitor tubing and IV site for leaks.
Use only Luer-Lok® connections.

(Continued on next page)

Figure 3-1. Antineoplastic Safe Handling Guidelines *(Continued)*

Administration (cont.)
Use sterile gauze pad to wipe outside of container.
Wear PPE and double latex gloves for workers handling bodily fluids for up to 48 hours after patient has received chemotherapy. See page 41 for individuals with latex allergies.
Wash hands before and after gloving.
Always don PPE.

Spills
Cytotoxic drugs are classed by OSHA as hazardous drugs (HDs). As such, care and caution should be taken to minimize exposure risk.
ASHP rates spills based on volume spilled.
- < 5 ml = small
- > 5 ml = large

Immediately contain the spill by placing absorbent plastic-backed pad over the spill.
Do not use hands to clean up spills involving broken glass.
Restrict access to the area surrounding the spill.
Don PPE.
Use spill kit.
Commercially available or on-site assembly as follows:
- Disposable plastic-backed absorbent pads or liners x 3
- Sealable plastic bag
- Splash goggles
- Latex gloves x 2
- Long-sleeved, cuffed disposable gown
- Disposable absorbent pads
- Detergent
- Scooper device with scraper (for glass)
- Sharps container
- Chemotherapy waste bucket
- HD contamination labels
- Plastic-lined linen bags x 2

Restrict access to the area until all exposure risk is removed.
Dispose of spill paraphernalia in chemotherapy waste container.

Disposal
PPE: place in specially marked disposal container.
Needles: place in approved sharps container; do not cut, grind, or recap needles.
Administration sets: dispose intact in chemotherapy waste bucket.
Linen: place in impervious, labeled laundry bags. Prewash prior to adding to other laundry for second wash. Laundry personnel should wear latex gloves while handling prewashed linens.
Have disposal equipment at the point of administration.
Any unused CD should be sealed and securely returned to pharmacy.
Reusable items: for example, wipe goggles with detergent, water, and disposable sterile gauze.
Wear face shield and N95 mask, gloves, and gown for all equipment clean up. DO NOT re-use gloves and gown.
    Waste buckets: Chemotherapy waste disposal containers with lid (some are commercially available); close and dispose when ¾ full.
Equipment: Wipe down reusable pumps and IV poles with detergent, and rinse with water.

Note. Based on information from AMA, 1985; ASPH, 1990; DHHS (NIOSH), 1988; NIH, 1999; OSHA, 1986, 1995, 1999; Varricchio, 1997; Welch & Silveria, 1997; Wilkes et al., 1999.

basic five rights of medication administration–(a) right patient, (b) right drug, (c) right dose, (d) right route, and (e) right time–are key to preventing medication variances. Other rights of the patient include the right to access health care and have that care provided by a competent oncology professional, the right to informed decision making, and the right to appropriate education regarding their disease, treatment options, and symptom management. Attention to these patient rights is the responsibility of the members of the oncology healthcare team.

Preparation and Administration

Chemotherapy dosage is most often based on calculation of the body surface area (BSA) of the patient or area under the pharmacokinetic curve (AUC). The AUC is the use of preclinical pharmacology to guide dose escalation during the conduct of Phase I clinical trials (Khleif & Curt, 2000). The AUC is expressed by calculating the plasma concentration of a drug over time and measuring the area beneath the plotted curve. AUC is expressed in concentration times units (Cleri & Berkery-Haywood, 1999). The BSA is derived from a calculation of the patient's height and weight. Based on the agent used and the health state of the patient, the physician may decide to use the ideal body weight rather than the actual body weight (i.e., cases of severe ascites or edema) (Dorr & von Hoff, 1994). As with all chemotherapy, the patient's drug and dose should be calculated, checked, and verified by more than one professional in preparation and prior to administration.

The degree of bone marrow suppression between chemotherapy cycles can be a dose-limiting side effect during the course of treatment. Therefore, in nonhematopoietic malignancies, the absolute neutrophil count (ANC) should be computed from the white blood cell (WBC) count and differential prior to preparing the dose for administration. Chapter 7 reviews computation of the ANC. The bone marrow may be compromised when several agents are given sequentially or concomitantly (Baquiran & Gallagher, 1998). With the addition of hematopoetic growth factor to some treatment regimens, many patients are now able to continue treatment at the standard dose to effect the most desired treatment outcome.

Cytotoxic agents that require reconstituting and mixing should be prepared using a Class II laminar air flow biological safety cabinet (BSC) and hood. Personal protective equipment (PPE) should be worn during preparation and administration of cytotoxic agents outside of the biologic safe cabinet. The following equipment should be used: (a) Luer-Lok® (Becton, Dickinson, & Co., Franklin Lakes, NJ) connections for tubing and syringes; (b) long-sleeved, cuffed, and closed-front gown; (c) nonsterile, powderless, 0.007–0.009-inch-thick, powder-free latex gloves (Nitrile or other nonlatex gloves may be used for people with latex allergies. In a recent study by Singleton and Connor (1999) most of the chemotherapy gloves on the market are either impermeable or minimally permeable to three drugs studied: BCNU, etoposide, and paclitaxel.); (d) goggles or face shields and a respirator if aerosolization is likely or when a BSC is not available; and (e) prep mats (Dorr & Griffin-Brown, 1990). Gloves should be changed regularly and changed immediately if punctured or torn. If skin comes in contact with the cytotoxic agent, the affected area should be washed thoroughly with soap and water. A scrub brush should not be used. If eye exposure occurs, eyes should be flushed with copious amounts of water for at least 15 minutes (U.S. Department of Labor, OSHA, 1986).

Chemotherapy Protective Agents

The mechanism of action of cytotoxic agents is a double-edged sword. The toxic benefit of antineoplastic agents on cancer cells poses a risk to normal cells related to the toxic effect. Within the last two decades, several agents have been introduced to selectively protect normal tissue and cells from specific toxic effects of several chemotherapy agents. These agents are referred to as chemoprotective agents. Presently, only a select number of chemoprotective agents are approved by the U.S. Food and Drug Administration (FDA). Table 3-1 lists several of the chemoprotectant agents that currently are FDA-approved.

Routes of Chemotherapy Administration

Chemotherapy can be effectively and safely administered through multiple routes. The route of administration is determined by the type and site of the cancer, the drug, and the overall treatment goal. However, most agents are administered via the intravascular and oral routes. Other routes include intramuscular, subcutaneous, intracavitary, and intrathecal. Vascular access is a key factor when parenteral routes of administration are planned. Chapter 4 addresses the assessment, selection, and maintenance of various vascular access devices used to administer antineoplastic therapy.

Oral Route

A number of antineoplastic agents may be given orally. When selecting the oral route, special considerations include drug availability, solubility, absorption, metabolism, and elimination. Advantages of oral administration include convenience to the patient, lower cost, often less toxicity, and fewer side effects (Dorr & von Hoff, 1994; OSHA, 1986). Table 3-2 includes a list of available agents that may be administered orally. The oral agents may be given alone or in combination with other routes of administration based on the treatment protocol.

Table 3-1. Chemoprotectant Agents		
Protective Agent	Chemotherapy Agent	Toxicity Modulated Effect
Amifostine	Cisplatin	Bone marrow suppression, nephrotoxicity, neurotoxicity
Dexrazoxane	Doxorubicin	Cardiotoxicity
Mesna	Ifosfamide	Uroepithelial

Note. Based on information from Foster-Nora & Siden, 1997; Kintzel, 2000; Shapiro et al., 1990.

Table 3-2. Oral Chemotherapeutic Agents

Generic Drug Name	Brand Name	Supplied Form	Cancer/Disease Indications
Altretamine	Hexalen[®n]	50 mg capsule	Ovarian
Aminoglutethimide	Cytadren[®d]	250 mg tablet	Adrenal, ectopic tumors producing adrenocortico-tropic hormone
Anastrozole	Arimidex[®b]	1 mg tablet	Advanced breast
Bexarotene	Targretin[®g]	75 mg capsule	Refractory cutaneous T cell lymphoma
Bicalutamide	Casodex[®b]	50 mg tablet	Prostate (stage D2)
Busulfan	Myleran[®e]	2 mg tablet	Chronic myelogenic leukemia (CML)
Capecitabine	Xeloda[®k]	2 mg tablet	Metastatic breast cancer resistant to paclitaxel and an anthracycline-containing regimen
Chlorambucil	Leukeran[®e]	100 mg, 500 mg oblong, film-coated tablets	Chronic lymphatic leukemia (CLL), Hodgkin's disease, non-Hodgkin's lymphoma
Cyclophosphamide	Cytoxan[®c]	25 mg, 50 mg tablets	Breast, ovarian, acute lymphatic leukemia (ALL), acute myelogenic leukemia (AML), CLL, neuroblastoma, Hodgkin's, non-Hodgkin's lymphoma, retinoblastoma
Estramustine phosphate sodium	Emcyt[®j]	140 mg capsule	Prostate
Etoposide	VePesid[®c]	50 mg capsule	Testicular, small cell lung carcinoma
Testolactone	Teslak[®h]	50 mg tablet	Advanced breast in post-menopausal women
Flutamide	Eulexin[®l]	125 mg capsule	Prostate
Hydroxyurea	Hydrea[®c]	500 mg capsule	Head and neck, CLL, ovarian, melanoma
Imatinib mesylate	Gleevec[®j]	100 mg capsule	Accelerated and refractory CML
Letrozole	Femara[®i]	2.5 mg tablet	Advanced breast
Leucovorin calcium	—	5 mg, 10 mg, 15 mg, 25 mg tablets	Antidote for methotrexate, megaloblastic anemia

(Continued on next page)

Table 3-2. Oral Chemotherapeutic Agents *(Continued)*

Generic Drug Name	Brand Name	Supplied Form	Cancer/Disease Indications
Levamisole	Ergamisol[®f]	50 mg tablet	Colon (stage III)
Lomustine	CeeNU[®c]	10 mg, 40 mg, 100 mg capsules	Hodgkin's disease, metastatic brain tumors
Megestrol acetate	Megace[®c]	20 mg, 40 mg tablet	Breast, endometrial, AIDS, cachexia
Melphalan	Alkeran[®e]	2 mg tablet	Ovarian, myeloma
Mercaptopurine	Purinethol[®e]	50 mg tablet	ALL, AML
Methotrexate	Mexate[®c], Folex[®a]	2.5 mg tablet	Acute leukemia, breast, head and neck, lung, lymphosarcoma, Burkitt's lymphoma
Mitotane	Lysodren[®c]	500 mg tablet	Adrenal cortex
Procarbazine	Matulane[®m]	50 mg capsule	Hodgkin's disease, anaplastic astrocytoma
Tamoxifen	Nolvadex[®b]	10 mg, 20 mg tablet	Breast
Temozolomide	Temodar[TMl]	5 mg, 20 mg, 100 mg, 250 mg capsules	Refractory anaplastic astrocytoma
Thioguanine	Tabloid[®e]	40 mg tablet	AML
Toremifene	Fareston[®l]	60 mg tablet	Breast
Tretinolin	Vesanoid[®j]	10 mg capsule	Acute promyelocytic leukemia

[a] Adria Laboratories, Dublin, OH
[b] AstraZeneca, Wilmington, DE
[c] Bristol-Myers Squibb Oncology/Immunology, Princeton, NJ
[d] Ciba-Geigy, Tarrytown, NY
[e] Glaxo Wellcome Inc., Research Triangle Park, NC
[f] Janssen Pharmaceutica Inc., Titusville, NJ
[g] Ligand Pharmaceuticals, San Diego, CA
[h] Mead Johnson-a Bristol Myers Squibb Co.
[i] Novartis Pharmaceuticals Corporation, East Hanover, NJ
[j] Pharmacia & Upjohn, Peapack, NJ
[k] Roche Laboratories Inc., Nutley, NJ
[l] Schering Corporation, Kenilworth, NJ
[m] Sigma-Tau Pharmaceuticals, Inc., Gaithersburg, MD
[n] U.S. Bioscience Inc., West Conshohocken, PA

Note. Based on information from Cleri & Berkery-Haywood,1999; Delmar Publishers & Medical Economics Co., 2000; Dorr & von Hoff, 1994; Murphy et al., 1995; PDR, 1998; Peters, 1998; Preston & Wilfinger, 1993.

The caregiver should use gloves when handling oral tablets because of the risk of absorption through the skin and concern related to long-term exposure. The patient receiving oral agents should be instructed to accurately document intake of medication to avoid under- or overdosing.

Intravenous Route

The most common route of administration of antineoplastic agents is intravenous (IV). When administering chemotherapy via the IV route, it is imperative that the line is secure and patent. Numerous venous access devices (VADs) are available for safe administration of chemotherapy agents. A detailed overview of VAD selection, function, and maintenance can be found in Chapter-4. Peripheral IV catheters carry a certain amount of inherent risk associated with leaking and infiltration of cytotoxic fluids. In the case of chemotherapy agents, particular attention must be paid to the location of the insertion site and skin and venous integrity prior to, during, and after administration as well as the type of chemotherapeutic agent to be infused. Leaking or infiltration of chemotherapeutic agents and IV fluid out of the vein and into the tissue is known as extravasation. When a vesicant inadvertently leaks out into the tissue during infusion, an initial tissue response usually results in pain, swelling, and redness at the site. With or without treatment, the extravasation of a vesicant agent could result in cellulitis, sloughing and blistering of the surrounding tissue, and tissue necrosis. A number of chemotherapeutic agents are known as irritants. An irritant agent causes local tissue aching, tightness of the skin, and phlebitis at and around the site of injection or infusion (McCune, Harvey, Pfeiffer, & Lindley, 1998). While administering chemotherapy agents, if signs and symptoms of extravasation are present, the infusion should be stopped immediately and an appropriate extravasation protocol/antidote initiated (see Table 3-3). If the patient complains of stinging or burning during the infusion, even if blood return is present, stop the infusion immediately, flush the line with compatible fluid, initiate extravasation protocol, and restart the IV at another site distal to the original site or in the opposite extremity. If extravasation occurs, the physician or practitioner should be notified immediately to determine the next appropriate intervention.

The type of IV infusion is determined by the regimen and duration of the infusion and may include one or more of the following: IV push infusion directly into the IV site with a syringe; side arm infusion given through a fast-flowing IV line with a compatible IV fluid; short-term infusion via a minibag; or a long-term continuous infusion. Continuous infusions of chemotherapeutic agents should be administered via a central line, especially in the case of known vesicants and irritants.

Intrathecal/Intraventricular Route

The location of some tumors requires regional drug delivery. The blood-brain barrier prevents most systemic agents from affecting the central nervous system and is the inherent protection of the brain and spinal column from harm. To get the maximal benefit from chemotherapy agents to treat brain

Table 3-3. Vesicant Chemotherapy Agents*

Class	Generic Drug Name	Brand Drug Name	Antidote
Antitumor antibiotic	Dactinomycin	Cosmegen[®f]	Apply ice compress for 15 minutes QID for 72 hours at the extravasation site.
	Daunorubicin	Daunomycin[®f], Cerubidine[®b]	
	Doxorubicin	Adriamycin[®g]	Apply ice. Topical dimethyl sulfoxide (DMSO), 1–2 ml DMSO 50%–100%; apply once topically at the site.
	Idarubicin	Idamycin[®g]	No antidote or local measures
	Plicamycin	Mithracin[®a]	Apply moderate heat
Alkylating agent	Mechlorethamine	Mustargen[®f]	Sterile isotonic sodium thiosulfate 1/6 molar, 4.14 g/100 ml sterile water.
			Dilute 4 ml of sodium thiosulfate 10% with 6.0 ml of sterile water for injection. Inject 2 ml into site through original needle.
	Mitomycin-C	Mutamycin[®c]	Some benefit with topical DMSO
	Menogaril		None known
Vinca alkaloid	Vinblastine	Velban[®d]	Apply warm compress to site for 15 minutes QID x two days.
	Vincristine	Oncovin[®d]	
	Vindesine	Eldisine[®d]	
	Vinorelbine	Navelbine[®e]	

*Cisplatin (Platinol[®c]) can cause tissue damage and ulceration; therefore, it is considered an irritant. If irritation occurs, apply an ice compress for 6–12 hours. If inflammation and pain persist, consult a plastic surgeon.
[a] Bayer Corporation Pharmaceuticals Division, West Haven, CT
[b] Bedford Laboratories, Bedford, OH
[c] Bristol-Myers Squibb Oncology/Immunology, Princeton, NJ
[d] Eli Lilly and Company, Indianapolis, IN
[e] Glaxo Wellcome Inc., Research Triangle Park, NC
[f] Merck & Co., Inc., West Point, PA
[g] Pharmacia & Upjohn, Peapack, NJ

Note. Based on information from Dorr, 1990; Finley & LaCivita, 1992; Gullatte & Graves, 1990; Kirkwood et al., 1994; Wilkes et al., 1999; Wood, 1998; Ziegfeld et al., 1998.

tumors and central nervous system metastases, it is necessary to access the intrathecal space. Infusion into the cerebrospinal space can be done via a spinal tap or with the use of an Ommaya® reservoir (American Hospital Supply Corporation, Evanston, IL). When repeated entry into the intrathecal space is necessary, either an Ommaya or Rickham® (Johnson & Johnson, New Brunswick, NJ) reservoir is the device of choice (Berkery, Cleri, & Skarin, 1997; Dorr & von Hoff, 1994; Wood, 1998).

Intra-arterial Route

Another regional delivery method is the arterial route. The benefit of the intra-arterial (IA) method is the ability to deliver a high concentration of the chemotherapeutic agent in close proximity to the tumor site. The IA route also reduces systemic side effects that the patient may experience from the chemotherapeutic agent. When the IA catheter is in place, circulation and sensation of the extremity should be monitored frequently. Patients should not receive anticoagulant therapy or platelet-interfering drugs prior to IA therapy. Once the IA catheter is in place and after it is removed, the site should be monitored for bleeding. A pressure dressing and sand bag should be used to maintain pressure on the arterial exit site until danger of bleeding has passed.

Intraperitoneal Route

Intraperitoneal administration is the delivery of chemotherapy into the abdominal-peritoneal space. The concept is the same as that of other regional delivery methods. Cancers that spread or seed into the peritoneal space are the target of this delivery method. Malignancies treated via this route include ovarian, liver, and other gastrointestinal cancers (Dorr & von Hoff, 1994).

Safe Handling and Disposal

OSHA first published guidelines for the management of cytotoxic drugs (CDs) in the workplace in 1986 (U.S. Department of Labor, OSHA, 1986). OSHA's revised recommendations include CDs and other hazardous drugs (HDs). For purposes of this handbook, the preparation, administration, safe handling, and disposal of the HDs will be limited to CDs. In an effort to minimize the exposure risk of healthcare workers to CDs, special precautions should be taken in all aspects of preparation, administration, and disposal. Precautions should be taken to avoid splattering, spraying, and aerosolization of CDs. Risks for these types of exposures include (a) withdrawal of needles from vials, (b) drug transfer using syringes and needles or filter straws, (c) breaking open of ampules, and (d) expulsion of air from a drug-filled syringe (OSHA). ASHP (1990) recommends the following safety provisions to be included in institutional HD safety programs: (a) establishment of a designated HD handling area, (b) use of BSCs to prepare CDs, (c) procedures for safe removal of contaminated waste, and (d) decontamination procedures. These institutional policies and procedures should be reevaluated annually and amended as new guidelines are published.

There should be no eating, drinking, or applying cosmetics or lotions in the CD preparation, administration, or disposal area. HDs should be clearly labeled and stored away from food and drink. Safe-handling precautions should be followed when exposed to body excreta of patients receiving chemotherapy; urine, feces, emesis, and sweat should be handled using appropriate PPE. Appropriate PPE should include a N95 mask and face shield or goggles; powder-free, 0.007–0.009-inch-thick latex gloves (nitrile if latex allergic); and a long-sleeved, cuffed-to-the-wrist, gown cover up. Avoid splashing when emptying excreta containers (U.S. Department of Labor, OSHA, 1986). Wear PPE when measuring output or cleaning up bodily waste or bathing a patient receiving chemotherapy. ASHP (1990) recommends that linens be placed in specially marked, nonpermeable laundry bags (Nevidjon & Travaglini, 1990; Reyman, 1993). Linens should be double-bagged and prewashed separate from other linens.

Workers handling linens contaminated with chemotherapy excreta should wear PPE. All chemotherapy administration sets, bags, and tubing should be disposed of in a leak-proof, puncture-resistant container. Chemotherapy waste containers are commercially available. OSHA (1995) supports the ASHP (1990) recommendation that sharps are not to be broken, cut, or crushed; they should be disposed of in approved sharps containers. NIH (1999) recommends covering the CD preparation safety cabinet work surface area with plastic-backed absorbent paper. If splashing in the eye occurs, flush the affected eye(s), while holding back the eye lid(s), with copious amounts of water for at least 15 minutes.

Healthcare professionals should educate patients and families about safety and exposure risks when handling body fluids of patients receiving chemotherapy. Workers who are of childbearing age or pregnant should be informed about exposure risk of hazardous drugs (Harrison, Godefroid, & Karanaugh, 1996; Langhorne, 1997; Shapiro, Gotfried, & Lishner, 1990).

Latex Sensitivity

Some individuals are allergic to the naturally occurring proteins found in latex. These proteins can be inhaled and absorbed through the skin and mucous membranes. Inhalation can occur via powders in the gloves that act as vectors that bind to the protein and become airborne. Latex sensitivity has gained increased attention over the past five years. The use of latex by sensitive individuals causes contact dermatitis and hypersensitivity. Gloves are required for handling cytotoxic agents, but synthetic gloves may be used by individuals with latex sensitivity. Burt (1999) recommends synthetic, nonlatex alternatives, such as nitrile, neoprene, styrene, and butyl.

Hazardous Drug Spills

OSHA classifies CDs as HDs, and care should be taken to avoid spills of these agents. ASHP and OSHA classify HD spills outside the BSC as follows: (a) small: < 5 ml volume or 5 g, (b) large: > 5 ml volume or 5 g. Institutional and workplace policies and procedures should be in place for the safe handling of CD spills. The OSHA/ASHP cleanup guidelines for small and large spills are outlined in Figure 3-1. As with any potential or actual exposure to CDs, PPE must be worn to clean up spills. If broken glass is involved, do not risk picking it up with gloved hands. Use a scoop to contain glass and pick it up for disposal in a sharps container (National Institute for Occupational Safety and Health, 1988; NIH, 1999; U.S. Department of Labor, OSHA, 1999).

Storage and Transport of Hazardous Drugs

ASHP (1995) recommends that storage areas for CDs be restricted to authorized personnel. Signs restricting entry to the area should be clearly posted. Containers of HDs should be placed securely to prevent risk of breakage. If a container is damaged, the healthcare worker should open it under a BSC while wearing the appropriate PPE. When transporting HDs, OSHA recommends that they be securely capped or sealed; placed in clear, sealed plastic bags; and transported in unbreakable, impervious containers (U.S. Department of Labor, OSHA, 1988, 1999). Any staff working with HDs should be knowledgeable regarding spills and containment of HDs and CDs.

Patient and Significant Other Education and Support

The diagnosis of cancer continues to strike fear and a sense of impending doom in patients and their significant others. The stages of grief, as espoused by Elizabeth Kübler-Ross (1969), are relived by the patient each time a diagnosis of cancer is confirmed. Oncology professionals must remember that a diagnosis of cancer is similar to dropping a pebble into a pond: there is a ripple effect; everyone who cares for and is close to the patient feels the emotional chill, fear, and anxiety. With this in mind, it is important to identify the patient's primary caregiver and support person and to include not only the patient but also the significant other(s) in the education, treatment plan, and support. Early and ongoing education of the patient can serve to allay fear and anxieties.

As the patient's physical, psychological, and social needs are assessed, level of understanding, comprehension, readiness to learn, and cultural perspectives should be considered. A complete baseline health assessment, including tumor markers, radiography, serum chemistry, hematologic studies, and nutrition status, should be completed and documented prior to initiation of chemotherapy. With each subsequent treatment, the clinician should complete the patient's history, physical, psychosocial, and emotional assessment. Health beliefs, practices, and decision making on the part of the patient and family are influenced by cultural, religious, and spiritual factors, so assessment of these factors should be included in patient care assessment and management.

Prior to treatment, an initial assessment of the patient's readiness to learn is made. Multifaceted teaching approaches should be used. The patient should be given materials written at an appropriate literacy level (usually fifth grade). Computer programs that convert text into the appropriate literacy level are available. Video, audio, and computer technology can be used once it has been established that the patient has access to the equipment needed to use the resources. Teaching strategies, while multifaceted, also must be culturally relevant as well as age- and linguistically appropriate. Teaching and learning needs should be addressed and reinforced throughout the cancer trajectory. Verbal reinforcement and return demonstrations will help when teaching psychomotor skills such as self-injection and venous access dressing changes. Teaching strategies should use both the cognitive and psychomotor domains.

Encourage the patient to maintain a treatment journal of questions, answers, appointments, treatment regimens, pertinent laboratory values, subjective symptoms, and effective management techniques for disease or treatment-related side effects. When to notify the physician, nurse, nurse practitioner, or physician's assistant of significant health-related events should be reinforced at each visit. The patient should be included in every aspect of care. The knowledgeable patient is better equipped to make informed decisions and choices about cancer care and symptom management. Support groups and survivor resources can be given to the patient and caregiver. Psychosocial and emotional support of the patient and significant other throughout the cancer experience are addressed in detail in Chapters 9 and 10.

Summary

CD administration requires a knowledgeable, skilled, and competent professional. Competency programs should minimally include information about neoplastic growth, treatment goals, drug information (vesicant, irritant, preparation, and administration), and safe handling and disposal guidelines. Cytotoxic agents should be prepared in an approved BSC. PPE, disposal containers, and spill kits must be available in the area of chemotherapy preparation, administration, and disposal. Education and consent of the patient prior to treatment are essential. Because of the teratogenic and carcinogenic effect of cytotoxic drugs, safe handling and protection of the worker, patient, and environment from unintentional exposure should be a priority. Institutional policies and procedures and employee surveillance should be in place and reviewed annually to minimize CD exposure risks.

Cytotoxic therapy guidelines should be developed to minimize and prevent errors related to dose calculations, preparation, and administration. Accurate and timely documentation of chemotherapy preparation, administration, and patient response are essential elements of safety for the patient. ONS has published *Cancer Chemotherapy Guidelines and Recommendations for Practice* (Mrozek-Orlowski, 1999) and *Safe Handling of Cytotoxic Drugs* (Welch & Silveira, 1997) to assist with the development of the necessary guidelines.

References

American Medical Association Council on Scientific Affairs. (1985). Guidelines for handling parental antineoplastics. *JAMA, 253,* 1590–1592.

American Society of Health-System Pharmacists. (1990). ASHP technical assistance bulletin on handling cytotoxic and hazardous drugs. *American Journal of Hospital Pharmacy, 47,* 1033–1049.

Baquiran, D.C., & Gallagher, J. (1998). *Lippincott's cancer chemotherapy handbook.* Philadelphia: Lippincott.

Berkery, R., Cleri, L.B., & Skarin, A.T. (1997). *Oncology pocket guide to chemotherapy* (3rd ed.). New York: Mosby-Wolfe Medical Communications.

Burt, S. (1999). The facts about latex allergy. *Nursing Management, 30*(8), 18–25.

Cleri, L.B., & Berkery-Haywood, R. (1999). *Oncology pocket guide to chemotherapy* (4th ed.). Philadelphia: Mosby-Wolfe Medical Communications.

Delmar Publishers & Medical Economics Company. (2000). *PDR®. A nurse's handbook™.* Montvale, NJ: Author.

Dorr, R.T. (1990). Antidotes to vesicant chemotherapy extravasation. *Blood Reviews, 4,* 41–60.

Dorr, R.T., & Griffin-Brown, J. (Eds.). (1990). *Reducing the risk of cytotoxic exposure.* Evansville, IN: Bristol-Myers Company.

Dorr, R.T., & von Hoff, D.D. (Eds.). (1994). *Cancer chemotherapy handbook.* Norwalk, CT: Appleton & Lange.

Finley, R.S., & LaCivita, C.L. (1992). Neoplastic diseases. In M.A. Koda-Kimble & L.Y. Young (Eds.), *Applied therapeutics: The clinical use of drugs* (5th ed.) (pp. 1–48). Vancouver, WA: Applied Therapeutics, Inc.

Fishman, M., & Mrozek-Orlowski, M. (Eds). (1999). *Cancer chemotherapy guidelines and recommendations for practice* (2nd ed.). Pittsburgh: Oncology Nursing Press, Inc.

Foster-Nora, J.A., & Siden, R. (1997). Amifostine for protection from antineoplastic drug toxicity. *American Journal of Health-System Pharmacy, 54,* 787–800.

Gullatte, M.M., & Graves, T. (1990). Advances in antineoplastic therapy. *Oncology Nursing Forum, 17,* 867–875.

Harrison, B.R., Godefroid, R.J., & Karanaugh, E.A. (1996). Quality assurance testing of staff pharmacists handling cytotoxic agents. *American Journal of Health-System Pharmacy, 53,* 402–407.

Khleif, S.N., & Curt, G.A. (2000). Animal models in developmental therapeutics. In R.C. Bast, D.W. Kufe, R.P. Pollock, R.R. Weichselbaum, J.F. Holland, & E. Frei (Eds.), *Cancer medicine* (pp. 573–584). London: B.C. Decker, Inc.

Kintzel, P.E. (2000). Guidelines for chemoprotectant agents. *Oncology Special Edition, 3,* 71–74.

Kirkwood, J.M., Lotze, M.T., & Yasko, J.M. (Eds.). (1994). *Current cancer therapeutics* (5th ed.). Philadelphia: Current Medicine.

Kübler-Ross, E. (1969). *On death and dying.* New York: Macmillan.

Langhorne, M. (1997). Chemotherapy. In S.E. Otto (Ed.), *Oncology nursing* (pp. 530–572). St. Louis, MO: Mosby.

McCune, J.S., Harvey, R.D., Pfeiffer, D., & Lindley, C.M. (Eds.) (1998). *1998 guide to cancer chemotherapeutic regimens.* New York: McMahon Publishing Group.

Murphy, G.P., Lawrence, W., & Lenhard, R.E. (Eds.). (1995). *Clinical oncology* (2nd ed.). Atlanta: American Cancer Society.

National Institutes of Health. (1999). *Safe preparation of cytotoxic drugs: Steps A, B, C. Recommendations for safe handling of cytotoxic drugs*. Bethesda, MD: Author. Retrieved March 19, 2001 from the World Wide Web: http:/www.nih.gov/od/ors/ds/pubs/cyto/stepl.htm

National Institutes for Occupational Safety and Health (1988). Guidelines for protecting the safety and health of health care workers (DHHS Publication No. [NIOSHJ88–110]). Cincinnati, OH: U.S. Department of Health and Human Services, Public Health Service, Centers for Disease Control and Prevention.

Nevidjon, B., & Travaglini, J. (1990). Complications related to cancer therapy. *Clinical Advances in Oncology Nursing, 2*, 1–12.

PDR: Oncology prescribing guide (2nd ed.). (1998). Montvale, NJ: Medical Economics Company.

Peters, B.G. (Ed.). (1998). *Pocket guide to injectable chemotherapeutic agents* (2nd ed.). Collegeville, PA: Rhône-Poulenc Rorer Pharmaceuticals, Inc.

Preston, F.A., & Wilfinger, C. (1993). *Memory bank for chemotherapy* (2nd ed.). Boston: Jones and Bartlett.

Reyman, P.E. (1993). Chemotherapy: Principles of administration. In S.L. Groenwald, M.H. Frogge, M. Goodman, & C.H. Yarbro (Eds.), *Cancer nursing: Principles and practice* (3rd ed.) (pp. 293–330). Boston: Jones and Bartlett.

Shapiro, J., Gotfried, M., & Lishner, M. (1990). Reduced cardiotoxicity of doxorubicin by a 6 hour infusion regimen: A prospective randomized evaluation. *Cancer, 65,* 870–873.

Singleton, L.C., & Connor, T.H. (1999). An evaluation of the permeability of chemotherapy gloves to three cancer chemotherapy drugs. *Oncology Nursing Forum, 26,* 1491.

U.S. Department of Labor, Occupational Safety and Health Administration. (1986). Work practice guidelines for personnel dealing with cytotoxic (antineoplastic) drugs. *American Journal of Hospital Pharmacy, 43,* 1193–1204.

U.S. Department of Labor, Occupational Safety and Health Administration. (1995). *Controlling occupational exposure to hazardous drugs. Directorate of Technical Support* (OSHA Instructional CPL 2–2.20B CH–4). Bethesda, MD: Author

U.S. Department of Labor, Occupational Safety and Health Administration. (1999). *OSHA Technical Manual: Section VI: Chapter 2. Controlling occupational exposure to hazardous drugs*. Retrieved March 4, 2001 from the World Wide Web: http://www.ishasic.gov/dis/osta/olm_vl/olm_vi_2.html

Varricchio, C. (Ed.). (1997). *A cancer source book for nurses*. Atlanta: American Cancer Society.

Welch, J., & Silveira, J.M. (Eds.). (1997). *Safe handling of cytotoxic drugs: An independent study module*. Pittsburgh: Oncology Nursing Press, Inc.

Wilkes, G.M., Ingwersen, K., & Burke, M.B. (1999). *1999 oncology nursing drug handbook*. Boston: Jones and Bartlett.

Wood, L. (1998). *New therapies: New nursing challenges. Newer therapeutic agents: Nursing management* (pp. 1–2). West Conshohocken, PA: Meniscus Limited.

Ziegfeld, C.R., Lubejko, B.G., & Shelton, B.K. (Eds.). (1998). *Manual of cancer care*. Philadelphia: Lippincott.

CHAPTER 4

Vascular Access Devices

Jennifer S. Webster, MN, RN, CS, AOCN®

Introduction

Infusion therapy in the oncology setting is increasingly complex, and the role of the oncology nurse is continually expanding. Administration of chemotherapeutic agents requires constant updating of knowledge and skills. The oncology nurse faces an ever-increasing array of vascular access devices (VADs) as advances in design have improved the options of chemotherapy delivery to people with cancer. The purpose of this chapter is to provide nurses caring for patients with cancer with an overview of the various central venous access devices, some devices used in alternate routes of chemotherapy administration, the advantages and disadvantages of each device, and their care requirements.

Brief History of Vascular Access Devices

Since the early 1900s, catheters have been inserted into the central circulation for the provision of short-term parenteral nutrition and for research into cardiac physiology (Andris & Krzywda, 1997). Percutaneous central venous catheters (CVCs) that could remain in place for several days or weeks have been commonly used in the hospital setting since the late 1960s (Roy, Wilkinson, & Bayliss, 1967; Wenzel & Edmond, 1999). The first long-term VAD (the Broviac® tunneled catheter [Evermed Corporation, Medina, WA]) was developed in 1973 to provide long-term parenteral nutrition (Broviac, Cole, & Scribner, 1973). In 1979, the Broviac catheter was modified by increasing the internal diameter, thus allowing for withdrawal of blood samples as well as for high-volume infusions (Hickman et al., 1979). The modified catheter (named the Hickman® catheter [Bard Access Systems, Inc., Salt Lake City, UT] for the physician who designed the changes) became the catheter of choice for long-term venous access (Andris & Krzywda; Hickman et al.). Further modifications led to the development of double- and triple-lumen Hickman catheters and to valve technology (Groshong® catheter, Bard Access Systems, Inc.) that reduced blood backup and negated the need for regular heparinization.

In the early 1980s, a totally implanted vascular access system (Port-a-Cath®, Pharmacia, Inc., Piscataway, NJ) was developed using a catheter attached to a subcutaneous port anchored in the chest wall (Niederhuber, Ensminger, & Gyves, 1982). The lack of an external catheter offered increased protection from infection and reduced the care needed to maintain the access. Developments in the past 15 years have included double-lumen ports, port septums that can be accessed from the side instead of the top, and smaller ports and catheters to allow for placement in the brachial vein (Camp-Sorrell, 1996; Greene, 1996; Hadaway, 1995).

Since the early 1990s, the use of peripherally inserted central catheters (PICCs) has become increasingly popular as a bridge between short-term percutaneous devices and surgically inserted long-term devices. PICCs are inserted by registered nurses with specialty training, thus allowing for hospital bedside or at-home insertion. PICCs usually remain in place four to six weeks, although some may last for several months and, occasionally, years. As ambulatory and homecare settings become increasingly prevalent in treating patients with cancer, devices such as PICCs that provide a safe alternative to a surgically inserted long-term VAD have become popular among patients and healthcare professionals (Goodman, 2000; Martin, Walker, & Goodman, 1996).

Central Venous Catheters
Percutaneous Central Venous Catheters

Percutaneous, or nontunneled, CVCs have been in use for decades in the hospital setting. Generally thought of as short-term, placement of these catheters is intended for use for days or weeks (Woolery-Antill, 1998). The catheters may be single- or multilumen and are commonly composed of silicone, polyurethane, or polyvinyl-chloride (Bacquiran & Gallagher, 1998; Camp-Sorrell, 1996; Gullatte, 1990). These materials are constructed to create a rigid catheter that is easy to insert, thus allowing for placement under local anesthesia at the bedside or in the emergency room instead of in the operating room (Goodman, 2000). Common veins in which percutaneous CVCs are placed include the internal jugular vein, the external jugular vein, and the subclavian vein (see Figure 4-1). The distal

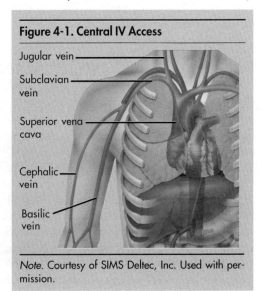

Figure 4-1. Central IV Access

Jugular vein

Subclavian vein

Superior vena cava

Cephalic vein

Basilic vein

Note. Courtesy of SIMS Deltec, Inc. Used with permission.

tip of the catheter rests in the superior vena cava or right atrium (see Figure 4-2). Correct placement is confirmed by chest x-ray. The catheter exit site is usually only a short distance (approximately one inch) from the entrance to the vein, thus providing an efficient means for bacteria to enter the venous system (Jones, 1998; Martin et al., 1996). The rigidity of the catheter also may cause damage to the inner lining of the vein, which increases the risk for thrombosis and infection. The introduction of antimicrobial surface coatings on the indwelling portion of the catheter has reportedly reduced the incidence of infection, however further clinical trials are needed (Gullatte, 1990; Wenzel & Edmond, 1999). Often used with patients

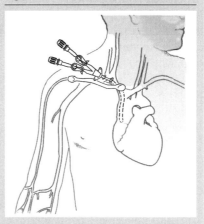

Figure 4-2. Subclavian Catheter

Note. Figure courtesy of Tri-State Hospital Supply Corporation. Used with permission.

with cancer for postoperative analgesic administration, acute care fluid management, and short-term total parenteral nutrition, these catheters rarely are inserted for chemotherapy administration alone. However, the nurse may encounter the patient who already has a percutaneous CVC for other therapies and now requires chemotherapy or the patient who is receiving a short-term yet complex antineoplastic regimen requiring multiple catheter lumens. Percutaneous catheters also may be inserted in the patient with cancer for renal dialysis or apheresis, but these catheters usually are dedicated solely for those procedures and are unavailable for chemotherapy administration (Goodman).

Daily maintenance of these catheters has been well defined. Figure 4-3 outlines the common care procedures.

These catheters most commonly are used in the hospital setting and are maintained by healthcare professionals. The healthcare team should discuss alternative devices with patients who require ongoing chemotherapy treatments or need to be discharged home with central venous access, as it is inappropriate to use these short-term acute care catheters as long-term venous access or in the home setting.

Figure 4-3. Care of Percutaneous (Nontunneled), Short-Term Vascular Access Devices

Dressing Change
Change gauze dressing QOD or 3x per week. Change transparent dressing every four to seven days. Use aseptic technique.

Flushing Procedure
Heparin 10 u/ml–100 u/ml, 1 ml per lumen, q 8–12 hours.

Cap Change
Every week and when leaking or soiled

Tunneled Central Venous Catheters

Central venous tunneled catheters are made of silicone, polyurethane, or a combination of the two and are available in single, double, or triple lumens in various gauges and lengths (see Figure 4-4). Every catheter has a Dacron® (E.I. du Pont de Nemours and Co., Wilmington, DE) polyester cuff designed to anchor in the subcutaneous tissue approximately one to two inches from the exit site and to reduce inadvertent dislodgment (see Figure 4-5). Certain catheters also may have a separate antibiotic-impregnated cuff just below the skin surface. These cuffs are designed to reduce infection by releasing an antimicrobial agent over a four- to six-week period and by providing a physical barrier to passage of bacteria from the skin into the vein. The catheters are inserted under local or general anesthesia into one of the central veins (the subclavian, jugular, or cephalic veins are the most common choices) with the catheter tip resting in the superior vena cava near the right atrium. The catheter is tunneled through subcutaneous tissue to a separate exit site, usually on the chest wall midway between the sternum and clavicle above the nipple line (see Figure 4-5). The subcutaneous tunnel acts as a barrier to bacteria traveling from the skin into the vein, reducing the potential for infection and allowing the catheter to remain in place for months to years (Camp-Sorrell, 1996; Goodman, 2000; Masoorli, 1997).

The distal tip of the tunneled catheter may be open- or close-ended in the vein. The open-ended catheter requires clamping at the proximal end during cap, syringe, or tubing changes to avoid air embolism. Open-ended catheters are at risk for blood backup and clotting; therefore, they must be flushed daily with a heparin solution when not in use and after each blood aspiration or fluid infusion (Camp-Sorrell, 1996; Goodman, 2000). The patented closed-end Groshong catheter has a two-way, pressure-sensitive valve that remains closed except during infusion or aspiration. Positive pressure

Figure 4-4. Double Lumen Tunneled Catheter (Hickman®)

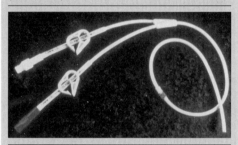

Note. Photo courtesy of Bard Access Systems, Inc. Used with permission.

Figure 4-5. Tunneled Catheter Position

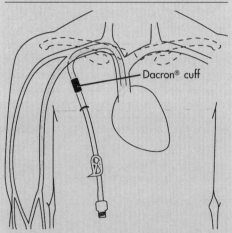

Dacron® cuff

Note. Figure courtesy of SIMS Deltec, Inc. Used with permission.

into the catheter will open the valve outward, allowing fluid infusion. Negative or vacuum pressure will cause the valve to open inward, allowing blood aspiration. When the catheter is not in use, the valve remains closed and potential for air embolism or blood backup into the catheter is virtually eliminated (see Figure 4-6). Catheter clamps are not needed, and the manufacturer recommends flushing only once a week with normal saline. However, anecdotal reports of occasional blood backup and clot formation resulted in a small prospective, nonrandomized study of Groshong catheters comparing normal saline flush to weekly heparinized flush of 2.5 cc of 1/100 u heparin (Mayo, Horne, Summers, Pearson, & Helsaveck, 1996). The authors of the study reported significantly fewer problems with the catheters in the heparin flush group and recommended addition of a weekly heparin flush to the plan of care.

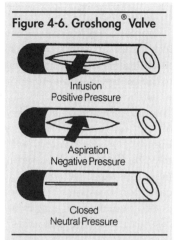

Figure 4-6. Groshong® Valve

Infusion
Positive Pressure

Aspiration
Negative Pressure

Closed
Neutral Pressure

Note. Figure courtesy of Bard Access Systems, Inc. Used with permission.

New pressure-sensitive valve technology, such as the PASV Catheter™ (Catheter Innovations, Inc., Salt Lake City, UT), is designed to reduce blood flow back up.

Another variation of the tunneled catheter has been the tunneled apheresis catheter (Pheres-Flow™, Neostar Medical Technologies Corporation, Atlanta, GA) developed in the early 1990s. Unlike the standard percutaneous apheresis catheters, the tunneled apheresis catheter can remain in place for months because of the subcutaneous tunnel. However, compared to the standard tunneled catheters, the Pheres-Flow has a larger diameter and is made of a stronger material able to withstand the aspiration pressure of a pheresis machine. This catheter is particularly useful in patients who may require apheresis or peripheral blood stem cell collection but who also will require long-term IV access. Figure 4-7 outlines the common care procedures for tunneled catheters.

Figure 4-7. Care of Tunneled Catheters

Dressing Change
Change gauze dressing QOD or 3x per week. Change transparent dressing every four to seven days. Use aseptic technique until exit site healed, then may use clean technique.

Flushing Procedure
- Heparin 100 u/ml, 1.8–2.5 ml per lumen, q 24h.
- **Groshong®:** Normal saline solution 10 ml weekly.
- **Tunneled apheresis:** Heparin 1,000 u/ml–5000 u/ml, 1ml per lumen, q 72h while used for apheresis. Heparin is withdrawn prior to use. Heparin 100 u/ml, 1.8–2.5 ml per lumen, q24h while in use for other fluid therapies or during routine catheter maintenance.

Cap Change
Every week and when leaking or soiled. During apheresis, caps are changed after each collection session. After completion of apheresis, sessions caps are changed weekly.

Implanted Ports and Reservoirs

Implanted ports consist of a soft silicone or polyurethane catheter attached to a reservoir with a raised silicone resealable septum surrounded by a titanium, stainless steel, or plastic base (see Figure 4-8). The catheter tip is placed in the central vein, and the port is implanted into a surgically created subcutaneous pocket, usually on the chest wall (see Figure 4-9). Implanted ports may be single- or double-lumen, and the distal end of the catheter may be open- or closed-ended. The port is accessed through the skin using a specialty, noncoring, 90° (or right-angle) Huber needle that pierces the self-sealing septum and enters the reservoir (see Figure 4-10). The needle may remain in place for up to seven days under aseptically applied transparent dressing; if further access is required, a new needle and dressing must be placed. Upon completion of treatment, the needle may be removed after flushing the port with heparinized saline; the port then only requires once-a-month flushing to maintain patency. During the time the port is not in use, it is completely subcutaneous; therefore, no dressings are required and patients may shower or swim without restrictions. Only a small circular lump under the skin reveals the location of the port, making it a more cosmetically pleasing VAD than external catheters. The lengthy time between maintenance flushing means that few patients have to learn how to flush the ports themselves. Therapy requirements usually entail seeing a physi-

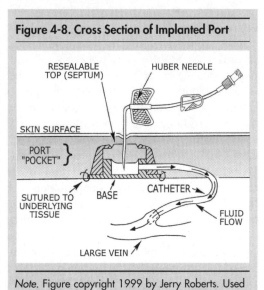

Figure 4-8. Cross Section of Implanted Port

RESEALABLE TOP (SEPTUM)
HUBER NEEDLE
SKIN SURFACE
PORT "POCKET"
SUTURED TO UNDERLYING TISSUE
BASE
CATHETER
FLUID FLOW
LARGE VEIN

Note. Figure copyright 1999 by Jerry Roberts. Used with permission.

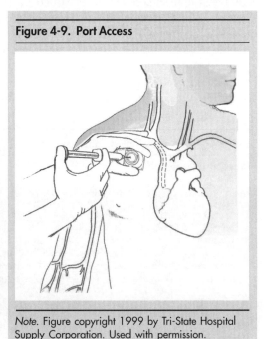

Figure 4-9. Port Access

Note. Figure copyright 1999 by Tri-State Hospital Supply Corporation. Used with permission.

cian or healthcare professional at least once a month, and the port can be flushed at that time. Disadvantages to the implanted port include the necessity of piercing the skin to access the port, the difficulty of palpating the port for access in an obese person, and the need for specialty training in port access for healthcare personnel (Andris & Krsywda, 1997; Camp-Sorrell, 1996; Fulton, 1997; Goodman, 2000; Gullatte, 1989; Gullatte, Koretz, & Sarma, 1991). The subcutaneous placement of the port and resulting lack of visibility may hinder troubleshooting of an occluded catheter or early detection of edema or drug extravasation (Schulmeister & Camp-Sorrell, 2000; Viale, Yamamoto, & Geyton, 1999).

A more recent addition to the selection of implanted ports is the P.A.S. Port™ (SIMS Deltec, St. Paul, MN) system. The P.A.S. Port has a smaller reservoir and base that allow for placement in the subcutaneous tissue of the upper or lower arm, with the catheter inserted at the antecubital fossa and threaded via the basilic, cephalic, or axillary vein into the superior vena cava (see Figure 4-11). The P.A.S. Port is more advantageous than the chest wall port because the surgical insertion procedure is less extensive and can be completed in a physician's office. An-

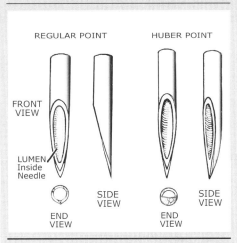

Figure 4-10. Comparison of Regular Needle Point to Huber Needle Point

REGULAR POINT   HUBER POINT

FRONT VIEW

LUMEN Inside Needle

SIDE VIEW   SIDE VIEW

END VIEW   END VIEW

Note. Figure copyright 1999 by Tri-State Hospital Supply Corporation. Used with permission.

Figure 4-11. P.A.S. Port™ Position

Note. Figure courtesy of SIMS Deltec, Inc. Used with permission.

other advantage is that the skin on the upper chest is spared a surgical incision and Huber needle insertions, making this catheter a good choice for patients with extensive chest surgeries or chest wall radiation (Goodman, 2000; Martin et al., 1996). The P.A.S. Port is accessed with a very short (0.5 inch) noncoring needle because of its proximity to the skin surface, but other aspects of care, such as flushing and dressing change, are similar to other implanted ports (see Figure 4-12).

Figure 4-12. Care of Implanted Ports

Dressing Change
Use only noncoring Huber needle to access port. During access, change needle and transparent dressing every week, or gauze dressing 3x per week. Use aseptic technique.

Flushing Procedure
Heparin 100 u/ml, 5 ml, once a month when not accessed. During access, after medication administration, 10 ml normal saline flush, followed by heparin 100 u/ml, 5 ml.

Cap Change
Every week with needle change and when leaking or soiled

Peripherally Inserted Central Catheters

The use of a PICC has become increasingly popular as a bridge between a short-term percutaneous device and a surgically inserted long-term device (Goodman, 2000). The PICC is a thin, flexible catheter inserted at the antecubital fossa into the basilic or cephalic vein and advanced to the superior vena cava (see Figure 4-13). The catheter may be inserted at the bedside or under fluoroscopy if necessary, thus negating the need for a surgical procedure. PICCs inserted at the bedside must have central venous placement confirmed by x-ray. Once confirmed, PICCs may be used for medications, including vesicants, and blood product infusion similar to any other CVC. Registered nurses with specialty training are allowed to insert PICCs in most states, although the legal parameters differ from state to state. PICCs are designed to remain in place four to six weeks, although they may be durable enough to last several months and, occasionally, years. Advantages of the PICC include its ease of placement at the bedside, relatively low complication rate, small size, and cost-benefit ratio. Disadvantages include the placement in the antecubital fossa, thereby limiting arm mobility, and a possible inability to draw blood because of the small diameter of the catheter. Patients who require frequent blood draws or intensive long-term therapy may not be appropriate PICC candidates (Berg, 1996; Goodman, 2000; Martin et al., 1996).

A modification of the PICC, the midline catheter, is a shortened catheter that is only inserted to the axillary vein (see Figure 4-14). A midline is not a central catheter, and care must be taken to distinguish it via labeling and documentation so that it is not confused with a PICC. Hyperalimentation and vesicant chemotherapeutic agents are not appropriate solutions for midline infusion (Kupensky, 1998). Nursing management of the PICC and midline are similar and are listed in Figure 4-15.

Central Venous Access Device Choices

As the choices of VADs continue to multiply, it may be difficult to explain to the patient the advantages and disadvantages of each option. Table 4-1 provides a brief description, the usual life span, and advantages and disadvantages of each major device category to assist the oncology nurse with comparison. Individual access devices may differ in their specific uses.

Figure 4-13. Central Catheter Placement

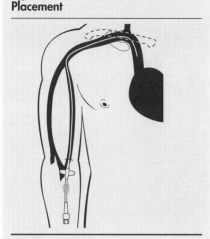

The tip of the peripherally inserted central catheter resides in a central vein.

Note. Figure courtsey of SIMS Deltec, Inc. Used with permission.

Figure 4-14. Midline Catheter Placement

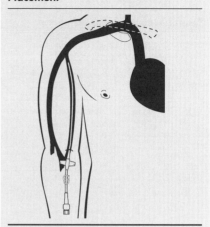

The tip of the Midline catheter is positioned in a peripheral vein.

Note. Figure courtsey of SIMS Deltec, Inc. Used with permission.

Figure 4-15. Care of Peripherally Inserted Central Catheters or Midline Catheters

Dressing Change
Change transparent dressing changed 24h after initial insertion, then every four to seven days, or gauze dressings 3x per week. Use aseptic technique.

Flushing Procedure
Heparin 100 u/ml, 1 ml per lumen, q 8–12h

Cap Change
Every week and when leaking or soiled

Central Venous Access Device Complications

Many CVC complications may be avoided with proactive nursing interventions; however, catheter complications such as occlusion, infection, and breakage do occur. Successful management of catheter complications may prevent interruption of therapy or catheter replacement. Table 4-2 lists the most common catheter complications, interventions, and prevention methods.

Alternative Administration Devices
Arterial Catheters

Intra-arterial drug administration involves the insertion of a catheter into an artery that provides blood supply to a tumor. The infusion of antineoplastic agents directly into the tumor bed increases drug concentration at the tumor site without increasing systemic drug concentration, thus reducing the potential for

Table 4-1. Comparison of Vascular Access Devices: Advantages, Disadvantages, and Recommendations

Central Venous Access Device	Description, Life Span	Advantages	Disadvantages
Percutaneous nontunneled	Rigid catheter inserted directly into a central vein Single-, double- or triple-lumen catheter available Life span: three to six weeks	Can be inserted at bedside Multiple lumens allow for concurrent infusion of several therapies May be used to obtain blood samples. Easy to remove Recommended for acute-care and critical-care situations	Insertion is a major invasive procedure requiring informed consent. Insertion is complex; may require multiple attempts. Insertion can lead to complications, such as pneumothorax, bleeding, and infection. Potential for infection is high; meticulous aseptic care of catheter is required. Not recommended for long-term or outpatient therapy because of potential for infection and care requirements.
Tunneled	Soft, flexible catheter inserted so tip is in superior vena cava and proximal end is tunneled through subcutaneous tissue to exit on the chest wall. Single-, double- or triple-lumen catheter available. Life span: months to years	Reliable, long-term source of venous access Multiple lumens allow for concurrent infusion of several therapies. Has potentially lower infection rates than percutaneous catheters May be used to obtain blood samples External catheter segment can usually be repaired with specialty kit. Recommended for long-term use or therapy that requires frequent IV access	Requires surgical procedure for placement Requires daily to weekly care, such as flushing with heparin and dressing changes Dressing and flush supplies may be expensive. Potential for infection, dislodgment, thrombosis External catheter may alter body image and restrict certain activities, such as swimming or showering. Not recommended for short-term or intermittent therapies

(Continued on next page)

Table 4-1. Comparison of Vascular Access Devices: Advantages, Disadvantages, and Recommendations *(Continued)*

Central Venous Access Device	Description, Life Span	Advantages	Disadvantages
Implanted port	Catheter is attached to a reservoir with a resealable silicone septum surrounded by a rigid base. Catheter tip is in a central vein; reservoir port is implanted in a subcutaneous pocket, usually on chest wall. Single- or double-lumen catheter available Life span: months to years	Port is completely subcutaneous; only a raised bump is visible. No dressings are required when not in use Monthly flush needed when not in use No restrictions on activities such as swimming or showering May be used to obtain blood samples Recommended for long-term use or therapy that requires intermittent or occasional IV access	Requires surgical procedure for placement Requires needle placement through skin to access May be difficult to access if port not easily palpable Noncoring needles must be used to access port. No triple-lumen access available May interfere with magnetic resonance imaging procedures Not recommended for therapies requiring frequent multiple access to the venous system over weeks to months
Peripherally inserted central catheter (PICC) or midline catheter	Thin flexible catheter inserted at the antecubital fossa into the basilic or cephalic vein and advanced to the superior vena cava (PICC) or axilla (midline). Single- or double-lumen catheter available Life span: weeks to months	Specially trained RN can insert. Can be inserted at bedside Easy to remove Provides safe, economical access to the venous system Small size is convenient for elderly and children. Less expensive than percutaneous, tunneled, or implanted port catheters Recommended for use in therapies lasting weeks to months that do not require a great deal of catheter manipulation	RN must be specially trained and maintain a high level of competence. May be unable to obtain blood samples May limit arm movement May kink or clot easily because of small catheter diameter Transfusion of red blood cells may be discouraged by manufacturer or agency policy. Not available in triple-lumen size Durability may be compromised with frequent use and manipulation. Not recommended for use in long-term therapies requiring frequent catheter manipulations, multiple blood samples, or blood transfusions

Table 4-2. Common Catheter Complications and Intervention Methods

Catheter Complication	Signs and Symptoms	Interventions
Pneumothorax, hemothorax: related to air or blood in the pleural cavity as a result of injury to a lung or vein during the catheter insertion process	Dyspnea, tachypnea, chest pain, tachycardia, decreasing or absent breath sounds in affected area, cyanosis	Notify physician, obtain chest x-ray, administer oxygen; patient may need needle aspiration or chest tube placement.
Air embolism: the introduction of air into the central venous device and thus into the patient's venous system; usually related to catheter breakage or loosened connections of IV tubing	Sudden respiratory difficulty, such as tachypnea and dyspnea, chest or pleuritic pain, tachycardia, hypotension, enlarged neck veins, cyanosis	Notify physician, place patient on left side, place patient bed in Trendelenburg position, and administer oxygen. If catheter is broken or leaking, place clamp between source of leak and patient.
Postinsertion bleeding at site: a result of traumatic insertion, thrombocytopenia, or other coagulopathies	Bloody discharge or frank bleeding at catheter exit site that may persist for hours. A hematoma may develop at exit site.	Apply pressure to exit site; may need small sandbags (three to five lbs.) applied to site. Change dressings as needed; may require topical thrombin or gel foam. If bleeding does not stop, catheter may need to be removed.
Difficulty aspirating blood, or complete occlusion: related to blood clot, fibrin sheath, drug precipitate, kinked catheter, catheter malposition, or venous obstruction	Difficulty obtaining blood return despite easy infusion of fluids or complete inability to aspirate and infuse fluids	Assess/correct possible causes: patient position, kink in IV tubing, malposition of implanted port needle. Attempt to aspirate and gently flush catheter.
Breakage or puncture: damage usually related to the use of hemostats, scissors, safety pins, or sharp clamps on the external catheter segment. Excessive force while flushing, such as attempting to flush during catheter occlusion or when clamps are inadvertently left closed, also will cause catheter breakage.	Visible leaking from catheter. When flushed, fluid leaks out of puncture site.	Instill a thrombolytic agent for catheter occluded by blood; if unsuccessful after two attempts, consider another source of occlusion, such as drug precipitate or catheter malposition. X-ray or dye study may be needed. Follow institutional policy for drug or lipid precipitate. If unable to resolve, catheter may need to be removed.

(Continued on next page)

Table 4-2. Common Catheter Complications and Intervention Methods *(Continued)*

Catheter Complication	Signs and Symptoms	Interventions
Infection Exit site	Redness, swelling, tenderness, discharge at exit site; may have positive cultures of exit site	Increase cleansing and dressing change frequency, and apply a topical antibacterial ointment to site. Assess catheter care technique of caregivers, and correct any poor technique. Patient may need IV antibiotics.
Catheter tunnel or port pocket	Redness, swelling, tenderness, or warmth tracking along catheter tunnel or above implanted port; may have positive blood culture of catheter	Patient will need IV antibiotics. Maintain meticulous aseptic technique when accessing port or catheter and when changing dressing. Catheter or port may need to be removed.
Systemic	Fever is the most common indicator of systemic infection. Patient may also have chills, tachycardia, diaphoresis, and hypotension and may have positive blood cultures.	Patient will need IV antibiotics. Monitor vital signs and urine output for signs of septic shock. Catheter or port may need to be removed.

Note. Based on information from Bacquiran & Gallagher, 1998; Camp-Sorrell, 1996; Woolery-Antill, 1998.

side effects (Goodman, 2000). The common hepatic artery is the most commonly used vessel, primarily to target liver metastases from colon carcinoma but also as a method to treat hepatocellular cancer. Antineoplastic agents used include floxuridine, fluorouracil, doxorubicin, and mitomycin C (Almadrones, Campana, & Dantis, 1995; West, 1998). Despite the use of this method of delivery for more than two decades, controversies regarding benefits versus risk and expense still remain (Camp-Sorrell, 1996; West).

Two types of intra-arterial catheters may be used. External catheters are inserted percutaneously in radiology and are temporary, usually remaining in place for less than seven days. An external catheter is used when a patient is unable to tolerate surgery for an internal/permanent catheter, the clinical protocol requires antineoplastic therapy of short duration, or to determine the efficacy of treatment before surgical insertion of a permanent device. The site of insertion is covered with a sterile transparent dressing and must be monitored closely for bleeding, infection, or dislodgment of the catheter. The advent of internal arterial catheters has reduced the use of percutaneous catheters (Almadrones et al., 1995; West, 1998).

The more common intra-arterial catheter is a permanent device attached to either an implanted port or infusion pump placed in the subcutaneous tissue of the lower abdomen or upper chest. Intra-arterial ports are designed like IV ports with a raised, resealable silicone septum surrounded by a titanium or plastic base. The port is accessed with a noncoring needle by a trained professional and attached to an ambulatory infusion pump. Arterial flow resistance may be quite strong, requiring a pump with adequate pounds-per-square-inch pressure and weekly flushing of the port with 5,000 u of heparin when not in use (Almadrones et al., 1995; Camp-Sorrell, 1996; West, 1998). The only mechanical difference between an intra-arterial port and an IV port is the anatomical placement of the catheter; therefore, dressing protocol should mimic the healthcare institution's established protocol for IV port care (Goodman, 2000; West). Chemotherapy usually is administered in the ambulatory care setting; therefore, the nurse must teach the patient the signs and symptoms of infection, needle dislodgment, catheter occlusion, and infiltration.

Intra-arterial pumps are totally implanted into a surgically created pocket of subcutaneous tissue and are designed for continuous, low-volume, long-term ambulatory therapy (Camp-Sorrell, 1996). There are two manufacturers of implantable pumps: Arrow International in Reading, PA, makers of the Arrow Model 3000™ Infusion Pump and Medtronic Neurological in Minneapolis, MN, makers of the SynchroMed and IsoMed Infusion Systems™. Both manufacturers offer a model with a secondary port that bypasses the pumping mechanism and allows for direct arterial injection of a medication. Each pump has a flat, circular-shaped septum, which is accessed with a noncoring pump needle using strict aseptic technique (see Figures 4-16, 4-17, 4-18, and 4-19). The septum is connected to a drug reservoir that delivers the medication via a vapor-pressured bellows system (Arrow) or a peristaltic roller pump powered by a lithium battery that lasts three to four years (Medtronic). Refill of the drug reservoir is required approximately every two weeks. The flow rates are either preset prior to implantation or adjustable via an external electronic wand that communicates with the internal pump

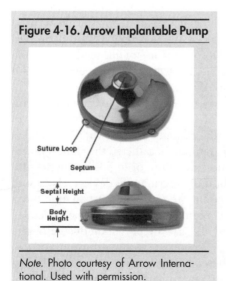

Figure 4-16. Arrow Implantable Pump	Figure 4-17. IsoMed Implantable Pump

Suture Loop

Septum

Septal Height

Body
Height

IsoMed™
Pump

Note. Photo courtesy of Arrow International. Used with permission.

Note. Photo courtesy of Medtronic, Inc. Used with permission.

(Berg, 1996; Goodman, 2000). Flow rates may increase with hypertension, fever, or travel to a higher altitude. Flow rates may decrease with hypotension, drop in body temperature, or travel to a lower altitude. Possible variations in flow rate, inability to change the flow rate, restriction of medication to 50 ml or less, and the high cost of insertion are all disadvantages of the implanted pumps (Camp-Sorrell). Patients must have an understanding of how the pump works, their travel restrictions, and their need to keep appointments to have the pump refilled (West, 1998). Table 4-3 lists the signs and symptoms of the most common catheter and pump complications.

Intraperitoneal Catheters

Antineoplastic agents may be directly administered into the peritoneal space to increase drug concentrations in the peritoneum while maintaining lower systemic blood concentrations. Ovarian and rectal carcinomas are the most common diagnoses for use of intraperitoneal chemotherapies (Bacquiran & Gallagher, 1998; West, 1998). Agents used include carboplatinum, cisplatinum, cytosine aribinoside, doxorubicin, etoposide, fluorouracil, and

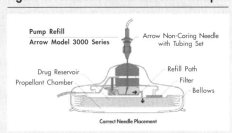

Figure 4-18. Internal View of Arrow Pump

Note. Photo courtesy of Arrow International. Used with permission.

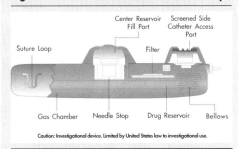

Figure 4-19. Internal View of IsoMed Pump

Note. Photo courtesy of Medtronic, Inc. Used with permission.

Table 4-3. Signs and Symptoms of Intra-arterial Catheter and Pump Complications

Signs	Symptoms
Infection	Pain, fever, redness, swelling, and/or drainage at insertion site
Catheter complications: dislodgment, infiltration, or occlusion	Pain or discomfort during infusion, inability to infuse or sluggish infusion, weak or absent peripheral pulse
Drug therapy effects	Site- and drug-specific; intrahepatic therapy may induce rising liver function tests, chemical hepatitis, biliary sclerosis, cholecystitis, pancreatitis
Ambulatory pump pocket infection or seroma	Pain, fever, redness, swelling, and/or drainage at pocket; fluid and/or edema above and around pump

Note. Based on information from West, 1998; Woolery-Antill, 1998.

methotrexate (Woolery-Antill, 1998). Side effects include not only toxicities associated with specific drugs but also those related to increased intra-abdominal pressure, such as abdominal pain, nausea, respiratory distress, and diarrhea. Raising the head of the bed to reduce intra-abdominal pressure on the diaphragm, instructing the patient to roll from side to side to evenly distribute the intra-abdominal fluid, and the administration of analgesics are all appropriate intervention strategies to reduce these side effects (Almadrones et al., 1995; West, 1998).

The two most common methods for delivery of chemotherapy to the peritoneal space are via an external Tenckhoff dialysis catheter or implantable peritoneal port. The Tenckhoff catheter is a silicone catheter inserted directly into the peritoneum via a subcutaneous tunnel. The catheter exits through the skin, extending approximately 10 inches, and is capped between infusions. One or two Dacron cuffs on the catheter act as barriers to infection and anchor the catheter to prevent dislodgment (Almadrones et al., 1995). The Tenckhoff catheter has a large internal diameter that allows for the rapid infusion of drugs and fluid (two liters in 10–15 minutes). Daily care of the catheter includes sterile dressing changes at the exit site until the site has completely healed and assessing for any bleeding, leaking, or signs of infection. Once the site has healed (approximately two to four weeks), daily clean dressings may replace the sterile dressing changes (see Table 4-4) (Woolery-Antill, 1998). Because of the potential for infection and daily maintenance needs, the use of the external Tenckhoff catheter has decreased in favor of the implantable port (Goodman, 2000; West, 1998).

The implantable peritoneal port uses a catheter similar in design to the Tenckhoff, but the end is attached to a titanium or silicone casing surrounding a reservoir and self-sealing septum that is placed in a surgically created subcutaneous pocket. The port is usually implanted over a lower rib to stabilize access and is accessed using a large-bore noncoring needle under aseptic technique. The noncoring needle restricts the flow of IV fluids or chemotherapy; therefore, flow rates are not as rapid as those that occur with the external Tenckhoff catheter, and two liters may require a 30–45-minute infusion time. The port is flushed

Table 4-4. Care of Intraperitoneal Catheters

Type of Intraperitoneal Catheter	Dressing Change	Flush Procedure	Cap Change
Tenckhoff (external)	Sterile dressing changed daily until site well healed, then switch to clean dressing daily or 3x per week	After completion of infusion, flush with 10–20 ml normal saline solution; no maintenance flush necessary	After completion of each therapy
Implanted port	Sterile transparent dressing and noncoring needle changed weekly during port access	Heparin 1/100 u, 5 ml after removal of needle; no maintenance flush necessary	Cap on attached intravenous tubing changed weekly or when soiled or leaking

with 10 ml normal saline solution after administration of medication. No maintenance care is required in between treatments (Camp-Sorrell, 1996). Potential for infection is lower than occurrence with the external Tenckhoff peritoneal catheter, and patients may swim or shower without restriction. Table 4-5 summarizes the signs and symptoms of intraperitoneal catheter complications.

Intraventricular Catheters

Certain cancer cells easily cross the blood-brain barrier, resulting in central nervous system (CNS) involvement of the malignancy. Acute lymphocytic leukemia is the malignancy most commonly associated with CNS involvement but other malignancies, such as breast cancer and lymphoma, may have meningeal invasion (Goodman, 2000; Martin et al., 1996). Immunocompromised patients also may experience fungal meningitis or brain abscesses that could benefit from direct delivery of antifungal drugs (Kosier & Minkler, 1999). Most antineoplastic agents do not cross the blood-brain barrier, so they must be delivered directly into the cerebrospinal fluid (CSF). The instillation of chemotherapy directly into the CSF is possible via lumbar puncture or the insertion of an Ommaya reservoir (American Hospital Supply Corporation, Evanston, IL). Prior to selecting the method of administration, the benefits and risks to the patient must be determined. Two factors must be weighed: the pain and possible complications of having a lumbar puncture performed for each treatment versus the potential complications of surgically inserting the Ommaya reservoir but having a permanent access to the CSF (Berg, 1996).

The Ommaya reservoir consists of a silicone catheter attached to a self-sealing dome-shaped reservoir. Placement of the Ommaya reservoir is a surgical procedure performed under local or general anesthesia. A burr hole is made in the skull

Table 4-5. Signs and Symptoms of Intraperitoneal Catheter Complications

Sign	Symptoms
Infection	Pain, fever, redness, swelling, and drainage at insertion site
Catheter complications: dislodgment, infiltration, or occlusion	Abdominal pain or discomfort during infusion, inability to infuse or sluggish infusion, inability to aspirate easily from catheter
Drug therapy effects	Gastrointestinal disturbances, such as nausea, vomiting, diarrhea, anorexia, gastroesophageal reflux; may be related to the agents used or the increased intra-abdominal pressure
Increased intra-abdominal pressure	Gastrointestinal disturbances, restlessness, abdominal pain, dyspnea
Peritonitis	Abdominal distension, rebound tenderness, fever, decreased or absent bowel sounds, gastrointestinal disturbances

Note. Based on information from West, 1998; Woolery-Antill, 1998.

and the catheter is threaded into the lateral ventricle of the brain. The reservoir is placed subcutaneously between the scalp and the skull, so once the surgical site is healed, only a small bulge underneath the scalp is visible (see Figure 4-20). Computerize tomography scan and clear return of CSF upon access of the reservoir confirm placement (Almadrones et al., 1995; Kosier & Minkler, 1999; West, 1998). The risk of infection is the primary complication of Ommaya insertion and remains relatively small. Antibiotics may be given prophylactically and for 72 hours after insertion (Woolery-Antill, 1998).

Selected chemotherapy agents, antibiotics, antifungal agents, and opiate an-

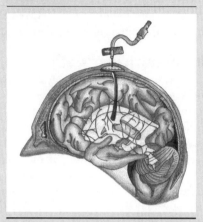

Figure 4-20. Position of Ommaya Reservoir

algesics are all appropriate medications that may be administered via the Ommaya reservoir. Antineoplastic agents that are commonly used include methotrexate, cytarabine, interferon, and thiotepa (Camp-Sorrell, 1996; Goodman, 2000). Ommaya reservoirs usually are only accessed and the selected medication instilled by specially trained nurses or physicians using aseptic technique. A small-gauge needle is inserted through the scalp into the reservoir and CSF is slowly removed (1 cc every 1–2 minutes) for a total amount equal to the volume of the medication to be instilled. The medication is then gently administered (1–2 cc/ minute) and the needle flushed with bacteriostatic saline or CSF to ensure that all medication has been instilled. No heparinization is necessary, as CSF continually flows through the reservoir (Kosier & Minkler, 1999; West, 1998). Responsibilities of the staff nurse include assessment of the site for signs and symptoms of local infection, bleeding, leakage of CSF, or shifting of the reservoir dome (see Table 4-6). The Ommaya reservoir may remain in place for months or years.

Ambulatory Infusion Pumps

Ambulatory infusion pumps have become increasingly popular in the therapy of patients with cancer and are now used for the administration of antineoplastic agents, total parenteral nutrition, antibiotics, analgesics, antiemetics, insulin, heparin, and hydration fluids. The advent of home IV therapy services, visiting nurse companies with expertise in home infusion devices, equipment maintenance, drug preparation and delivery, and 24-hour availability, has had a dramatic impact on the ability to deliver ambulatory infusion therapy safely and efficiently. Before initiating ambulatory pump therapy, several patient and treatment parameters must be assessed. The patient must have adequate venous access and may require CVC placement. The drug infusion procedure, number of doses, and length of treatment time affect how frequently the patient

Table 4-6. Signs and Symptoms of Intraventricular Catheter Complications

Sign	Symptoms
Infection	Pain, fever, redness, swelling, drainage at insertion site, headache, nausea, general malaise, stiff neck, cerebrospinal fluid (CSF) not clear
Reservoir complications: dislodgment or occlusion	Reservoir does not fill with CSF; dome of catheter does not depress easily or refill when depressed
Drug therapy effects	Chemotherapy: headache, fever, nausea, vomiting, ataxia, blurred vision, stomatitis
	Analgesia: dizziness, excessive sedation, nausea, vomiting, constipation, urinary retention, respiratory depression

Note. Based on information from West, 1998; Woolery-Antill, 1998.

must return to the ambulatory care setting or how much drug and nursing time a home infusion company must provide. The ability of the patient and family to participate in patient care, to manipulate the pump, and to troubleshoot problems must be considered. Healthcare personnel should assess the patient's living environment to ensure that it includes clean, readily available handwashing facilities, electricity, a refrigerator, a telephone, and readily available transportation to a healthcare facility (McNally, 1997; Yuska & Nedved, 2000). Finally, the cost of the therapy must be considered, as some insurance companies and Medicare have strict reimbursement guidelines for the types of therapies they will approve. Only with careful assessment and planning will home infusion therapy be successful (Bacquiran & Gallagher, 1998; Rapsilber & Camp Sorrell, 1995).

Ambulatory infusion pumps are classified by their mechanism of operation: elastomeric reservoir, syringe, and peristaltic. Table 4-7 provides a brief comparison of the mechanism of action, advantages, and disadvantages of each infusion pump. The mechanism of action, size, weight, power source, alarm mechanisms, cost, advantages, and disadvantages vary by individual pump. Each of these factors, along with reimbursement issues, level of service provided by the manufacturer, amount of teaching required, and availability of knowledgeable staff should be considered when selecting an infusion device.

Pertinent Documentation for All Vascular Access Devices

Documentation of the daily nursing assessment and care of a VAD is an integral part of the plan of care. The oncology nurse should assess the dressing on the catheter insertion/exit site at least once a day to ensure that it is dry and intact. Routine care of the catheter, such as dressing changes, flushes, and cap changes should be documented, and any problems should be noted. The catheter insertion/exit site should be assessed at each dressing change for redness,

Table 4-7. Comparison of Ambulatory Infusion Pumps

Type of Ambulatory Infusion Pump	Mechanism of Action	Advantages	Disadvantages
Elastomeric	Balloon pump: balloon is filled with fluid; deflates by gravity or exerted positive pressure. Single-dose volume capacity is from 50–500 ml; infusion time is 30 minutes to 5 hours.	Disposable, lightweight, portable, small No batteries or programming required Easy for patients to use	Limited infusion rates No system alarms Not for infusions longer than five hours or volume > 500 ml Difficult to fill Costly
Syringe	Disposable syringe is filled with fluid, plunger is pushed forward by a spring or electronically powered battery.	Lightweight, compact No drug calculations required Some do not require batteries. Some have alarms. Easy for patients to use Cost-effective	Limited infusion volumes and rates Some require batteries. Some do not have alarms. Requires manual dexterity to manipulate syringe and tubing
Peristaltic	Disposable cassette with 50–100 ml reservoir is attached to pump. Fluid is propelled forward by appendages that move in a wavelike motion across intravenous tubing or by a cylinder that rotates attached intravenous tubing.	Flexible programming: intermittent or continuous flow rates ranging from 0.1 ml–400 ml/hour Compact Have alarms	Requires programming Requires batteries Pump and large-volume infusion bags can be heavy. Requires high level of skill/knowledge to use Costly

Note. Based on information from Baquiran & Gallagher, 1998; Camp-Sorrell, 1996; Rapsilber & Camp-Sorrell, 1995.

swelling, local warmth, rash, hematoma, clear or purulent drainage, bleeding, and tenderness. Any of these findings should be documented in the patient care record, and follow-up action should be noted.

Complications with use of the device, such as partial or complete occlusion, breakage, pain upon infusion, or leakage at exit site as medications are infused, should be described in detail in the medical record. Physician notification, strategies used to manage the complications, and effectiveness of those strategies must be documented. Completion of appropriate agency documentation and notification of the risk management department also may be required (Camp-Sorrell, 1996).

Patient/Family Education Regarding Vascular Access Devices

Education of the patient and family regarding the purpose and care of the selected VAD is critical for the successful long-term management of the device. Components of any teaching plan should include
- Indications for the access device, and other options
- Type of device to be inserted
- Potential complications and troubleshooting
- Care and maintenance of the device, including demonstration of self-care skills
- Activity limitations, if any
- Signs and symptoms of complications and how to report complications
- Community resources for supplies and assistance
- Emergency resources.

Teaching may be accomplished with written materials, videos, model demonstration, or patient return demonstration. All pertinent teaching should be documented in the medical record (Bacquiran & Gallagher, 1998, Camp-Sorrell, 1996; Goodman, 2000).

Liability Issues and the Role of the Oncology Nurse

Increasingly complex and sophisticated delivery methods and devices accompany the expanding role of the nurse in infusion therapy. As the responsibilities of the nurse increase, legal accountability also rises (Schulmeister, 1998). Schulmeister wrote that a nurse can reduce the likelihood of being directly named in a lawsuit by following the listed guidelines.
- Maintaining clinical competency
- Being familiar with, and adhering to policies, procedures, and standards of care
- Making a conscious effort to communicate effectively
- Displaying care and concern
- Thoroughly documenting care

Annual review and update of institutional policies and procedures is recommended. Clarity and comprehensiveness of all policies, up-to-date information, and appropriateness to the setting are important components to assess during the annual review. Involvement of the staff nurse or IV therapy specialist ensures that the experiences of personnel using the VADs are considered in the annual review. More information on legal issues is covered in Chapter 6.

Research Questions

Many questions and controversies remain regarding VADs. Selection of dressings and cleansing agents, prevention of infection, and prevention of other catheter complications are some of the areas studied by nurse researchers. Unfortunately, faulty research designs, small sample size, inconsistent definition and measurement of outcome variables, and failure to address extraneous variables limit the application and generalization of most of these studies (Camp-Sorrell, 1996; Fulton, 1997). Fulton wrote that "future research should focus on settings, unique conditions, and population variables that ultimately lead to successful use of long-term access devices" (p. 255) and recommends the following directions for investigators.

- Design device-specific research that captures unique features of each device.
- Design longitudinal studies that follow devices for the entire period of placement.
- Specify the patient population; examine nuances within patient subgroups.
- Address under-represented populations and settings, such as home care, extended care, and rural settings.
- Increase confidence in outcome measures by giving greater attention to reliability of laboratory methods, diagnostic criteria, and interrater reliability.
- Consider extraneous and interacting variables in the research design and statistical analysis.

Summary

Patients with cancer frequently require long-term, reliable VADs. Oncology nurses can help patients to assess their options in device selection by weighing the advantages and disadvantages of each device. Clinical care of the catheters, patient and family education, and support for the patient with a VAD are integral components of nursing care for the patient with cancer. To provide up-to-date care, oncology nurses need to become familiar with the newest devices, the controversies in care, and the latest research findings.

References

Almadrones, L., Campana, P., & Dantis, E.C. (1995). Arterial, peritoneal, and intraventricular access devices. *Seminars in Oncology Nursing, 11,* 194–202.

Andris, D.A., & Krzywda, E.A. (1997). Central venous access: Clinical practice issues. *Nursing Clinics of North America, 32,* 719–740.

Bacquiran D.C., & Gallagher, J. (1998). *Lippincott's cancer chemotherapy handbook.* Philadelphia: Lippincott-Raven.

Berg, D. (1996). Drug delivery systems. In M.B. Burke, G.M. Wilkes, & K. Ingwersen (Eds.), *Cancer chemotherapy: A nursing process approach* (2nd ed.) (pp. 561–595). Boston: Jones and Bartlett.

Broviac, J.W., Cole, J.J., & Scribner, B.H. (1973). A silicone rubber atrial catheter for prolonged parenteral alimentation. *Surgery, Gynecology and Obstetrics, 136,* 602–606.

Camp-Sorrell, D. (1996). *Access device guidelines: Recommendations for nursing practice and education.* Pittsburgh: Oncology Nursing Press, Inc.

Fulton, J.S. (1997). Long-term vascular access devices. *Annual Review of Nursing Research, 15,* 237–259.

Goodman, M. (2000). Chemotherapy: Principles of administration. In C.H. Yarbro, M.H. Frogge, M. Goodman, & S.L. Groenwald (Eds.), *Cancer nursing: Principles and practice* (5th ed.) (pp. 385–443). Boston: Jones and Bartlett.

Greene, J.N. (1996). Catheter-related complications of cancer therapy. *Infectious Disease Clinics of North America, 10,* 255–292.

Gullatte, M.M. (1989). Managing an implanted infusion device. *RN, 52*(1), 45–49.

Gullatte, M.M. (1990, July/August). Nursing management of external central venous catheters (CVCs). *Advancing Clinical Care,* pp. 12–17.

Gullatte, M.M., Koretz, M.J., & Sarma, P.R. (1991). Managing implanted venous access devices. *Journal of Medical Association of Georgia, 80,* 169–171.

Hadaway, L. (1995). Comparison of vascular access devices. *Seminars in Oncology Nursing, 11,* 154–166.

Hickman, R.O., Buckner, C.D., Clift, R.A., Sanders, J.E., Stewart, P., & Thomas, E.D. (1979). A modified right atrial catheter for access to the venous system in marrow transplant recipients. *Surgery, Gynecology and Obstetrics, 148,* 871–875.

Jones, G.R. (1998). A practical guide to evaluation and treatment of infections in patients with central venous catheters. *Journal of Intravenous Nursing, 21*(5S), S134–S142.

Kosier, M.B., & Minkler, P. (1999). Nursing management of patients with an implanted Ommaya reservoir. *Clinical Journal of Oncology Nursing, 3,* 63–67.

Kupensky, D.T. (1998). Applying current research to influence clinical practice: Utilization of midline catheters. *Journal of Intravenous Nursing, 21*(5), 271–274.

Martin, V.R., Walker, F.E., & Goodman, M. (1996). Delivery of cancer chemotherapy. In R. McCorkle, M. Grant, M. Frank-Stromborg, & S. Baird (Eds.), *Cancer nursing: A comprehensive textbook* (2nd ed.) (pp. 395–433). Philadelphia: W.B. Saunders.

Masoorli, S. (1997). Managing complications of central venous access devices. *Nursing, 27*(8), 59–63.

Mayo, D.J., Horne, M.K., III, Summers, B.L., Pearson, D.C., & Helsaveck, C.B. (1996). The effects of heparin flush on patency of the Groshong catheter: A pilot study. *Oncology Nursing Forum, 23,* 1401–1405.

McNally, J.C. (1997). Home care. In S.L. Groenwald, M.H. Frogge, M. Goodman, & C.H. Yarbro (Eds.), *Cancer nursing: Principles and practice* (4th ed.) (pp. 1501–1530). Boston: Jones and Bartlett.

Niederhuber, J.E., Ensminger, W., & Gyves, J.W. (1982). Totally implanted venous and arterial access system to replace external catheters in cancer treatment. *Surgery, 92,* 706–712.

Rapsilber, L.M., & Camp-Sorrell, D. (1995). Ambulatory infusion pumps: Application to oncology. *Seminars in Oncology Nursing, 11,* 213–220.

Roy, R.B., Wilkinson, R.H., & Bayliss, C.E. (1967). The utilization of long nylon catheters for prolonged intravenous infusions. *Canadian Medical Association Journal, 96*(2), 94–97.

Schulmeister, L. (1998). A complication of vascular access device insertion. *Journal of Intravenous Nursing, 21,* 197–202.

Schulmeister, L., & Camp-Sorrell, D. (2000). Chemotherapy extravasation from implanted ports. *Oncology Nursing Forum, 27,* 531–538.

Viale, P.H., Yamamoto, D.S., & Geyton, J.E. (1999). Extravasation of infusate via implanted ports: Two case studies. *Clinical Journal of Oncology Nursing, 3,* 145–151.

Wenzel, R.P., & Edmond, M.B. (1999). The evolving technology of venous access. *New England Journal of Medicine, 340,* 48–50.

West, V.L. (1998). Alternate routes of administration. *Journal of Intravenous Nursing, 21,* 221–231.

Woolery-Antill, M. (1998). Parenteral therapy: Access and delivery. In B.L. Johnson & J. Gross (Eds.), *Handbook of oncology nursing* (pp. 171–217). Boston: Jones and Bartlett.

Yuska, C.M., & Nedved, P.G. (2000). Home care. In C.H. Yarbro, M.H. Frogge, M. Goodman, & S.L. Groenwald (Eds.), *Cancer nursing: Principles and practice* (5th ed.) (pp. 1661–1680). Boston: Jones and Bartlett.

CHAPTER 5

Antineoplastic Agents

Mary Jensen Camp, PharmD, BCPS, BCOP
Mary Magee Gullatte, RN, MN, ANP, AOCN®, FAAMA
James W. Gilmore, PharmD
Donald A. Hutcherson, RPh

History

The introduction of chemotherapy in the early 1900s has resulted in the development of curative therapeutic interventions for several types of solid tumors and hematologic malignancies. The first modern chemotherapeutics, the alkylating agents, were the product of a secret war gas program in both world wars. It was the exposure of seamen to mustard gas that led to the observation that these agents cause lymphoid and marrow hypoplasia. During the past five years, a new level of understanding of the mechanisms through which chemotherapy induces cell death and by which genetic changes can lead to resistance has opened the door to new paradigms for the treatment of cancer incorporating molecular, genetic, and biologic therapies. The greatest progress in recent years has not been the discovery of new, useful chemotherapeutic agents but rather the design of more effective regimens.

Principles of Chemotherapy

For anticancer drug therapy to be effective, several features must be present. The drug must reach the cancer cells; sufficient toxic amounts of drug, or its active metabolite, must enter the cells and remain there for a long enough period of time; and the cancer cells must be sensitive to the toxic effects of the drug. In addition, all of this must occur before the emergence of resistance. The patient also must be able to withstand the adverse effects of the drug. Principles of chemotherapy include cure, prolongation of survival, palliation, and chemoprevention.

Classification

Agents used in cancer chemotherapy are commonly categorized, in several different classification systems, by their mechanism of action or by their origin.

Chemotherapeutic agents generally are divided into seven categories, which include alkylating agents (nitrogen mustard derivatives, nitrosoureas, nonclassic alkylators, and a miscellaneous group), antimetabolites (fluorinated pyrimidines, purine analogues, cytidine analogues, and folate antagonists), anthracene derivatives (anthracyclines and anthracenediones), antitumor antibiotics, antimicrotubule agents, heavy metal compounds (also called platinum analogues), and miscellaneous agents. In addition to the chemotherapeutic drugs listed, a number of hormonal agents are used in the treatment of patients with cancer. The primary use of these agents is in hormonally responsive cancers such as prostate, breast, and endometrial cancers. Hormonal therapies include antiestrogens, estrogens, aromatase inhibitors, gonadotropin-releasing hormone analogues, and antiandrogens. Biologic therapy also has emerged as an important modality of cancer treatment. These agents produce antitumor effects primarily through the action of natural host defense mechanisms.

Chemotherapy (A–Z)

The goal of this section is to provide the reader with a quick and clinically pertinent chemotherapy drug information resource. The reader is referred to other resources for more detailed information. Each drug monograph is divided into several sections as described below. This drug information reference serves solely as a reference and does not take the place of sound clinical judgment or the manufacturer's recommendations as outlined in the product package insert.

Drug Name	The generic, chemical, or nonproprietary name of the drug.
Other Name	Names, including the U.S. brands, to which the drug may be commonly referred.
Classification	The classification of the drug, based on mechanism of action or origin of derivation.
Mechanism	The mechanism of action of the drug.
Vesicant Information	Whether or not the drug is an irritant or vesicant and any antidote information.
Preparation and Mixture	General guidelines for reconstitution and dilution.
Administration	General administration guidelines for commonly used regimens.
Storage and Stability	The manufacturer's recommendations for storage and stability as discussed in the product package insert or information from reputable sources.
How Supplied	The commercial availability of the drug.
Dosage	Commonly used dosages and dosing regimens are described; refer to other sources or the manufacturer for more detailed information.

Compatibility Information	Known admixture information is described; refer to other sources or the manufacturer if specific admixture information is unknown or not listed.
Contraindications/ Precautions	Circumstances indicating inappropriateness or caution warranted for treatment or use.
Drug Interactions	Clinically pertinent drug interactions are described; not necessarily inclusive; refer to other sources or the manufacturer for more detailed information.
Toxicity/Side Effects	Drug-induced toxicity or adverse events classified as acute and/or potentially life-threatening, serious, and other.
Special Considerations	Any unusual or unique circumstances relating to the drug.
Indications	Uses of the drug as indicated by the U.S. Food and Drug Administration (FDA), commonly used drug compendia (USP DI, American Hospital Formulary System [AHFS], or drug evaluations), or the literature.
Dosage Adjustment Recommendations	Guidelines to drug specific dosage adjustments (e.g., adjustments for renal and hepatic impairment, drug toxicity).
Pharmacokinetics	Clinically pertinent pharmacokinetics.
Manufacturer	Drug manufacturer.

Abbreviations Used in Chapter 5

5'-DFUR—5'-deoxy-5-fluorouridine
5-FU—5-fluorouracil
AHFS—USP-DI, American Hospital Formulary System
ALT—alanine aminotransferase
AML—acute myelogenous leukemia
ANC—absolute neutrophil count
ANLL—acute nonlymphocytic leukemia
APL—acute promyelocytic leukemia
AST—aspartate aminotransferase
AUC—area under the curve
AV—atrioventricular
B_6—pyridoxin
BCG—bacillus Calmette-Guérin
BSA—body surface area
BUN—blood urea nitrogen
BW—body weight
CBC—complete blood count
CHF—congestive heart failure
CLL—chronic lymphocytic leukemia
CML—chronic myelogenous leukemia
CR—complete remission
CrCl—creatinine clearance
CSF—cerebrospinal fluid
CXR—chest X-ray
D5W—5% dextrose in water
DEET—N, N-diethyl-m-toluamide
DEHP—di-(2-ethylhexyl) phthalate
DLCO—diffusing capacity of the lung for carbon monoxide
DMSO—dimethyl sulfoxide
DNA—deoxyribonucleic acid
DOE—dyspnea on exertion
ECG—electrocardiogram
EDTA—edetate calcium disorder
EEG—electroencephalogram
FDA—U.S. Food and Drug Administration
FFP—fresh frozen plasma
FSH—follicle-stimulating hormone
FVC—forced vital capacity
GI—gastrointestinal
G-CSF—granulocyte-colony-stimulating factor
GM-CSF—granulocyte-macrophage-colony-stimulating factor
HAI—hepatic artery infusions
HCT—hematopoietic cell transplantation

HER2—human epidermal growth factor receptor 2 protein
IBW—ideal body weight
IM—intramuscular
INR—international normalized ratio
IT— intrathecal
IV—intravenous
IVP—IV push
IVPB—intravenous piggyback
KS—Kaposi's sarcoma
LDH—lactate dehydrogenase
LDL—low-density lipoprotein
LH—luteinizing hormone
LHRH—luteinizing hormone-releasing hormone
LVEF—left ventricular ejection fraction
MAO—monoamine oxidase
MDS—myelodysplastic syndrome
MTIC—monomethyl 5-triazino imidazole carboxamide
MTX—methotrexate
MUGA—multiple gated acquisition
NCI—National Cancer Institute
NS—normal saline
PEG—monomethoxy-polyethelene glycol
PML-RAR$_a$—promyelocytic leukemia-retinoic acid receptor-alpha
PT—prothrombin time
PTT—partial thromoplastin times
PVC—polyvinylchloride
RBCs—red blood cells
RNA—ribonucleic acid
SBP—systolic blood pressure
SC—subcutaneous
SCr—serum creatinine
SGOT—serum glutamic oxalacetic transaminase
SGPT—serum glutamic pyruvic transaminase
SIADH—syndrome of inappropriate antidiuretic hormone
SOB—shortness of breath
TEPA—triethylenephosphoramide
ULN—upper limit of normal
w/v—weight/volume
w/w—weight to weight
WBC—white blood cell

Chemotherapeutic Agents

Alitretinoin

Other Name	Panretin®, 9-*cis*-retinoic acid
Classification	Miscellaneous; retinoid.
Mechanism	A naturally occurring endogenous retinoid that binds to and activates intracellular retinoid receptors. These receptors, once activated, function as transcription factors that regulate gene expression important in cellular differentiation and proliferation in both normal and neoplastic cells.
Vesicant Information	Not classified as a vesicant or an irritant. Alitretinoin is commercially available as a topical preparation.
Preparation and Mixture	No preparation or admixture necessary. Alitretinoin is commercially available as a topical preparation.
Administration	Topical.
Storage and Stability	Store gel at 25°C (77°F).
How Supplied	Panretin® is supplied as a 0.1% alitretinoin gel in tubes containing 60 g.
Dosage	Alitretinoin should be applied sufficiently to cover lesions with a generous coating two times a day. The gel should be allowed to dry for three to five minutes before covering with clothing. The frequency of application can be gradually increased to three or four times a day according to individual lesion tolerance. If application site toxicity occurs, application frequency can be reduced. Occlusive dressings should not be used with alitretinoin gel. Responses to gel may occur as soon as two weeks after initiation of therapy, with further benefit attained with continued application. The therapy should be continued as long as the patient benefits.
Compatibility Information	No information is available on the compatibility of alitretinoin gel physically combined with other topical products.
Contraindications/ Precautions	Contraindicated in patients with a known hypersensitivity to retinoids or to any of the ingredients in the product. Alitretinoin therapy may cause fetal harm if significant absorption were to occur in a pregnant woman.

Drug Interactions	**Agent**	**Effect**
	DEET (N,N-diethyl-m-toluamide)	Animal toxicology studies showed increased DEET toxicity; DEET is a common component of insect repellent products.

No drug interaction data are available on concomitant administration of alitretinoin and systemic anti-Kaposi's sarcoma (KS) agents.

Toxicity/Side Effects	Adverse events in clinical trials of KS patients occurred almost exclusively at the application site. Toxicity usually begins with treatment site erythema; continued application may lead to increased erythema and edema. Dermal

	toxicity may become treatment-limiting with intense erythema, edema, and vesiculation. Usually, however, most adverse events are mild to moderate in severity and include rash, pain, pruritus, exfoliative dermatitis (e.g., flaking, peeling, desquamation, exfoliation), skin disorders (e.g., excoriation, cracking, scab, crusting, drainage, eschar, fissure, oozing), paresthesia, and edema.
Special Considerations	Should severe irritation occur, therapy may be temporarily discontinued for a few days until symptoms subside. Because of potential dermal toxicity, avoid application to normal skin surrounding lesions. In addition, do not apply gel on or near mucosal surfaces of the body. Occlusive dressings should not be used. Although there are no reports of alitretinoin gel causing photosensitivity reactions, patients should be advised to minimize exposure of treated areas to sunlight and sunlamps during therapy. In addition, patients should not concurrently use products that contain DEET, a common component of insect repellents.
Monitoring Parameters	Monitor for signs and symptoms of dermal toxicity.
Indications	Alitretinoin is indicated in the topical treatment of cutaneous lesions in patients with AIDS-related KS. It is not indicated when systemic anti-KS therapy is required (e.g., more than 10 new lesions in the prior month, symptomatic lymphedema, symptomatic pulmonary KS, symptomatic visceral involvement).
Dosage Adjustment Recommendations	Alitretinoin is initially applied twice daily and gradually increased to three or four times a day based on lesion tolerance. If application site toxicity occurs, the frequency of application may be reduced. In the event of severe dermal toxicity, therapy can be temporarily discontinued until symptoms subside.
Pharmacokinetics	Indirect evidence suggests alitretinoin absorption into the plasma is not extensive. Plasma levels of 9-*cis*-retinoic acid were evaluated during clinical trials with the range of plasma concentrations similar to the range of circulating, naturally occurring 9-*cis*-retinoic acid plasma concentrations.
Manufacturer	Stiefel Laboratories, Inc., Coral Gables, FL, for Ligand Pharmaceuticals Incorporated, San Diego, CA

Altretamine

Other Name	Hexalen®, hexamethylmelamine
Classification	Alkylating agent; nonclassic alkylator.
Mechanism	Metabolized to an active metabolite that covalently binds to microsomal proteins and deoxyribonucleic acid (DNA); further breakdown to formaldehyde also may mediate some of the cytotoxicity of this agent.
Vesicant Information	Not classified as a vesicant or an irritant. Altretamine is available commercially as an oral product.
Preparation and Mixture	No preparation or admixture necessary. Altretamine is available commercially as an oral product.

Administration	Oral.
Storage and Stability	Store in tightly sealed bottles at controlled room temperature (15°–30°C; 59°–86°F). The intact capsules are stable for at least two years.
How Supplied	Commercially available in 50-mg clear, hard gelatin capsules in bottles of 100. The capsules are imprinted with the following: USB001.
Dosage	Doses calculated based on body surface area (BSA). Several dosing schedules have been used. The approved dose for single-agent therapy of advanced ovarian cancer is 260 mg/m^2/day administered in four divided daily doses for 14–21 days of a 28-day treatment cycle. In other regimens, the dose as a single agent usually ranges from 4–12 mg/kg/day in four divided daily doses, after meals and at bedtime. When given in combination, altretamine is typically dosed as 150 mg/m^2/day for 14 days of a 28-day treatment cycle.
Compatibility Information	Not applicable. Altretamine is available commercially as an oral product.
Contraindications/ Precautions	Contraindicated if known hypersensitivity to the product. Risk versus benefit should be considered in patients with preexisting severe bone marrow depression or severe neurologic toxicity.

Drug Interactions	**Agent**	**Effect**
	Monoamine oxidase inhibitor (MAO) (phenelzine [Nardil®, Parke-Davis, Morris Plains, NJ], tranylcypromine [Parnate®, SmithKline Beecham Pharmaceuticals, Philadelphia, PA], selegiline [Eldepryl®, Somerset Pharmaceuticals, Inc., Tampa, FL], and procarbazine [Matulane®, Sigma-Tau Pharmaceuticals, Inc., Gaithersburg, MD]).	Concomitant use may cause severe orthostatic hypotension.
	Phenobarbital	Concomitant use decreases metabolism of altretamine (potential to increase toxicity of altretamine).
	Cimetidine	Concomitant use increases metabolism of altretamine (potential to decrease effectiveness of altretamine).
	Tricyclic antidepressants	Concomitant administration may cause incapacitating dizziness and syncopal episodes.

Toxicity/Side Effects	**Acute and/or Potentially Life-Threatening:** None noted.
	Serious: Progressive peripheral and central neurotoxicity reported in 21% of patients (e.g., paresthesia, hyperesthesia, hyperreflexia, decreased sensory and proprioceptive sensations, hallucinations, confusion); reversible upon discontinuation of the drug. Progressive peripheral and central

neurotoxicity may be ameliorated by pyridoxine (B$_6$), but tumor response may be compromised.

Other: Mild to moderate myelosuppression (e.g., anemia, thrombocytopenia, leukopenia) in > 10% of patients. Nadir occurs usually three to four weeks after initiation of therapy with recovery two to three weeks thereafter. Nausea and vomiting may occur in up to one-third of patients; usually mild in nature and occasionally dose-limiting. Diarrhea, loss of appetite, and abdominal cramps occur less frequently.

Special Considerations	Take after meals to reduce stomach upset. Moderately emetogenic (30%–60%); consider serotonin antagonist in combination with dexamethasone. Take missed dose as soon as possible unless almost time for next dose; do not double-dose.
Monitoring Parameters	Monitoring recommended prior to initiation of therapy and at periodic intervals during therapy unless otherwise specified. • Complete blood count (CBC) with differential: Recommended prior to initiation of therapy, prior to each subsequent dose, and at periodic intervals during therapy. • Hemoglobin and/or hematocrit: Recommended prior to initiation of therapy, prior to each subsequent dose, and at periodic intervals during therapy. • Platelet count: Recommended prior to initiation of therapy, prior to each subsequent dose, and at periodic intervals during therapy. • Neurologic examinations.
Indications	Altretamine is indicated for use as a single agent in the palliative treatment of patients with persistent or recurrent epithelial ovarian cancer. Off-label uses include cancers of the breast, colon, cervix, endometrium, and lung and non-Hodgkin's lymphoma.
Dosage Adjustment Recommendations	Altretamine should be temporarily discontinued (for 14 days or longer) if any of the following occur. 1. Gastrointestinal (GI) intolerance unresponsive to symptomatic measures 2. White blood cell (WBC) count < 2,000/mm^3 or granulocyte count < 1,000/m^3 3. Platelet count < 75,000/mm^3 4. Progressive neurotoxicity Therapy may be reinitiated at a reduced dose of 200 mg/m^2/day. If neurotoxicity continues even after dosage reduction, it is recommended that altretamine be discontinued.
Pharmacokinetics	Well absorbed orally, undergoes rapid and extensive metabolism in the liver, has a half-life of approximately 13 hours, and is eliminated in the urine (< 1% unchanged).
Manufacturer	U.S. Bioscience, Inc., West Conshohocken, PA

Amifostine

Other Names	Ethyol®, 2-[(3-aminopropyl)amino] ethanethiol dihydrogen phosphate, WR-2721
Classification	Miscellaneous; chemoprotectant.
Mechanism	A prodrug that is dephosphorylated by alkaline phosphatase in tissues to a pharmacologically active free thiol metabolite. It is preferentially taken up by normal cells because of higher capillary alkaline phosphatase activity, higher pH, and better vascularity of normal tissues relative to tumor. The protectant effects appear to be mediated by scavenging of free radicals, competition with oxygen, promotion of repair of damaged macromolecules, and formation of mixed disulfides to protect normal tissue.
Vesicant Information	Not classified as a vesicant or an irritant.
Preparation and Mixture	Reconstitute with 9.7 ml of sterile 0.9% Sodium Chloride for Injection, USP, for a final concentration of 500 mg/10 ml.
Administration	Intravenous (IV) infusion (see dosage for specific infusion durations).
Storage and Stability	The lyophilized powder should be stored at controlled room temperature (20°–25°C; 68°–77°F). The reconstituted solution is chemically stable for up to five hours at room temperature or up to 24 hours under refrigeration. The solution also may be stored in polyvinylchloride (PVC) bags.
How Supplied	Supplied as a sterile lyophilized powder containing 500 mg of amifostine in 10-ml single-use vials. Packaged as three vials per carton.
Dosage	For reduction of cumulative renal toxicity with chemotherapy: 910 mg/m^2 IV once daily as a 15-minute infusion starting 30 minutes prior to chemotherapy administration. Patients should be adequately hydrated prior to amifostine therapy. For reduction of moderate to severe xerostomia from radiation: 200 mg/m^2 administered once daily as a three-minute infusion starting 15–30 minutes prior to radiation therapy.
Compatibility Information	The reader is referred to *Handbook on Injectable Drugs* (Trissel, 2001), for a comprehensive listing of compatibility.
Contraindications/ Precautions	Contraindicated in patients with a known sensitivity to amifostine, aminothiol compounds, or mannitol. Risk versus benefit should be assessed because of possibility of reduced antitumor efficacy, reduced effectiveness of definitive radiotherapy, profound hypotension, and severe nausea and vomiting. The safety of amifostine has not been established in patients with preexisting cardiovascular or cerebrovascular conditions. Patients who are hypotensive, are dehydrated, or cannot have antihypertensive medications stopped for 24 hours preceding therapy should not receive amifostine.
Drug Interactions	Special caution should be taken in patients receiving antihypertensives or other medications that could cause or potentiate hypotension.
Toxicity/Side Effects	**Acute and/or Potentially Life-Threatening:** Transient and profound hypotension may occur during or shortly after amifostine administration.

Patients should be adequately hydrated prior to administration and kept in a supine position during administration. Blood pressure should be monitored every five minutes during infusion and as clinically indicated thereafter. If hypotension occurs, place patient in Trendelenburg position, administer IV infusion of normal saline (NS), and consider interrupting amifostine administration (see guidelines under dosage adjustment recommendations). Short-term reversible loss of consciousness rarely has been reported. Nausea and vomiting may occur and are generally mild to moderate in severity; often subsides within 30 minutes. Pretreatment with an antiemetic (serotonin antagonist in combination with dexamethasone) is warranted. Other effects that may occur acutely during or immediately following infusion are flushing/feeling of warmth, fever, dizziness, somnolence, chills, hiccups, and sneezing. Rarely, anaphylactoid reactions have been reported, including hypoxia, laryngeal edema, chest tightness, and possible cardiac arrest.

Serious: Rare reports of seizures.

Other: Hypocalcemia and hypomagnesemia.

Special Considerations	Patients should be adequately hydrated prior to amifostine therapy and kept in a supine position during administration. Blood pressure should be monitored before, during (at five-minute intervals), and immediately after administration and thereafter as clinically indicated. Patients also should be instructed to drink plenty of fluids during the 24 hours before administration. Premedication with an antiemetic (serotonin antagonist in combination with dexamethasone) is warranted.
Monitoring Parameters	Monitoring is recommended prior to initiation of therapy and at periodic intervals during therapy unless otherwise specified. • Blood pressure should be monitored before, during (at five-minute intervals), and immediately after administration and thereafter as clinically indicated. • Serum calcium and magnesium levels should be monitored before administration and thereafter as clinically indicated.
Indications	Indicated to reduce the cumulative renal toxicity associated with repeated administration of cisplatin in patients with advanced ovarian cancer or non-small cell lung cancer. Amifostine also is indicated to reduce the incidence of moderate to severe xerostomia in patients with head and neck cancer who are undergoing postoperative radiation treatment in which the radiation port includes a substantial portion of the parotid glands. Other unapproved uses include reducing neutropenia and thrombocytopenia as well as preventing cisplatin-induced neuro- and ototoxicity, paclitaxel-induced neurotoxicity, and mucositis associated with radiation therapy.
Dosage Adjustment Recommendations	The infusion of amifostine should be interrupted if the systolic blood pressure (SBP) drops according to chart below or the patient is symptomatic.

Baseline SBP (mmHg)	Drop in SBP
Less than 100	20
100–119	25
120–139	30
140–179	40
>/=180	50

	If the blood pressure returns to normal within five minutes of discontinuing amifostine and the patient is asymptomatic, the infusion may be restarted and the full dose of amifostine may be subsequently administered. If the full dose cannot be administered, subsequent doses of amifostine should be reduced to 740 mg/m^2.
Pharmacokinetics	Following IV infusion, drug is rapidly dephosphorylated in tissues to active free thiol metabolite. The elimination half-life is nine minutes. Only small amounts of amifostine and its metabolites are excreted in the urine.
Manufacturer	USB Pharma B.V.; marketed by U.S. Bioscience, Inc., West Conshohocken, PA, and Alza Pharmaceuticals, Mountain View, CA

Arsenic trioxide

Other Names	Trisenox®
Classification	Miscellaneous.
Mechanism	Not completely understood; causes morphological changes and DNA fragmentation characteristic of apoptosis in vitro. In addition, arsenic trioxide causes damage or degradation of the fusion protein promyelocytic leukemia-retinoic acid receptor-alpha (PML-RAR$_a$).
Vesicant Information	Not classified as a vesicant or an irritant, although injection site pain and edema have been reported.
Preparation and Mixture	Dilute immediately after withdrawing from ampule in 100–250 ml 5% Dextrose Injection, USP, or 0.9% Sodium Chloride for Injection, USP. Ampules are for single-use only and do not contain a preservative. Discard unused portions.
Administration	IV infusion over one to two hours.
Storage and Stability	Diluted solutions are chemically and physically stable for 24 hours at room temperature and for 48 hours under refrigeration.
How Supplied	Supplied as a clear, colorless, sterile solution in 10-ml single-use glass ampules in packages of 10.
Dosage	Induction regimen for acute promyelocytic leukemia (APL) is 0.15 mg/kg/day until bone marrow remission. Total number of doses for induction remission should not exceed 60. Consolidation treatment should begin three to six weeks following induction therapy. Consolidation regimen is 0.15 mg/kg/day for 25 doses over a period up to five weeks.
Compatibility Information	Arsenic trioxide should not be mixed with other medications.
Contraindications/ Precautions	Contraindicated in patients with a known hypersensitivity to arsenic trioxide. Risk versus benefit should be considered in patients with preexisting cardiac abnormalities as electrocardiogram (ECG) abnormalities including QT prolongation and complete atrioventricular (AV) block have been reported. Arsenic trioxide is considered teratogenic and may cause fetal harm if administered to a pregnant woman.

Drug Interactions	No formal interaction studies have been conducted. Caution is advised when administering arsenic trioxide with other agents, particularly those that can prolong the QT interval or lead to electrolyte abnormalities.
Toxicity/Side Effects	Most patients experience drug-related toxicity, most commonly leukocytosis, GI abnormalities, fatigue, edema, hyperglycemia, headache, dizziness, edema, skin manifestations (rash, itching), and respiratory events (cough, dyspnea). Although common, they are reversible and usually do not require interruption of therapy.
	Acute and/or Potentially Life-Threatening: Reports of patients with APL treated with arsenic trioxide developing a retinoic acid APL-like syndrome or APL differentiation syndrome have occurred. This syndrome, which may be fatal, is characterized by fever, weight gain, dyspnea, and pulmonary and/or pleural infiltrates with or without hyperleukocytosis. Steroids (e.g., dexamethasone 10 mg IV twice a day) should be initiated immediately upon first sign of syndrome and continued for three days or longer until symptoms have subsided.
	Serious: Cardiac abnormalities including QT prolongation, atrial dysrhythmias, and AV block
	Other: Cardiovascular: As noted above and tachycardia, palpitations and other ECG abnormalities, hypo- and hypertension. Dermatologic: Dermatitis, pruritus, petechiae, nonspecific erythema, dry skin, hyperpigmentation, and urticaria. GI: Nausea/vomiting, diarrhea, constipation, anorexia, abdominal pain, dyspepsia, sore throat, GI hemorrhage, and fecal incontinence. Hematologic: Leukocytosis, anemia, thrombocytopenia, neutropenia, and disseminated intravascular coagulation. Musculoskeletal: Arthralgia, myalgia, bone pain, neck and back pain. Neurologic: Dizziness, headache, insomnia, tremor, anxiety, depression, agitation, paresthesias, somnolence, convulsions, and coma. Miscellaneous: Fatigue, rigors, injection site pain, weakness, hypersensitivity, dry mouth, hypo- or hyperkalemia, hypomagnesemia, hypocalcemia, hyperglycemia, increase in hepatic transaminases, cough, wheezing, rales, dyspnea, infections, pallor, flushing, eye irritation, blurred vision, renal impairment/failure, and earache.
Special Considerations	May cause fetal harm when administered to pregnant women. Women of childbearing age should be advised of potential risk to unborn child if to become pregnant while on arsenic trioxide therapy. Notify physician immediately if symptoms of retinoid-APL syndrome develop.
Monitoring Parameters	Monitoring is recommended prior to initiation of therapy and twice weekly during induction therapy and weekly during consolidation therapy unless otherwise specified. • CBC with differential: Should be monitored more frequently if clinically unstable. • Electrolytes: Should be monitored more frequently if clinically unstable. • Coagulation tests: Prothrombin time (PT) and International Normalized Ratio (INR); should be monitored more frequently if clinically unstable.

- ECG: Monitor weekly during induction and consolidation therapy; monitor more frequently if clinically unstable.
- Liver function tests: Aspartate amino transferase (AST), alanine amino transferase (ALT); monitor at baseline and periodically during therapy.
- Pregnancy testing: Obtain prior to initiating therapy and periodically thereafter as clinically indicated.

Indications	Indicated for the induction of remission and consolidation in patients with APL who are refractory to, or have relapsed from, retinoid and anthracycline chemotherapy and whose APL is characterized by the presence of the t (15,17) translocation or PML-RAR$_a$ gene expression. Under clinical investigation for front-line therapy for APL as well as in the treatment of multiple myeloma, myelodysplastic syndromes, and other forms of AML.
Dosage Adjustment Recommendations	Use caution in patients with renal failure as renal excretion is the primary route of elimination.
Pharmacokinetics	Arsenic trioxide undergoes reduction and methylation (primary site in liver). The drug is stored in the liver, kidney, heart, lung, nails, and hair. The trivalent form is excreted in the urine.
Manufacturer	Cell Therapeutics, Inc., Seattle, WA

Asparaginase

Other Names	Elspar®, L-Asparaginase, pegaspargase (Oncaspar®)
Classification	Miscellaneous; enzyme.
Mechanism	Enzyme that deaminates asparagine to aspartic acid and ammonia, thereby depriving tumor cells of the amino acid for protein synthesis. Asparaginase is available from two different purified microbiological sources, *E. coli* (most used in clinical practice) and *Erwinia* (not cross-reactive; reserved for patients with allergic reactions to *E. coli* preparation).
Vesicant Information	Not classified as a vesicant or an irritant.
Preparation and Mixture	IV administration: lyophilized powder should be reconstituted with 5 ml Sterile Water for Injection, USP, or Sodium Chloride for Injection, 0.9%, USP, without preservative; shake to dissolve (vigorous shaking may cause excessive foaming); only clear, colorless solutions should be used. May be used for direct IV administration over no less than 30 minutes into side port of a running IV or further diluted into 50–250 ml NS or 5% dextrose in water (D$_5$W) for IV infusion. If gelatinous fiber-like particles develop, a 5-micron in-line filter is recommended (use of a 0.2-micron filter may result in loss of potency).
	Intramuscular (IM) administration: Reconstitute 10,000 U vial with 2 ml of Sodium Chloride for Injection, 0.9%, USP.
	Elspar® should be a clear and colorless solution once reconstituted. Discard solutions that are or become cloudy.

Administration	May be administered intramuscularly or intravenously. IV infusions should be given over a period of at least 30 minutes through a side arm of an already running infusion of NS or 5% Dextrose Injection, USP. When administering intramuscularly, volume of injection should not exceed 2 ml. If greater than 2 ml are needed, two injection sites should be used. An intradermal test dose is recommended prior to the initial administration of the drug and when a week or more has elapsed between doses (see Special Considerations).
Storage and Stability	Vials should be stored under refrigeration. Reconstituted solutions, whether further diluted or not, are stable for eight hours at room temperature; discard solutions that become cloudy.
How Supplied	Elspar® for injection is supplied as a white lyophilized plug or powder in sterile 10-ml vials containing 10,000 IU of asparaginase.
Dosage	Single agent: 200 IU/kg IV daily for 28 days. Most commonly used in combination chemotherapy regimens dosed at 1,000–6,000 IU/m² given in various dosing schedules (e.g., every three days, every other day, daily). Higher dosages given less frequently also have been used.
Compatibility Information	Compatible with 5% Dextrose Injection, USP, Sodium Chloride for Injection, 0.9%, USP, or Sterile Water for Injection.
Contraindications/ Precautions	Elspar® should not be used in patients with pancreatitis or a history of pancreatitis or in patients with a known history of anaphylaxis to the drug. Risk versus benefit should be considered in patients with gout or a history of gout, significant hepatic impairment, active infection, or history of uric acid nephropathy.

Drug Interactions	**Agent**	**Effect**
	Methotrexate (MTX)	Asparaginase can diminish or abolish MTX antineoplastic activity when used concomitantly.
	Prednisone	Concomitant therapy increases likelihood of hyperglycemia.
	Vincristine	Asparaginase administered before vincristine can increase neurotoxic effects of vincristine.
	Drugs metabolized by the liver	Asparaginase may affect liver function, thus increasing toxicity of other drugs metabolized by the liver.

Toxicity/Side Effects	**Acute and/or Potentially Life-Threatening:** Hypersensitivity, anaphylaxis (e.g., respiratory distress, hypotension, laryngeal constriction, diaphoresis, bronchospasm, loss of consciousness, death) can occur in 10%–40% of patients; more common with single-agent therapy and IV administration. Intradermal test dose recommended with initial administration of the drug and when a week or more has elapsed between doses (see Special Considerations), although a negative skin test does not preclude the possibility of an allergic reaction. If anaphylaxis occurs, consider changing to *Erwinia* preparation. Coagulation defects (e.g., disseminated

intravascular coagulation; prolongation of factors V, VII, VIII, IX; prothrombin; fibrinogen) may lead to fatal bleeding. Fulminant and/or fatal pancreatitis, although uncommon, may develop.

Serious: Hepatotoxicity (e.g., elevations of serum glutamic oxalacetic transaminase [SGOT], serum glutamic pyruvic transaminase [SGPT], alkaline phosphatase, bilirubin), hyperglycemia with glucosuria and polyuria, diabetic ketoacidosis, neurotoxicity (e.g., depression, fatigue, coma, confusion, agitation, hallucinations, Parkinson-like syndrome), and renal insufficiency.

Other: Mild nausea and vomiting, myelosuppression (uncommon and usually mild), skin rash, urticaria, arthralgia, fever, and chills.

Special Considerations	Intradermal test dose: Reconstitute 10,000 IU vial with 5 ml of diluent (Sterile Water for Injection, USP, or Sodium Chloride for Injection, 0.9%, USP; final concentration 2,000 IU/ml); withdraw 0.1 ml and inject into another vial containing 9.9 ml of diluent (final concentration 20 IU/ml); use 0.1 ml or 2 IU of this solution for the intradermal test dose. Skin test area should be observed for one hour for erythema and wheal reaction. A negative skin test does not preclude the possibility of an allergic reaction on administration of full-dose therapy. **Be prepared** to treat anaphylaxis (with antihistamine, corticosteroid, epinephrine, oxygen) at each administration. Desensitization should be considered for patients with a positive reaction to the intradermal skin test; refer to product package insert for further details and desensitization protocol. For moderately low emetogenic potential, premedication with a phenothiazine should be adequate. Monitor fibrinogen, if below 100 mg/dl; contact physician for possible administration of coagulation factors (i.e., fresh frozen plasma [FFP]).
Monitoring Parameters	Monitoring is recommended prior to initiation of therapy and at periodic intervals during therapy unless otherwise specified. • CBC with differential: Recommended prior to initiation of therapy, prior to each subsequent dose, and at periodic intervals during therapy. • Hemoglobin and/or hematocrit: Recommended prior to initiation of therapy, prior to each subsequent dose, and at periodic intervals during therapy. • Liver function tests: ALT, AST, alkaline phosphatase, total bilirubin, lactate dehydrogenase (LDH). • Serum amylase • PT • Vital signs during administration • Fibrinogen (if < 100 mg/dl, contact physician prior to administration) • Uric acid • Renal function tests: Creatinine clearance (CrCl), actual or calculated, and/or serum creatinine (SCr) recommended prior to initiation of therapy, prior to each subsequent dose, and at periodic intervals during therapy • Glucose
Indications	Elspar® is indicated the treatment of acute lymphocytic leukemia (ALL), although it also may be used in the treatment of acute myelogenous leukemia (AML) and chronic myelogenous leukemia (CML), lymphoma, and soft-tissue sarcoma.

Dosage Adjustment Recommendations	Desensitization should be performed before administering the first dose of Elspar® in patients who had a positive intradermal skin test and on retreatment of patients with a previous mild hypersensitivity reaction when continuation of therapy is deemed necessary. Refer to product package insert for further details and desensitization protocol.
Pharmacokinetics	Not absorbed after oral administration. Half-life of 8–30 hours. Large volume of distribution (70%–80% of plasma volume). Cerebrospinal fluid (CSF) levels 1% of corresponding plasma levels. Trace amounts excreted in urine.
Manufacturer	Merck & Co., Inc., West Point, PA

Bexarotene

Other Names	Targretin®
Classification	Miscellaneous; retinoid.
Mechanism	Selectively binds and activates retinoid X receptor subtypes (RXRa, RXRb, RXRg). These receptors, once activated, function as transcription factors that regulate gene expression important in cellular differentiation and proliferation in both normal and neoplastic cells.
Vesicant Information	Not classified as a vesicant or an irritant. Bexarotene is available commercially as an oral and topical product.
Preparation and Mixture	No preparation or admixture necessary. Bexarotene is available commercially as an oral and topical product.
Administration	Oral and topical.
Storage and Stability	Store capsules at 2°–25°C (36°–77°F). Store the gel at room temperature. Avoid exposure of capsules and gel to high temperatures and humidity, and protect from light.
How Supplied	Bexarotene capsules are supplied as 75-mg off-white, oblong, soft gelatin capsules. The capsules are imprinted with the following: Targretin. The gel contains 1% bexarotene and is supplied as a 60-g tube.
Dosage	The recommended initial dose for the treatment of cutaneous T cell lymphoma, which is refractory to one prior systemic therapy, is 300 mg/m^2/day taken as a single daily dose (see table below). The dose should be taken with or immediately following a meal. Therapy should be continued as long as patient is deriving clinical benefit. The daily dosage based on initial dose of 300 mg/m^2/day is illustrated in the following table.

BSA (m^2)	Total Daily Dose (mg/day)	Number of 75-mg Capsules
0.88–1.12	300	4
1.13–1.37	375	5
1.38–1.62	450	6
1.63–1.87	525	7
1.88–2.12	600	8
2.13–2.37	675	9
2.38–2.62	750	10

Bexarotene gel is applied once every other day for the first week and is then increased in application frequency at weekly intervals to two, three, and four times daily, based on individual lesion tolerance. Most patients tolerate application two to four times per day. Most responses were seen in clinical trials at dosing frequencies of two times per day or higher.

Compatibility Information	No information is available on the compatibility of bexarotene gel physically combined with other topical products.
Contraindications/ Precautions	Contraindicated in patients with a known hypersensitivity to bexarotene or other components of the product. May cause fetal harm; must not be given to a pregnant women or a woman who intends to get pregnant. In addition, contraindicated in patients with cutaneous T cell lymphoma with risk factors for pancreatitis (e.g., uncontrolled hyperlipidemia, excessive alcohol intake, biliary tract disease, uncontrolled diabetes, prior pancreatitis and/or on medications known to increase triglyceride levels or associated with pancreatic toxicity). Risk versus benefit should be considered in patients with hepatic insufficiency; diabetic patients using insulin, agents enhancing insulin secretion, or insulin sensitizers (e.g., troglitazone); or patients with hypothyroidism.
Drug Interactions	No formal drug interaction studies have been performed. However, on the basis of the metabolism of bexarotene by the cytochrome P450 enzyme system, drugs that inhibit this enzyme system (e.g., itraconazole, ketoconazole, erythromycin, gemfibrozil) or grapefruit juice would be expected to lead to increased plasma concentrations and possible toxicity. Concomitant administration of gemfibrozil and bexarotene resulted in substantial increases in bexarotene plasma concentrations. Concomitant therapy with these agents is not recommended. Furthermore, drugs that induce the P450 enzyme system (e.g., rifampin, phenobarbital, phenytoin) would be expected to decrease plasma concentrations. In addition, bexarotene is highly bound to plasma proteins (> 99%). The protein to which it binds, as well as the ability for bexarotene to displace or be displaced by other protein-bound drugs, has not been studied.
Toxicity/Side Effects	**Capsules:**

Acute and/or Potentially Life-Threatening: Fatal events in clinical studies were rare and include acute pancreatitis, subdural hematoma, and liver failure.

Serious: Moderately severe and severe adverse events occur most frequently in patients receiving > 300 mg/m^2 and include asthenia, headache, hyperlipidemia, hypercholesteremia, leukopenia, and GI symptoms (e.g., anorexia, diarrhea, vomiting, pancreatitis).

Other:
Cardiovascular: Peripheral edema.
Dermatologic: Rash, dry skin, pruritus, alopecia, and exfoliative dermatitis.
Endocrine: Hypothyroidism.
Hematologic: Leukopenia and anemia.
Miscellaneous: Insomnia, infection, LDH increase, chills, fever, back pain, and flu-like syndrome.

	Gel: The most common reported adverse events were application site toxicity, including rash, pain, pruritus, exfoliative dermatitis (e.g., flaking, peeling, desquamation, exfoliation), skin disorder (e.g., excoriation, cracking, scab, crusting, drainage, eschar, fissure, oozing), paresthesia, and edema.
Special Considerations	Take bexarotene capsules with or immediately following a meal. Bexarotene gel should be applied in sufficient quantity to cover the lesion with a generous coating. The gel should be allowed to dry before covering with clothing. Avoid contact with normal healthy skin. Do not apply gel in areas near mucosal surfaces. Occlusive dressing should not be used. Bexarotene gel is intended for topical use only. In addition, patients on bexarotene topical therapy should not concurrently use products that contain DEET, a common component of insect repellents. Women of child-bearing potential should be advised not to become pregnant during bexarotene therapy. A negative pregnancy test should be obtained one week prior to initiation of therapy and monthly thereafter. Effective contraception must be used one month prior to treatment initiation and throughout bexarotene therapy. Male patients with sexual partners who are pregnant, possibly pregnant, or who could become pregnant must use condoms during sexual intercourse. Because the retinoids have been associated with photosensitivity reactions, patients should be advised to minimize exposure to sunlight and artificial ultraviolet light while receiving bexarotene therapy. CA 125 assay values may be increased in patients with ovarian cancer while on bexarotene therapy.
Monitoring Parameters	Monitoring is recommended prior to initiation of therapy and at periodic intervals during therapy unless otherwise specified. **Capsules:** • CBC with differential. • Liver function tests: Obtain at baseline and after one, two, and four weeks of treatment; if stable, periodically thereafter. • Thyroid function tests. • Lipid studies: Obtain at baseline and weekly for two to four weeks until the lipid response to bexarotene has been established, then at eight-week intervals (fasting triglycerides should be normal or normalized with appropriate intervention prior to initiation of bexarotene therapy). **Gel:** • Monitor for signs and symptoms of dermal toxicity.
Indications	Indicated for the treatment of cutaneous manifestations of cutaneous T cell lymphoma in patients who are refractory to at least one prior systemic therapy. Bexarotene gel is indicated in the topical treatment of cutaneous lesions in patients with Stage IA or IB cutaneous T cell lymphoma who have refractory or persistent disease after other therapies or who have not tolerated other therapies.
Dosage Adjustment Recommendations	Dosage reduction to 200 mg/m^2/day, then to 100 mg/m^2/day or temporarily discontinued if necessitated by the development of toxicity. Doses may be carefully titrated up to 300 mg/m^2/day once toxicity is manageable. If

	no tumor response is seen after eight weeks of therapy at the 300 mg/m²/day dose level and the patient is tolerating therapy, the dose may be escalated to 400 mg/m²/day with careful monitoring. If application site toxicity occurs with the use of the gel, the frequency of application may be reduced or temporarily discontinued until symptoms subside.
Pharmacokinetics	After oral administration, maximum plasma concentrations are reached at about two hours, and half-life is approximately seven hours. Administration with or immediately following a fat-containing meal increases plasma area under the pharmacokinetic curve (AUC) concentrations and maximum concentrations by 35% and 48%, respectively. After topical therapy, generally low plasma concentrations are detected in patients receiving low- to moderate-intensity therapy. Quantifiable plasma concentrations increase with increasing percent of body area treated and with increasing intensity of therapy. Bexarotene is highly plasma protein-bound (> 99%), although it is unclear as to which proteins it binds.
Manufacturer	R.P. Scherer for Ligand Pharmaceuticals Incorporated, San Diego, CA

Bleomycin

Other Names	Blenoxane®
Classification	Antitumor antibiotic.
Mechanism	Exact mechanism unknown; thought to bind to DNA, leading to single- and double-strand breaks, thereby inhibiting DNA synthesis. Also thought to inhibit ribonucleic acid (RNA) and protein synthesis to a lesser degree.
Vesicant Information	Minor irritant; IV administration should be given slowly over 10 minutes; may cause pain at injection site for subcutaneous (SC) or IM administration.
Preparation and Mixture	IM or SC administration: Reconstitute 15 U vial with 1–5 ml and 30 U vial with 2–10 ml of Sterile Water for Injection, USP, Sodium Chloride for Injection, 0.9%, USP, or Bacteriostatic Water for Injection, USP. IV administration: Reconstitute 15 U or 30 U vial with 5 ml or 10 ml, respectively, of Sodium Chloride for Injection, 0.9%, USP. Intrapleural administration: 60 U (most common dose) of bleomycin is dissolved in 50–100 ml Sodium Chloride for Injection, 0.9%, USP. Bleomycin should not be reconstituted or diluted with D₅W or other dextrose-containing solution because of potential loss of potency.
Administration	May be SC, IM, IV (slow IV push [IVP] not to exceed 1 unit/minute; IV infusion in 50–100 ml NS over 15 minutes or longer), or intrapleural (via a thoracostomy tube). In investigational trials, bleomycin has been administered intralesionally, topically, by bladder instillation, and intra-arterially. Lymphoma patients should be treated with a test dose of 2 U with the first two doses, usually given intravenously in 50 ml NS over 15 minutes; monitor vital signs every 15 minutes, and wait a minimum of one hour. If no reaction occurs, then the regular dosing regimen may be followed.

Storage and Stability	Store vials under refrigeration 2°–8°C (36°–46°F). Reconstituted solutions are stable for 24 hours at room temperature and 14 days under refrigeration.
How Supplied	Commercially available as a white or yellowish lyophilized powder in 15 U and 30 U sterile bleomycin sulfate, USP, per vial.
Dosage	Standard dose of bleomycin as a single agent is 10–20 U/m^2 IV, SC, or IM given once or twice per week. Not to exceed 30 U per dose or 400–450 U total lifetime dose. The most common intrapleural dose is 60 U diluted in 100 ml NS and instilled into the pleural cavity via a thoracostomy tube.
Compatibility Information	Compatibility information is available for a number of drugs, including chemotherapeutics, supportive-care agents, and antibiotics. The reader is referred to other resources on admixture (e.g., Trissel, 2001) for detailed information. Common admixture compatibilities include cyclophosphamide, vincristine, vinblastine, doxorubicin, and mesna. Bleomycin is incompatible with solutions containing divalent and trivalent cations because of chelation. In addition, bleomycin is inactivated by MTX, hydrogen peroxide, mitomycin, and ascorbic acid.
Contraindications/ Precautions	Contraindicated if known hypersensitivity or idiosyncratic reaction to the drug. Risk versus benefit should be considered in patients with hepatic impairment (lower dosages recommended), pulmonary function impairment, peripheral vascular disease, or severe renal impairment (lower dosages recommended).

Drug Interactions	**Agent**	**Effect**
	Cisplatin	Concomitant use may result in delayed bleomycin elimination and increased toxicity of bleomycin.
	Digoxin	Concomitant use may decrease plasma levels and renal excretion of digoxin.
	Phenytoin	Concomitant use may cause decreased phenytoin levels.

Toxicity/Side Effects	**Acute and/or Potentially Life-Threatening:** Pulmonary toxicity, interstitial pneumonitis that can progress to fibrosis and cause death from hypoxia, can be related to single doses or cumulative doses. Doses above 450 U, advanced age, preexisting pulmonary disease, previous chest irradiation, and exposure to high oxygen concentrations all increase risk. One hallmark finding recommended for halting therapy is end-inspiratory crackles. Hypersensitivity reactions, idiosyncratic reactions, although uncommon (1%), manifest as hypotension, mental confusion, fever, chills, and wheezing. Treatment is symptomatic and includes volume expansion, pressor agents, antihistamines, and corticosteroids. **Serious:** See above. **Other:** Not myelosuppressive. Dermatologic: Bleomycin concentrates in the skin and causes mild stomatitis, hyperpigmentation, thickening of the nail beds, alopecia, and a syndrome of skin erythema, rash, and edema.

	GI: Nausea and vomiting (rare). Miscellaneous: Fever (most often occurs 4–10 hours after administration, lasts for 4–12 hours and decreases in incidence with subsequent administration) and chills.
Special Considerations	Monitor for signs/symptoms of pulmonary toxicity (e.g., shortness of breath [SOB], dyspnea on exertion [DOE], crackles). As bleomycin is given mid-cycle in many regimens, it is important to check CBC with differential (recommended prior to initiation of therapy, prior to each subsequent dose, and at periodic intervals during therapy) regularly as it may be difficult to determine if fever on day of bleomycin administration is strictly a drug fever or if patient may be experiencing an episode of febrile neutropenia. Acetaminophen 650 mg every four to six hours for four doses may be used to prevent or treat bleomycin-induced fever. Moderately low emetogenic potential; phenothiazine or dexamethasone premedication should be adequate.
Monitoring Parameters	Monitoring is recommended prior to initiation of therapy and at periodic intervals during therapy unless otherwise specified. • Pulmonary function tests (e.g., diffusing capacity of the lung for carbon monoxide [DLCO]): Perform at initiation of bleomycin and monthly to every two months thereafter. A 30%–35% decrease from pretreatment value indicates need for cessation of drug. • Chest x-ray: Monitor at regular intervals, particularly if not monitoring pulmonary function by DLCO. • Renal function tests: CrCl, actual or calculated, and/or SCr; recommended prior to initiation of therapy, prior to each subsequent dose, and at periodic intervals during therapy.
Indications	Hodgkin's and non-Hodgkin's lymphomas, testicular cancer, and squamous cell cancers of the head, neck, and uterine cervix. It is widely used for intracavitary instillations in the management of malignant effusions. Off-label indications include Kaposi's, soft-tissue, and osteo-sarcomas; mycosis fungoides; and bladder, esophageal, endometrial, ovarian, and skin cancers.
Dosage Adjustment Recommendations	Adjustments for renal impairment are necessary (see Appendix B). It is not recommended to give bleomycin if the patient's CrCl is < 10 ml/minute.
Pharmacokinetics	Absorption from intrapleural and IM routes of administration approximates 30% of serum levels produced from IV administration. SC route produces serum concentrations equal to those of IV. Half-life depends on renal function; three to five hours for patients with normal renal function and up to 30 hours in severe renal impairment. Bleomycin concentrates in the skin, kidneys, lungs, and heart, and 50%–70% of the drug is excreted in the urine as active drug that cannot be removed by hemodialysis.
Manufacturer	Bristol-Myers Squibb Oncology/Immunology Division, Princeton, NJ

Busulfan

Other Names	Myleran®, Busulfex®
Classification	Alkylating agent; nitrogen mustard derivative.
Mechanism	Interferes with the normal function of DNA by alkylation and cross-linking the strands of DNA; marked effect on myeloid cells.
Vesicant Information	No data are available from the manufacturer on the vesicant status of Busulfex® IV.
Preparation and Mixture	Busulfan IV is diluted with Sodium Chloride for Injection, 0.9%, USP or 5% Dextrose Injection, USP. The diluent quantity should be 10 times the volume of busulfan, ensuring the final concentration is approximately ≥ 0.5 mg/ml. Once calculated volume of diluent is known, place diluent in syringe or IV bag, add the busulfan to the diluent, and mix thoroughly by inverting solution several times.
Administration	Oral and IV. IV solutions should be administered via a central catheter over two hours.
Storage and Stability	Store tablets at room temperature (15°–25°C; 59°–77°F) and in a dry place. Unopened ampules of injectable busulfan are stable until date indicated on the package when stored under refrigeration. Busulfan diluted in NS or D$_5$W is stable at room temperature (25°C) for up to eight hours, but the infusion must be completed within that time (eight hours from admixture). Busulfan diluted in NS is stable at refrigerated conditions (2°–8°C) for up to 12 hours, but the infusion must be completed within that time (12 hours from admixture).
How Supplied	Myleran® is commercially available as a white, scored tablet containing 2 mg of busulfan in bottles of 25 and imprinted with the following: K2A. Busulfex® is supplied as a sterile solution in 10-ml single-use, clear glass ampules, each containing 60 mg busulfan at a concentration of 6 mg/ml for IV use. Busulfex® is packaged in eight ampules of 10 ml and includes eight compatible 25-mm, 5.0-micron nylon membrane syringe filters.
Dosage	The usual adult dose of Myleran® for CML remission induction is 4–8 mg, total dose daily until WBC count falls below 15,000 cells per cubic millimeter. Maintenance doses range from 2 mg/week to 4 mg/day. Dosing for hematopoietic cell transplantation (HCT) preparative regimens ranges from 8–16 mg/kg (common regimen: 1 mg/kg/dose [ideal body weight (IBW)] every six hours for 16 doses). Busulfex® is dosed at 0.8 mg/kg of IBW or actual body weight, whichever is less, intravenously via a central venous catheter over two hours administered every six hours for four consecutive days (total of 16 doses). Obese or severely obese patients should be dosed on an adjusted body weight (Adj BW = IBW + 0.25x (actual weight–IBW).
Compatibility Information	Busulfex® IV is compatible with NS and D$_5$W only. No other data are available from the manufacturer regarding IV compatibilities.

Contraindications/ Precautions	Contraindicated in patients with known hypersensitivity to busulfan or any component, patients who failed to respond to previous courses, or patients who are pregnant or lactating. Risk versus benefit should be considered in patients with significant bone marrow depression, active infection, gout or a history of gout, or history of uric acid nephropathy or in patients receiving high doses of busulfan with a previous head trauma or seizure disorder.

Drug Interactions	**Agent**	**Effect**
	Acetaminophen	Use prior to or concurrently with busulfan may result in reduced busulfan clearance.
	Itraconazole	Concomitant use decreases busulfan clearance by up to 25%.
	Phenytoin	Concomitant use increases clearance of busulfan by 15% or more.
	Thioguanine	Long-term, continuous concomitant therapy may cause esophageal varices and hepatotoxicity.

Toxicity/Side Effects	**Acute and/or Potentially Life-Threatening:** Pulmonary: Bronchopulmonary dysplasia progressing to pulmonary fibrosis (busulfan lung) and pneumonitis may begin 1–10 years following therapy (average four years); cumulative toxicity greatest if dose exceeds 500 mg. Corticosteroids may be helpful; however, usually fatal within six months of onset, related to rapid, diffuse fibrosis. Neurologic: Seizures with high-dose regimens (HCT), begin prophylactic phenytoin prior to administration of busulfan. Caution should be exercised when administering Busulfex® in recommended doses to patients with a history of seizure disorder or head trauma or who are receiving other potentially epileptogenic drugs. High-dose regimen (HCT) may be associated with hepatic veno-occlusive disease in the setting of high AUC values (>1,500 µM minute); may be fatal. **Serious:** Severe bone marrow suppression, which may lead to bone marrow fibrosis or aplasia; myeloablative in high doses. **Other:** Dermatologic: Skin hyperpigmentation, urticaria, erythema, and alopecia. Endocrine: Ovarian suppression, amenorrhea, and sterility. GI: Nausea and vomiting, diarrhea, and loss of appetite. Miscellaneous: Confusion, weakness and fatigue, blurred vision, elevated liver enzymes (bilirubin, SGOT/SGPT), hyperuricemia, and uric acid nephropathy (associated with initial treatment of leukemia).

Special Considerations	Dosage of oral busulfan for the treatment of leukemia needs to be adjusted based on clinical response and degree of bone marrow suppression. Instruct patients to not take more than prescribed, take each dose at the same time each day, drink plenty of fluids, and not to take missed doses or double-up on doses. Antiemetics may be needed to ensure patient compliance. High-dose regimens (HCT) need qualified individuals for monitoring of busulfan exposure (AUC), prophylactic phenytoin,

	and close monitoring of hepatic function. Consider serotonin antagonists for antiemetic prophylaxis during high-dose busulfan therapy.
Monitoring Parameters	Monitoring is recommended prior to initiation of therapy and at periodic intervals during therapy unless otherwise specified. • Liver function tests: ALT, AST, alkaline phosphatase, total bilirubin, LDH. • CBC with differential: Recommended prior to initiation of therapy, prior to each subsequent dose, and at periodic intervals during therapy. • Platelet count: Recommended prior to initiation of therapy, prior to each subsequent dose, and at periodic intervals during therapy. • Hemoglobin and/or hematocrit: Recommended prior to initiation of therapy, prior to each subsequent dose, and at periodic intervals during therapy. • Pulmonary function tests: Recommended if pulmonary toxicity is suspected. • Uric acid. • Renal function tests: CrCl, actual or calculated, and/or SCr recommended prior to initiation of therapy, prior to each subsequent dose, and at periodic intervals during therapy.
Indications	Myleran is indicated in the palliative treatment of CML. Off-label uses include the treatment of AML and brain tumors. Busulfex® is indicated for use in combination with cyclophosphamide as a conditioning regimen prior to allogeneic HCT for CML.
Dosage Adjustment Recommendations	Dosage of oral busulfan for the treatment of leukemia needs to be adjusted based on clinical response and degree of bone marrow suppression. When the total leukocyte count has declined to approximately 15,000 cells per cubic millimeter, the drug should be withheld. As the leukocyte count may continue to fall for one month after drug discontinuation, it is important that busulfan be discontinued prior to the total leukocyte count falling into the normal range. High-dose regimens (HCT) require monitoring for busulfan exposure by AUC measurements with dosage adjustments usually necessary for an AUC value >1,500 μM/minute or as dictated by specific protocol.
Pharmacokinetics	Myleran (oral busulfan) is well absorbed by mouth. The drug is extensively metabolized into several metabolites, which are excreted in the urine. Peak plasma concentrations occur within four hours, and the oral product has a half-life of approximately two hours. Studies of distribution, metabolism, and elimination of IV busulfan (Busulfex) have not been done; however, the literature on oral busulfan is relevant.
Manufacturer	Myleran®, Glaxo Wellcome Inc., Research Triangle Park, NC; Busulfex®, Orphan Medical Inc., Ben Venue Laboratories, Bedford, OH

Capecitabine

Other Names	Xeloda®
Classification	Antimetabolite.

Mechanism	Prodrug of 5'-deoxy-5-fluorouridine (5'-DFUR), which is enzymatically converted to 5-fluorouracil (5-FU) in vivo. Specific to the S phase of the cell-cycle, 5-FU inhibits the formation of the DNA-specific nucleoside base thymidine, which is essential for DNA synthesis.
Vesicant Information	Not classified as a vesicant or an irritant. Capecitabine is available commercially as an oral product.
Preparation and Mixture	No preparation or admixture necessary. Capecitabine is available commercially as an oral product.
Administration	Oral.
Storage and Stability	Store in tightly sealed bottles at controlled room temperature 15°–30°C (59°–86°F). Keep out of reach of children.
How Supplied	Commercially available as biconvex, oblong, film-coated tablets packaged as follows: 150-mg, light-peach colored tablets in bottles of 120 (imprinted with Xeloda® on one side, 150 on the other); 500-mg, peach-colored tablets in bottles of 240 (imprinted with Xeloda on one side, 500 on the other).
Dosage	2,500 mg/m^2/day, in two divided doses (12 hours apart) at the end of a meal. This dose is given for two weeks (14 days) followed by a one-week (seven-day) rest period and repeated as three-week cycles.
Compatibility Information	Not applicable. Capecitabine is available commercially as an oral product.
Contraindications/ Precautions	Contraindicated if known hypersensitivity to 5-FU. Risk versus benefit should be considered in patients with a history of coronary artery disease or hepatic function impairment (lower dosages recommended).

Drug Interactions	**Agent**	**Effect**
	Antacids	Potential increase in capecitabine and 5'-DFCR blood concentrations.
	Leucovorin	Concurrent use may increase the therapeutic and toxic effects of fluorouracil.

Toxicity/Side Effects	**Acute and/or Potentially Life-Threatening:** Severe diarrhea and necrotizing enterocolitis (rare); replete fluids and electrolytes; immediate discontinuation of therapy for grade 2 or greater diarrhea (National Cancer Institute [NCI] Common Toxicity Criteria) until resolution or decrease in intensity to grade 1 (see dosage adjustment recommendations and special considerations). **Serious:** Stomatitis (painful erythema, edema, and ulcers of mouth, lips, or tongue) and hand-and-foot syndrome (also called palmar-plantar erythrodysesthesia and includes painful erythema, blistering, desquamation, and numbness or tingling and swelling of the palms of hands or bottoms of feet); patients experiencing grade 2 or greater (NCI Common Toxicity Criteria) of either should be instructed to stop taking capecitabine immediately (see dosage adjustment recommendations and special considerations sections).

Other:
Dermatologic: Skin rash or itching, changes in fingernails or toenails, photosensitivity, and radiation recall syndrome.
Cardiovascular: Rare; includes angina, cardiomyopathy, hypotension, and/or hypertension.
GI: Nausea (53%), vomiting, anorexia, constipation, and abdominal pain.
Hematologic: Neutropenia (26%), thrombocytopenia (24%), and anemia (72%).
Neurologic: Headache (9%), dizziness, and insomnia.
Miscellaneous: Fatigue (41%), myalgia, hyperbilirubinemia (22%), hepatitis, and edema (9%).

Special Considerations	Take within 30 minutes after a meal. Swallow tablets with water. Do not take missed doses or double-up doses. Consider symptomatic treatment for the development of nausea/vomiting (antiemetics [prochlorperazine]), diarrhea (antidiarrheals [loperamide]), and stomatitis (topical anesthetics). Withdrawal of capecitabine is recommended for the development of NCI grade 2 or higher toxicity; dosage adjustment may be necessary if treatment is reinstituted (see dosage adjustment recommendations).
Monitoring Parameters	Monitoring is recommended prior to initiation of therapy and at periodic intervals during therapy unless otherwise specified. • Liver function tests: ALT, AST, alkaline phosphatase, total bilirubin, LDH. • CBC with differential: Recommended prior to initiation of therapy, prior to each subsequent dose, and at periodic intervals during therapy. • Platelet count: Recommended prior to initiation of therapy, prior to each subsequent dose, and at periodic intervals during therapy.
Indications	Capecitabine is indicated for the treatment of patients with metastatic breast cancer resistant to both paclitaxel and an anthracycline-containing chemotherapy regimen or resistant to paclitaxel and for whom further anthracycline therapy is not indicated (e.g., patients who have received cumulative doses of 400 mg/m^2 of doxorubicin or doxorubicin equivalent). Capecitabine is being investigated in other settings in which 5-FU has been established as efficacious (e.g., colorectal and head and neck cancers).
Dosage Adjustment Recommendations	Patients should be monitored carefully for toxicity. Toxicity may be managed with symptomatic treatment, temporary interruptions in dosing, or dosage adjustments. Once the dose of capecitabine has been reduced, it should not be increased at a later time. Guidelines for dosage adjustments are as follows (based on NCI Common Toxicity Criteria): Grade 1 toxicity: No interruption or modification necessary. Grade 2 toxicity: Therapy should be interrupted until the effect has resolved or improved to the level of grade 1. Use the following as guidelines if therapy is to be resumed: after a first occurrence, treatment may be reinstituted at 100% of starting dose; after second occurrence, treatment may be reinstituted at 75% of starting dose; after third occurrence, treatment may be reinstituted at 50% of starting dose; and after fourth occurrence, treatment should not be reinstituted.

Grade 3 toxicity: Therapy should be interrupted until the effect has re-solved or improved to the level of grade 1. Use the following as guidelines if therapy is to be resumed: after a first occurrence, treatment may be reinstituted at 75% of starting dose; after second occurrence, treatment may be reinstituted at 50% of starting dose; and after third occurrence, treatment should not be reinstituted.

Grade 4 toxicity: Based on clinical judgment, treatment may be discontin-ued permanently or, after the effect has resolved or improved to the grade 1 level, treatment may be reinstituted at 50% of starting dose.

Hepatic impairment: Use with caution and monitor patients carefully; patients with severe hepatic dysfunction have not been studied.

Renal impairment: Insufficient data are available to recommend dosage adjustments for patients with renal insufficiency; use with caution.

Geriatrics: Elderly patients are more sensitive to the toxic side effects of 5-FU; monitor patients carefully.

Pharmacokinetics	Capecitabine is biotransformed in the liver and tissues into 5-FU in vivo. Fluorouracil is further metabolized in normal and tumor cells to active metabolites 5-fluoro-2-deoxyuridine monophosphate and 5-fluorouridine triphosphate. Capecitabine and 5-FU have a half-life of approximately 45 minutes, and most of the dose of capecitabine as a drug-related species is recovered in the urine.
Manufacturer	Roche Laboratories Inc., Nutley, NJ

Carboplatin

Other Names	Paraplatin®
Classification	Heavy metal compound; second-generation platinol.
Mechanism	Cell-cycle nonspecific; inhibits RNA, DNA, and protein synthesis through cross-linking of DNA strands.
Vesicant Information	Irritant.
Preparation and Mixture	Reconstitute with sterile water, NS or D_5W to 10 mg/ml; further dilution for infusion with NS or D_5W.
Administration	IV; do not use aluminum needles for mixing or administration.
Storage and Stability	Light-sensitive; unopened vials to be stored at room temperature. After reconstitution, stable at room temperature for eight hours. Does not con-tain preservatives.
How Supplied	For injection, 50-mg, 150-mg, and 450-mg vials of lyophilized white powder containing carboplatin and mannitol.
Dosage	As a single agent, 350–400 mg/m² IV and repeat dose every four weeks; dilute with sterile water, D_5W, or NS to obtain a final concentration of 10 mg/ml (e.g., 50 mg/5 ml diluent).

Compatibility Information	Incompatible with aluminum.
Contraindications/ Precautions	Hypersensitivity to carboplatin, mannitol, or platinol; bone marrow suppression, lactation, bleeding tendency.

Drug Interactions	**Agent**	**Effect**
	Aluminum-containing products	Causes loss of potency and forms a precipitate.
	Carboplatin	Decreases serum levels of phenytoin and reduces effectiveness.
	Aminoglycoside	Use with caution if given with aminoglycosides because of potential nephrotoxicity.

Toxicity/Side Effects	**Acute and/or Potentially Life-Threatening:** Mild to moderate nausea and vomiting from 6–24 hours after administration.
	Serious: Hematologic toxicity may be severe and prolonged with high-dose carboplatin. Thrombocytopenia with nadir occurs on day 14–21 with recovery on day 28. Leukocyte nadir occurs on day 21 with recovery in five to six weeks.
	Other: Cardiovascular: Embolism, stroke, and heart failure. Dermatologic: Alopecia (mild), skin rash, urticaria, and pruritus. GI: Anorexia, diarrhea, constipation, and weight loss. Hematologic: Anemia. Neurologic: Mild paresthesias and peripheral neuropathy. Miscellaneous: Elevated SGOT/SGPT, electrolyte abnormalities, bronchospasms, hematuria, and renal dysfunction.
Special Considerations	Do not use aluminum needles; causes formation of a black precipitate and decreases potency. Monitor hydration, emetic control (premedication with a serotonin antagonist in combination with dexamethasone for high-dose carboplatin), thrombocytopenia, cardiac status, and neuropathies in patients previously treated with CDDP (cisplatin).
Monitoring Parameters	Monitoring is recommended prior to initiation of therapy and at periodic intervals during therapy unless otherwise specified. • CBC with differential: Recommended prior to initiation of therapy, prior to each subsequent dose, and at periodic intervals during therapy. • Platelet count: Recommended prior to initiation of therapy, prior to each subsequent dose, and at periodic intervals during therapy. • Hemoglobin and/or hematocrit: Recommended prior to initiation of therapy, prior to each subsequent dose, and at periodic intervals during therapy. • Liver function tests: ALT, AST, alkaline phosphatase, total bilirubin, LDH. • Renal function tests: CrCl, actual or calculated, and/or SCr recommended prior to initiation of therapy, prior to each subsequent dose, and at periodic intervals during therapy.

Indications	FDA-approved for advanced ovarian cancer. Off-label uses include endometrial, non-small cell and small cell lung cancer, head and neck cancer, relapsed and refractory acute leukemia.
Dosage Adjustment Recommendations	Platelets > 100,000, dose at 125%; < 50,000, reduce dose to 75%.
Pharmacokinetics	Terminal half-life is about two-and-one-half to six hours; initial half-life is one to two hours. Distributes into the liver, kidneys, and large and small bowel. Ninety percent is bound in plasma protein; 70% is excreted renally as unchanged drug.
Manufacturer	Bristol-Myers Squibb Oncology/Immunology Division, Princeton, NJ

Carmustine

Other Names	BiCNU®, BCNU, bischloronitrosourea
Classification	Alkylating agent; nitrosourea.
Mechanism	Carmustine and/or its metabolites alkylate and interfere with the function of DNA and RNA and also are capable of cross-linking DNA.
Vesicant Information	Classified as an irritant; dilution of drug reduces pain and burning on administration and local injection site reactions.
Preparation and Mixture	Reconstitute with 3 ml of sterile diluent (dehydrated alcohol solution) supplied by manufacturer to dissolve lyophilized powder. Dilute with 27 ml sterile water for injection to produce a clear, colorless solution containing 3.3 mg carmustine per ml. Reconstituted solutions may be further diluted with Sodium Chloride for Injection, 0.9%, USP, or 5% Dextrose Injection, USP. Must use glass or other manufacturer-approved containers for administration. Protect from light.
Administration	IV in 100 ml or more of NS or D_5W over 15–45 minutes; longer infusion times are recommended (one to two hours) to alleviate venous pain and irritation. Also administered intra-arterially, topically, and intratumorally.
Storage and Stability	Intact vials should be stored under refrigeration. Vials are stable at room temperature for seven days. If exposed to heat, the powder may become oily and should be discarded. Reconstituted solutions are stable for eight hours at room temperature (25°C; 77°F) and 24 hours under refrigeration (2°–8°C; 36°–46°F). Solutions further diluted with NS or D_5W are stable for eight hours at room temperature and 48 hours at refrigeration in glass or other manufacturer-approved containers and protected from light.
How Supplied	Each package contains a vial of 100 mg carmustine as a sterile, white, lyophilized powder and a vial containing 3 ml sterile diluent.
Dosage	The usual dose is 150–200 mg/m² as a single dose or divided over two days every six to eight weeks. Subsequent dosing depends on hematologic response to previous dose (see dosage adjustment recommenda-

tions). As part of a preparative regimen prior to HCT, doses up to 300–900 mg/m^2 have been used (these doses are fatal without peripheral blood stem cell or marrow support).

| **Compatibility Information** | Incompatibilities include PVC infusion bags and sodium bicarbonate. Solutions of carmustine (1.5 mg/ml) and cisplatin (0.86 mg/ml) are compatible for four hours at room temperature in a glass container. |

Contraindications/Precautions

Contraindicated if known hypersensitivity to carmustine; risk versus benefit should be considered in patients with severe hepatic or renal function impairment (lower dosages recommended), active infection, existing or history of pulmonary function impairment, or significant bone marrow depression.

Drug Interactions

Agent	Effect
Cimetidine	Concomitant use may increase toxicity of carmustine.
Amphotericin	Concomitant use may enhance cellular uptake of carmustine.
Etoposide	Concomitant use reported to cause severe hepatic dysfunction with hyperbilirubinemia, ascites, and thrombocytopenia.

Toxicity/Side Effects

Acute and/or Potentially Life-Threatening: Pulmonary toxicity of BCNU can be dose-limiting and life-threatening and is reported to occur nine days to years after treatment. Patients present with SOB, tachypnea, and nonproductive cough. Usually characterized as interstitial pneumonia and fibrosis, which may be progressive and fatal. Patients who receive ≥ 1,000 mg/m^2 are at higher risk, although other factors (e.g., past history of lung disease, smoking, prior mediastinal irradiation, concurrent administration of other agents associated with pulmonary toxicity) may play a role. It is recommended that a cumulative dose of ≥ 1,400 mg/m^2 not be exceeded. Pulmonary function tests should be obtained at baseline and repeated during treatment. Patients with a baseline below 70% of predicted forced vital capacity (FVC) or DLCO are particularly at risk.

Serious: Renal toxicity and failure, although rare, usually are associated with high cumulative doses and prolonged therapy.

Other:
Dermatologic: Facial flushing if infused too rapidly, hyperpigmentation and alopecia.
GI: Nausea and vomiting (occurs within two to four hours of administration and is dose-related), diarrhea; and reversible elevation of liver enzymes.
Hematologic: Delayed, dose-related, and cumulative myelosuppression; occurs four to six weeks after administration and may be prolonged lasting for one to two weeks.
Miscellaneous: Pain (phlebitis) along the vein during infusion (can be lessened by application of ice), hypotension, dizziness, ataxia, and

	possible second malignancy; seizures, blindness, and severe retinal toxicity associated with intracarotid use.
Special Considerations	It is recommended that a cumulative dose of $\geq 1,400$ mg/m^2 not be exceeded because of pulmonary toxicity. Pulmonary function tests should be obtained at baseline and repeated during treatment. Moderately high to highly emetogenic depending on dose; prophylactic antiemetics, a serotonin antagonist in combination with dexamethasone, are necessary. Must protect reconstituted/diluted solutions from light. Application of ice may lessen pain/burning on administration. Repeat doses should not be administered sooner than every six weeks because of prolonged and delayed myelosuppression.
Monitoring Parameters	Monitoring is recommended prior to initiation of therapy and at periodic intervals during therapy unless otherwise specified. • CBC with differential: Recommended prior to initiation of therapy, prior to each subsequent dose, and at periodic intervals during therapy. • Platelet count: Recommended prior to initiation of therapy, prior to each subsequent dose, and at periodic intervals during therapy. • Hemoglobin and/or hematocrit: Recommended prior to initiation of therapy, prior to each subsequent dose, and at periodic intervals during therapy. • Liver function tests: ALT, AST, alkaline phosphatase, total bilirubin, LDH. • Renal function tests: CrCl, actual or calculated, and/or SCr recommended prior to initiation of therapy, prior to each subsequent dose, and at periodic intervals during therapy. • Pulmonary function tests: Recommended prior to therapy and at frequent intervals thereafter. • Blood pressure: During administration.
Indications	Carmustine is FDA-approved as a single agent or in combination for the treatment of brain tumors, non-Hodgkin's and Hodgkin's lymphoma, and multiple myeloma. It also is used in the treatment of melanoma, Ewing's sarcoma, and cancers of the breast, colon, rectum, liver, and stomach.
Dosage Adjustment Recommendations	Doses subsequent to the initial dose should be adjusted according to the hematologic response of the patient to the preceding dose. The following schedule is suggested by the manufacturer as a guide to dosage adjustment:

Nadir After Prior Dose

Leukocytes/mm^3	Platelets/mm^3	Percentage of Dose to be Given
> 4,000	>100,000	100%
3,000–3,999	75,000–99,999	100%
2,000–2,999	25,000–74,999	70%
< 2,000	< 25,000	50%

Hepatic impairment: Dosage adjustments may be necessary; however, no specific guidelines are available.

| **Pharmacokinetics** | Highly lipid soluble; rapidly distributes into the tissues and readily crosses blood-brain barrier. Carmustine is metabolized by the liver, has a short |

	half-life (active metabolites may persist for days), and approximately 70% of the drug and its metabolites are eliminated by the kidneys.
Manufacturer	Bristol-Myers Squibb Oncology/Immunology Division, Princeton, NJ

Chlorambucil

Other Name	Leukeran®
Classification	Alkylating agent; nitrogen mustard derivative.
Mechanism	Interferes with and prevents DNA, RNA, and protein synthesis by causing strand breaks and cross-links in DNA.
Vesicant Information	Not classified as a vesicant or an irritant. Chlorambucil is available commercially as an oral product.
Preparation and Mixture	No preparation or admixture necessary. Chlorambucil is available commercially as an oral product.
Administration	Oral.
Storage and Stability	Store at room temperature 15°–25°C (59°–77°F) and in a dry place.
How Supplied	White, sugar-coated tablet containing 2 mg chlorambucil in bottles of 50 and imprinted with the following: 635.
Dosage	The usual dose is 0.1–0.2 mg/kg body weight daily for three to six weeks as required. Average dose is between 4–10 mg/day. The dosage is carefully adjusted to the response of the patient and must be reduced as soon as there is an abrupt fall in WBC count. Alternate dosing schedules employing intermittent, biweekly, or once-monthly pulse dosing have been utilized in a number of clinical scenarios (e.g., chronic lymphocytic leukemia [CLL]).
Compatibility Information	Not applicable. Chlorambucil is available commercially as an oral product.
Contraindications/Precautions	Chlorambucil should not be used in patients who have demonstrated hypersensitivity or previous disease resistance to the agent. Cross-hypersensitivity between chlorambucil and other alkylating agents may occur. Risk versus benefit should be considered in patients with significant bone marrow depression, active infection, history of head trauma or seizure disorder, gout or a history of gout, or history of uric acid nephropathy.
Drug Interactions	Drugs, such as the tricyclic antidepressants, MAO inhibitors, and phenothiazines, which lower the seizure threshold, may increase the risk of chlorambucil-induced seizures.
Toxicity/Side Effects	**Acute and/or Potentially Life-Threatening:** Focal and/or generalized seizures (rare); pulmonary fibrosis, although rare, may develop with chronic, long-term use. **Serious:** Skin rash, which may progress to erythema multiforme, epidermal necrolysis, and Stevens-Johnson syndrome.

Other:	
	GI: Nausea, vomiting, anorexia, diarrhea, and hepatotoxicity (relatively uncommon).
	Hematologic: Dose-related leukopenia, lymphopenia, and thrombocytopenia; may be cumulative and dose-limiting.
	Miscellaneous: Hyperuricemia (possible uric acid nephropathy), neurotoxicity (e.g., confusion, agitation, weakness), diplopia, sterility, immunosuppression, and increased risk for infection, as well as possible secondary malignancy.
Special Considerations	Do not give in full doses before four weeks after a full course of radiation therapy or chemotherapy because of potential for profound bone marrow toxicity. If missed dose on once-daily schedule, take scheduled dose as soon as possible if remembered same day; if not remembered until next day, skip missed dose and take next regularly scheduled dose at specified time. If missed dose on multiple-dosing-per-day regimen, take as soon as remembered; however, if almost time for next dose, skip missed dose and take next regularly scheduled dose at specified time. Do not double-up on doses. Low probabilities of emetogenicity; however, consider prescribing an as-needed antiemetic.
Monitoring Parameters	Monitoring is recommended prior to initiation of therapy and at periodic intervals during therapy unless otherwise specified. • CBC with differential: Recommended prior to initiation of therapy, prior to each subsequent dose, and at periodic intervals during therapy. • Platelet count: Recommended prior to initiation of therapy, prior to each subsequent dose, and at periodic intervals during therapy. • Hemoglobin and/or hematocrit: Recommended prior to initiation of therapy, prior to each subsequent dose, and at periodic intervals during therapy. • Uric acid. • Liver function tests: ALT, AST, alkaline phosphatase, total bilirubin, LDH.
Indications	FDA-approved in the treatment of CLL and malignant lymphomas, including lymphosarcoma, giant follicular lymphoma, and Hodgkin's disease. Off-label uses include breast, testicular, and ovarian carcinomas, choriocarcinoma, and multiple myeloma.
Dosage Adjustment Recommendations	Dosage must be adjusted to meet the individual requirements of the patient, based on clinical response and degree of bone marrow depression.
Pharmacokinetics	Well absorbed orally with peak plasma concentrations within one hour of administration. Food may decrease oral bioavailability by approximately 10%. Chlorambucil is extensively bound to plasma proteins and is almost entirely hepatically metabolized.
Manufacturer	Glaxo Wellcome Inc., Research Triangle Park, NC

Cisplatin

Other Name	Platinol®, Platinol AQ®, CDDP
Classification	Heavy metal compound.
Mechanism	Cell-cycle nonspecific; prevents protein, DNA, and RNA synthesis by the formation of DNA cross-links, denaturing of the double helix, and binding to DNA base pairs and other proteins.
Vesicant Information	Irritant.
Preparation and Mixture	Reconstitute 10-mg vial to a concentration of 1 mg/ml. Infuse in NS solution (0.9%, 0.45%, or 0.225%). Do not use aluminum needles. Use stainless steel or venous catheters. May prep patient with mannitol (12.5 g) IV bolus as a preinfusion to CDDP.
Administration	IV (IVP, short-term, or continuous infusion). Infusion rate is 1 mg/minute. Intraperitoneal: dose in 2 l warmed NS infused over 10–15 minutes and dwell for four hours.
Storage and Stability	Once reconstituted, CDDP stable for 20 hours at room temperature. Do not refrigerate, and avoid exposure to light.
How Supplied	Available in 10-mg or 50-mg powder vial or as an aqueous solution (1 mg/ml in 50- and 100-ml vials).
Dosage	Varies based on disease regimen. Standard dose is 20–120 mg/m² every three to four weeks; high dose, 200 mg/m² given with 250 ml of 3% NS; intraperitoneal, 60–270 mg/m² as single dose.
Compatibility Information	Compatible with saline solutions for infusion. Incompatible with aluminum; use stainless steel.
Contraindications/ Precautions	Renal impairment, hearing loss, neuropathy, allergic or hypersensitivity to CDDP, lactation, myelosuppression
Drug Interactions	Aluminum and platinol forms a precipitate with loss of efficacy of CDDP. Use caution with drugs that cause renal function impairment.
Toxicity/Side Effects	**Acute and/or Potentially Life-Threatening:** Cisplatin is one of the most severe emetogens. Severe nausea and vomiting, manifesting in one to four hours, occurs in up to 90% of patients receiving cisplatin doses > 75 mg. Premedication with a serotonin antagonist in combination with dexamethasone (and possibly other agents) is warranted. Delayed nausea and vomiting may occur days (up to 96 hours) after therapy. Home medications should include a regimen to prevent delayed emesis. Acute renal failure may occur because of renal tubular damage. Vigorous hydration prior to and during therapy is necessary. Forced diuresis may be warranted in some situations. Avoid concomitant use of other nephrotoxic medications (e.g., aminoglycosides, amphotericin B). **Serious:** Peripheral neuropathy (motor and sensory) is dose- and duration-dependent; progressive with continued therapy. Ototoxicity, which occurs in 10%–30% of patients, is manifested by high-frequency hearing loss and tinnitus.

	Other:
	Cardiovascular: Postural hypotension, hypertension, bradycardia, ST-T wave changes, bundle branch block, and atrial fibrillation. GI: Anorexia, constipation, and diarrhea. Hematologic: Mild leukopenia (nadir 18–23 days) and thrombocytopenia; chronic and often significant anemia. Miscellaneous: Papilledema, tonic-clonic seizures, sensory loss (e.g., taste, speech), electrolyte abnormalities (e.g., hypomagnesemia, hypokalemia, hypophosphatemia, hypocalcemia), and pulmonary fibrosis.
Special Considerations	Do not use IV sets and needles containing aluminum parts. Hearing loss and peripheral neuropathies occur with prolonged and high-dose therapy. Highly emetogenic; premedication with a serotonin antagonist in combination with dexamethasone warranted. Pre- and post-CDDP IV hydration necessary. Mannitol may be necessary. Encourage fluid intake during therapy and for a few days after therapy. Magnesium and potassium supplementation may be necessary because of electrolyte abnormalities.
Monitoring Parameters	Monitoring is recommended prior to initiation of therapy and at periodic intervals during therapy unless otherwise specified. • CBC with differential: Recommended prior to initiation of therapy, prior to each subsequent dose, and at periodic intervals during therapy. • Platelet count: Recommended prior to initiation of therapy, prior to each subsequent dose, and at periodic intervals during therapy. • Hemoglobin and/or hematocrit: Recommended prior to initiation of therapy, prior to each subsequent dose, and at periodic intervals during therapy. • Liver function tests: ALT, AST, alkaline phosphatase, total bilirubin, LDH. • Renal function tests: CrCl, actual or calculated, and/or SCr recommended prior to initiation of therapy, prior to each subsequent dose, and at periodic intervals during therapy. • Serum chemistry profile (particularly magnesium and potassium): Recommended prior to initiation of therapy, prior to each subsequent dose, and at periodic intervals during therapy. • Neurologic examination. • Auditory testing. • Intake and output.
Indications	Cisplatin is FDA-approved for cancer of the bladder, testes, and ovaries. Off-label uses include endometrial, non-small cell and small cell lung cancer, and squamous cell cancer of the head and neck.
Dosage Adjustment Recommendations	Dose reduction is necessary for renal impairment (see Appendix B).
Pharmacokinetics	50%–100% absorbed systemically; 90% protein-bound. Eliminated unchanged in the urine. Triphasic half-life; terminal half-life of 73–290 hours.
Manufacturer	Bristol-Myers Squibb Oncology/Immunology Division, Princeton, NJ

Cladribine

Other Name	Leustatin®, 2-CDA, 2-chlorodeoxyadenosine
Classification	Antimetabolite; purine nucleoside analogue.
Mechanism	Phosphorylated to a 5'-triphosphate derivative that is incorporated into susceptible cells and into DNA, resulting in strand breaks and shutdown of DNA synthesis.
Vesicant Information	Not classified as a vesicant or an irritant.
Preparation and Mixture	Cladribine injection must be diluted prior to administration. Aseptic technique and environmental precautions are necessary because of the lack of preservative or bacteriostatic agent in the product. For admixture of a single 24-hour infusion, add the calculated daily dose (0.09–0.1 mg/kg) to an infusion bag containing 500 ml of Sodium Chloride for Injection, 0.9%, USP. For a seven-day continuous infusion, add the calculated seven-day dose to the infusion reservoir through a sterile 0.22-micron disposable hydrophilic syringe filter (to minimize the risk for microbial contamination). Then, add the appropriate amount of Bacteriostatic 0.9% Sodium Chloride Injection, USP (0.9% benzyl alcohol preserved) also through the filter to bring the total volume of the solution to 100 ml.
Storage and Stability	Store intact vials under refrigeration (2°–8°C; 36°–46°F) and protected from light. The 24-hour infusion solution (24-hour dose/500 ml NS) is stable for 24 hours at room temperature. The seven-day infusion solution (seven-day dose/q.s. to 100 ml bacteriostatic NS) is stable for seven days at room temperature. Once diluted, solutions should be administered promptly or stored in the refrigerator for no more than eight hours prior to the start of the infusion.
How Supplied	Clear, colorless, sterile, preservative-free, isotonic solution available in single-use vials containing 10 mg (1 mg/ml) of cladribine and packaged in a treatment set of seven vials.
Dosage	Patients with hairy cell leukemia receive a single seven-day course of cladribine dosed at 0.09–0.1 mg/kg/day or 4 mg/m^2/day as a continuous infusion. Regimens for other malignancies have utilized doses of 0.1–0.3 mg/kg/day for seven days. Daily doses should not exceed 0.3 mg/kg/day.
Compatibility Information	Incompatible with D$_5$W because of increased degradation of the product. Because compatibility testing has not been performed, solutions containing cladribine should not be mixed with other IV drugs or additives or infused simultaneously via a common IV line.
Contraindications/ Precautions	Contraindicated in patients with a hypersensitivity to cladribine or any of its components. Risk versus benefit should be considered in patients with gout or a history of gout, active infection, significant bone marrow depression, or uric acid nephropathy.
Drug Interactions	No known drug interactions. Caution should be used when cladribine is administered before, after, or in conjunction with other drugs or treatments known to cause immunosuppression or myelosuppression (including radiation therapy).

Toxicity/Side Effects	**Acute and/or Potentially Life-Threatening:** Myelosuppression and immunosuppression. Patients, particularly those with baseline hematologic impairment, are at increased risk from infection because of the neutropenic and immunosuppressive side effects of cladribine. Mean neutrophil count recovery is reported to be five weeks. Depressed CD_4 counts up to one year after treatment have been reported. Bacterial, viral, protozoal, or fungal infections, which may occur in the absence of neutropenia, can be life-threatening.
	Serious: Severe anemia in up to 37% of patients requiring increased blood transfusion requirements during the first month of therapy.
	Other: Dermatologic: Rash, pruritus, and erythema. GI: Nausea and vomiting (usually mild and not requiring prophylactic antiemetics), abdominal pain, and constipation. Neurologic: Headache, insomnia, fatigue (weakness, tiredness), and dizziness. Miscellaneous: Fever (temperature above 100°F usually begins between the fifth and seventh day of treatment and lasts for a few days), myalgia, arthralgia, pain or redness at the injection site, SOB, and tachycardia.
Special Considerations	If fever occurs, it is recommended that the patient be evaluated for possible infection.
Monitoring Parameters	Monitoring is recommended prior to initiation of therapy and at periodic intervals during therapy unless otherwise specified. • CBC with differential: Recommended prior to initiation of therapy, prior to each subsequent dose, and at periodic intervals during therapy. • Platelet count: Recommended prior to initiation of therapy, prior to each subsequent dose, and at periodic intervals during therapy. • Hemoglobin and/or hematocrit: Recommended prior to initiation of therapy, prior to each subsequent dose, and at periodic intervals during therapy. • Uric acid. • CD_4 and CD_8 counts: Prior to initiation of therapy and periodic intervals during and after therapy.
Indications	Cladribine is FDA-approved for the treatment of hairy cell leukemia. It may also be used in the treatment of non-Hodgkin's lymphoma, CLL, and Waldenstrom's macroglobulinemia.
Dosage Adjustment Recommendations	Specific risk factors predisposing to increased toxicity have not been defined. It is prudent to proceed carefully in patients with known or suspected renal insufficiency or severe bone marrow impairment of any etiology. Consider delaying or discontinuing the drug if neurotoxicity or renal toxicity occurs. Dosage reduction may be required when two or more bone marrow depressants, including radiation, are used concurrently or consecutively.
Pharmacokinetics	Rapidly distributed after IV administration with an elimination half-life of seven hours. Cladribine can cross the blood-brain barrier and achieve

	detectable CSF concentrations. Median time to achieve response in patients with hairy cell leukemia is approximately four months.
Manufacturer	Ortho Biotech Products, L.P., Raritan, NJ

Cyclophosphamide

Other Name	Cytoxan®, Neosar®, Endoxan®
Classification	Alkylating agent; nitrogen mustard derivative.
Mechanism	Cell-cycle phase nonspecific. Interferes with DNA replication by cross-linking DNA strands and interferes with RNA transcription. Both methods result in disruption of nucleic acid, causing cell death.
Vesicant Information	Not classified as a vesicant or an irritant. Extravasation may cause mild and transient skin discomfort.
Preparation and Mixture	Reconstitute with sterile or bacteriostatic water. Further dilute doses in excess of 600 mg in 50 ml D_5W or NS to infuse over 30 minutes to three hours.
Administration	Oral, IV, intraperitoneal. Infuse slow IVP through side arm of fast-flowing IV of D_5W. Intraperitoneal administration can be warmed prior to infusion. Oral dose taken should be taken with food to decrease nausea.
Storage and Stability	Store vials and tablets below 25°C (77°F). Reconstituted solution is stable for 24 hours at room temperature or six days when refrigerated.
How Supplied	Oral and parenteral; tablets, 25 mg and 50 mg; IV, 100-, 200-, 500-mg, 1-g, and 2-g vials of powder.
Dosage	Regimens vary based on disease entity; oral, 50–100 mg/m²/day as continuous therapy; IV, 400–1,800 mg/m² per treatment course; intraperitoneal, 200–500 mg dose.
Compatibility Information	Compatible with D_5W and NS for infusion.
Contraindications/ Precautions	Contraindicated in patients with hypersensitivity to cyclophosphamide and patients with severe marrow depression. Use with caution in patients with impaired renal or hepatic function or who are lactating.

Drug Interactions	**Agent**	**Effect**
	Corticosteroids	Inhibit metabolism of cyclophosphamide.
	Succinylcholine	Respiratory distress, apnea.
	Barbiturates and phenytoin	Increase cyclophosphamide metabolism.
	Doxorubicin	Potentiates effects of doxorubicin, increasing cardiotoxic effect.
	Anticoagulants	Increase effect of anticoagulants.

Toxicity/Side Effects	**Acute and/or Potentially Life-Threatening:** Highly emetogenic with high doses (> 1 g); onset within six to eight hours lasting for up to 24 hours. Acute hemorrhagic cystitis because of chemical irritation of the bladder

by the metabolite acrolein can be severe and even fatal. Encourage aggressive hydration with frequent voiding. Mesna and continuous bladder irrigation may be necessary. High-dose cyclophosphamide can cause cardiac dysfunction manifested by congestive heart failure (CHF) or cardiac necrosis that is rare but fatal.

Serious: Syndrome of inappropriate antidiuretic hormone (SIADH) and renal tubular necrosis.

Other:
Dermatologic: Alopecia, skin rash, hives, pruritus, and diaphoresis.
GI: Nausea (severity is dose-dependent), vomiting, and diarrhea.
Hematologic: Thrombocytopenia, leukopenia, and anemia.
Neurologic: Headache and dizziness.
Pulmonary: Pulmonary fibrosis and pneumonitis.
Miscellaneous: Myxedema, facial flushing, and nasal congestion.

Special Considerations	Use caution with concomitant succinylcholine. Provide IV hydration pre- and post-cyclophosphamide infusion to prevent or minimize hemorrhagic cystitis. Force oral fluids to 2 l/day with oral doses. In the high-dose cyclophosphamide setting, mesna also may be administered to prevent hemorrhagic cystitis. Oral cyclophosphamide should be taken with food. Advise patient regarding bleeding precautions.
Monitoring Parameters	Monitoring is recommended prior to initiation of therapy and at periodic intervals during therapy unless otherwise specified. • CBC with differential: Recommended prior to initiation of therapy, prior to each subsequent dose, and at periodic intervals during therapy. • Platelet count: Recommended prior to initiation of therapy, prior to each subsequent dose, and at periodic intervals during therapy. • Hemoglobin and/or hematocrit: Recommended prior to initiation of therapy, prior to each subsequent dose, and at periodic intervals during therapy. • Liver function tests: ALT, AST, alkaline phosphatase, total bilirubin, LDH. • Renal function tests: CrCl, actual or calculated, and/or SCr recommended prior to initiation of therapy, prior to each subsequent dose, and at periodic intervals during therapy. • Serum chemistry profile: Recommended prior to initiation of therapy and at periodic intervals thereafter. • Urinalysis: Recommended if hemorrhagic cystitis is suspected.
Indications	Cyclophosphamide is FDA-approved for AML, ALL, CML, chronic lymphoytic leukemia (CLL), Hodgkin's and non-Hodgkin's lymphoma, breast and ovarian carcinoma, myeloma, neuroblastoma, mycosis fungoides, and retinoblastoma.
Dosage Adjustment Recommendations	See Appendices A and B. Dose is reduced for myelosuppression based on treatment protocol or regimen.
Pharmacokinetics	Well-distributed; 50% bound in plasma proteins. Crosses the blood-brain barrier. Metabolized by the liver; primarily eliminated in the urine. Half-life is four to six and one-half hours; 75%–90% is absorbed in the GI tract.
Manufacturer	Cytoxan®, Bristol-Myers Squibb Oncology/Immunology Division, Princeton, NJ; Neosar®, Adria Laboratories, Kalamazoo, MI

Cytarabine

Other Name	Cytosar-U®, ARA-C, cytosine arabinoside
Classification	Antimetabolite; pyrimidine analogue.
Mechanism	Exhibits cell-cycle specificity, primarily killing cells undergoing DNA synthesis (S-phase). Although mechanism is not clearly understood, it appears to act through inhibition of DNA polymerase.
Vesicant Information	Not classified as a vesicant or an irritant; however, thrombophlebitis has occurred at the site of drug injection or infusion in some patients. Rarely, pain and inflammation have been noted with SC injections.
Preparation and Mixture	Diluents containing benzyl alcohol should be avoided in preparation of experimental high-dose therapy. For IV use, reconstitute with bacteriostatic water for injection with benzyl alcohol 0.945% weight/volume (w/v) added as preservative. Add 5 ml to 100-mg vial for a final concentration of 20 mg/ml; add 10 ml to the 500-mg vial for a final concentration of 50 mg/ml; add 10 ml and 20 ml to the 1-g and 2-g vials, respectively, for a final concentration of 100 mg/ml. May be further diluted with sterile water for injection, D_5W, or NS. Standard dilutions for IVP is 100 mg/ml in no larger than 30-ml syringe that is ≤ 75% full; for IV piggyback (IVPB), dose per 100 ml D_5W or NS; continuous IV, dose per 250–1,000 ml D_5W or NS. For SC use, reconstitute with sterile water or saline to a concentration of 50–100 mg/ml. Do not use bacteriostatic water for injection, USP, or solutions containing benzyl alcohol for reconstitution for IT use. May reconstitute intrathecal (IT) doses with preservative-free sodium chloride for injection, 0.9%, USP, or lactated Ringer's solution. Must use prepared IT doses immediately. The volume administered should correspond to an equal volume of CSF removed. Standard dilution for IT administration is dose in 3–5 ml lactated Ringer's solution or preservative-free sodium chloride for injection, 0.9% USP, ± MTX (12 mg) ± hydrocortisone (15–50 mg).
Administration	May be given by IV infusion (over 1–24 hours) or bolus injection SC or IT.
Storage and Stability	Vials should be stored at room temperature 20°–25°C (68°–77°F). Reconstituted solutions with Bacteriostatic Water for Injection, USP with Benzyl Alcohol 0.945% w/v are stable at room temperature for 48 hours and seven days under refrigeration. Diluted solutions containing up to 0.5 mg/ml are stable at room temperature for seven days. Solutions that develop a slight haze should be discarded. Solutions for IT use should be used immediately after preparation. IT doses of cytarabine with MTX and hydrocortisone in lactated Ringer's solution or preservative-free NS are stable at room temperature for 24 hours.
How Supplied	Sterile, lyophilized powder in multidose vials containing 100 mg, 500 mg, 1 g, and 2 g of cytarabine.
Dosage	Induction remission for acute nonlymphocytic leukemia (ANLL): 100 mg/m²/day continuous IV (CIV) days 1–7 or 100 mg/m²/day IV every 12 hours days 1–7. High-dose therapies include 1–3 g/m²/day IV over one to three

hours every 12 hours for two to six days. Other common regimens include 60–200 mg/m^2/day CIV for 5–10 days; 100 mg/m^2 IV or SC twice a day for five consecutive days every 28 days; 10 mg/m^2 SC every 12 hours for 15–21 days. IT doses usually in range of 10–30 mg/m^2, although doses up to 75 mg/m^2 up to three times per week have been used.

Compatibility Information	Cytarabine (0.26 mg/ml), daunorubicin (0.03 mg/ml), and etoposide (0.4 mg/ml) are stable in D$_5$W/0.45% NaCl for 72 hours at room temperature. Also compatible with MTX, potassium chloride, vincristine, hydrocortisone, sodium chloride, calcium, and magnesium sulfate. IT cytarabine compatible with MTX and hydrocortisone in lactated Ringer's solution or NS for 24 hours at room temperature. Incompatible with carbenicillin, penicillin G sodium, 5-FU, heparin sodium, oxacillin, and nafcillin.
Contraindications/ Precautions	Contraindicated in patients with a known hypersensitivity to cytarabine or any component. Risk versus benefit should be considered in patients with significant hepatic or renal function impairment (lower dosages recommended), significant bone marrow depression, active infection, gout or a history of gout, or history of uric acid nephropathy.

Drug Interactions	**Agent**	**Effect**
	Gentamicin	Concomitant use may cause possible decreased therapeutic effect against strains of *K. pneumoniae*.
	Flucytosine	Concomitant use may cause possible decreased flucytosine efficacy.
	Digoxin	Reversible decrease in digoxin steady-state plasma concentrations; monitor digoxin levels.
	MTX	Possible synergistic cytotoxic effect.
	Cyclophosphamide	Concurrent use with high-dose cytarabine in transplant setting has been reported to increase cardiac toxicity.

Toxicity/Side Effects	**Acute and/or Potentially Life-Threatening:** Severe, usually reversible but at times fatal CNS (e.g., reversible corneal toxicity, hemorrhagic conjunctivitis, cerebral and cerebellar toxicity, including coma), GI (e.g., severe GI ulceration, peritonitis, bowel necrosis, necrotizing colitis), or pulmonary toxicity (e.g., sudden respiratory distress, pulmonary edema) has been reported in experimental high-dose regimens. Nausea/vomiting may be severe with high doses with an acute onset one to three hours after administration. Antiemetic prophylaxis is needed (e.g., serotonin antagonist in combination with dexamethasone). **Serious:** Capillary leak syndrome may occur 2–21 days after treatment; more common with continuous infusion and higher doses; characterized by sudden onset of respiratory distress. High dose (> 200 mg/m^2) for fevers, flu-like syndrome, conjunctivitis (tearing, photophobia, pain and blurred vision: ophthalmic corticosteroid prophylaxis warranted). In ad-

dition, CNS toxicity (16%–40%) manifested mainly by cerebellar toxicity is dose-limiting. Onset is approximately six to eight days after dose and is characterized by slurred speech, ataxia, confusion, and nystagmus. Risk factors include cumulative dose (48 g/m^2), gender (men more than women), poor renal function (CrCl less than 60 ml/min), hepatic dysfunction, infusion rate (one-hour > three-hour), and age > 50.

Other:

Dermatologic: Skin rash, oral/anal inflammation, skin freckling, cellulitis at injection site, and alopecia.

GI: Anorexia, diarrhea, metallic taste, and stomatitis.

Hematologic: Myelosuppression is dose-limiting. Biphasic leukocyte nadir occurs at day 7–9 and a deeper fall at day 15–24. Thrombocytopenia nadir occurs at day 12–15 and anemia also is common.

Hypersensitivity (cytarabine syndrome): Flu-like syndrome of fevers, arthralgia, rash on palms of hands, soles of feet, neck, and chest (especially with concomitant use of allopurinol). Rash on palms and soles may have bullae formation and desquamation. Syndrome usually occurs 6–12 hours following drug administration. Corticosteroids have been shown to be beneficial in treating or preventing this syndrome.

Neurologic: Dizziness, headache, somnolence, and confusion.

Miscellaneous: Conjunctivitis (usually occurs on day 1–3), keratitis, photophobia, transient elevation in liver enzymes, and urinary retention.

After IT administration, the most common adverse effects include headache, nausea, vomiting, and fever. Rarely, meningism, paresthesia, paraplegia, seizures, blindness, and necrotizing encephalopathy occur.

Special Considerations	IV doses > 200 mg/m^2 may produce conjunctivitis that can be ameliorated with prophylactic use of a corticosteroid eye drop (e.g., dexamethasone 0.1% 1–2 drops each eye every six hours for two to seven days after cytarabine). Antiemetic prophylaxis with a serotonin antagonist in combination with dexamethasone for doses > 250 mg.
Monitoring Parameters	Monitoring is recommended prior to initiation of therapy and at periodic intervals during therapy unless otherwise specified. • CBC with differential: Recommended prior to initiation of therapy, prior to each subsequent dose, and at periodic intervals during therapy. • Platelet count: Recommended prior to initiation of therapy, prior to each subsequent dose, and at periodic intervals during therapy. • Hemoglobin and/or hematocrit: Recommended prior to initiation of therapy, prior to each subsequent dose, and at periodic intervals during therapy. • Renal function tests: CrCl, actual or calculated, and/or SCr recommended prior to initiation of therapy, prior to each subsequent dose, and at periodic intervals during therapy. • Liver function tests: ALT, AST, alkaline phosphatase, total bilirubin, LDH. • Uric acid.
Indications	Cytarabine is FDA-approved in combination with other agents for remission induction of ANLL. It also has been used in the treatment of ALL and CML in blast phase. IT administration is indicated in prophylaxis and

	treatment of meningeal leukemia. Off-label uses include non-Hodgkin's lymphoma, myelodysplastic syndrome, and carcinomatous meningitis.
Dosage Adjustment Recommendations	Adjustment is necessary in patients receiving high-dose cytarabine therapy who have renal impairment (see Appendix B). It is not recommended to give high-dose cytarabine if the patient's CrCl is 30 ml/minute or less. Dosage adjustment also is recommended in the setting of hepatic impairment, although no guidelines are available.
Manufacturer	Pharmacia & Upjohn, Peapack, NJ

Cytarabine liposome

Other Name	DepoCyt®, DTC 101
Classification	Antimetabolite; pyrimidine analogue.
Mechanism	DepoCyt® is a formulation of cytarabine with sustained release properties. Once absorbed inside the cell, cytarabine is converted to cytarabine-5'-triphosphate, which interferes with cell division during the S-phase.
Vesicant Information	Not a vesicant or an irritant.
Preparation and Mixture	After warming vials to room temperature, the solution should be gently agitated to resuspend DepoCyt®. DepoCyt® should be withdrawn from the vial and administered without further dilution.
Administration	DepoCyt® is administered through an intraventricular reservoir or by direct injection into the lumbar sac over a period of one to five minutes. Patients should receive concurrent oral dexamethasone with each treatment.
Storage and Stability	Unopened vials should be stored under refrigeration. After withdrawal from vial, doses should be administered within four hours.
How Supplied	Commercially available as white to off-white suspension in 5 ml single-use vials.
Dosage	DepoCyt® 50 mg is administered IT once every 14 days for two doses.
Compatibility Information	Further dilution of Depocyt® or admixture with other solutions is not recommended.
Contraindications/ Precautions	DepoCyt® should not be administered to patients who demonstrate hypersensitivity to cytarabine or have active CNS infections.
Drug Interactions	No formal studies of DepoCyt® and other medications were conducted.
Toxicity/Side Effects	**Acute and/or Potentially Life-Threatening:** None. **Serious:** Chemical arachnoiditis was observed in 100% of treatments without dexamethasone prophylaxis but only in 33% of treatments with prophylaxis. **Other:** Confusion, somnolence, abnormal gait, headache, fever, back pain, and nausea and vomiting also have been observed.

Special Considerations	All patients should be given prophylaxis for arachnoiditis with oral dexamethasone 4 mg twice daily for five days beginning on the day of DepoCyt® administration. After administration, CSF fluid will appear slightly cloudy to milky white on future samplings. DepoCyt® particles may be misread as WBCs on some automated cell counters but can easily be differentiated from cells by microscopic examination.
Monitoring Parameters	Evaluations of CSF fluid to monitor disease response should be performed.
Indications	DepoCyt® is indicated for the IT treatment of lymphomatous meningitis.
Dosage Adjustment Recommendations	None
Pharmacokinetics	Preliminary studies demonstrate peak levels of cytarabine are reached within five hours of administration. Elimination from the CSF is biphasic with a terminal half-life of 100–263 hours in doses ranging from 12.5–75 mg. The slow transfer of cytarabine from the CSF to the plasma allows negligible systemic exposure following treatments.
Manufacturer	Chiron Therapeutics, Emeryville, CA

Dacarbazine

Other Name	DTIC-Dome®, DTIC, dimethyl-triazeno-imidazole-carboxamide
Classification	Alkylating agent; miscellaneous (tetrazine).
Mechanism	Exact mechanism is unknown, although hypothesized to inhibit DNA synthesis through alkylation causing cross-linking and strand breaks in DNA, as well as through interaction with sulfhydryl groups.
Vesicant Information	Classified as an irritant, although is capable of causing tissue necrosis if extravasated. Aspirate any extravasated drug in surrounding tissue, and place ice on area for 20–30 minutes every few hours for 48 hours. Elevate limb as often as possible during first 48 hours, and protect exposed tissue from light following extravasation. Protecting the solution from light usually reduces the venous irritation and discomfort during administration.
Preparation and Mixture	Reconstitute with sterile water for injection, NS, or D_5W to a final concentration of 10 mg/ml using 9.9 ml with the 100-mg vial and 19.7 ml with the 200-mg vial. Further dilute with 250–500 ml NS or D_5W and infuse over 15–30 minutes.
Administration	May be administered as an IVP (over 1–2 minutes into freely running IV) or an infusion (over 15–30 minutes).
Storage and Stability	Store intact vials under refrigeration 2°–8°C (36°–46°F), and protect from light. Reconstituted solutions are stable for 24 hours at room temperature and 96 hours under refrigeration. Solutions that have been further diluted are stable for 24 hours at room temperature or under refrigeration. Protect reconstituted and/or diluted solutions from light. Dacarbazine rapidly deactivates (50% at four hours) if not protected from light. Decomposed drug turns pink.

How Supplied	Sterile, colorless to an ivory-colored, light-sensitive powder packaged in boxes of 12 and supplied in 10-ml vials containing 100-mg or 20-ml vials containing 200 mg dacarbazine.
Dosage	Common regimens include 375 mg/m^2 on days 1 and 15 of a 28-day cycle; 150–250 mg/m^2/day for five days repeated every three to four weeks; 75–125 mg/m^2/day for 10 days repeated every 28 days.
Compatibility Information	Incompatible with heparin, lidocaine, and hydrocortisone.
Contraindications/ Precautions	Contraindicated in patients with a history of hypersensitivity. Risk versus benefit should be considered in patients with renal and hepatic function impairment (lower dosages recommended), active infection, or significant bone marrow depression.

Drug Interactions	Agent	Effect
	Hepatic enzyme inducers (phenytoin, phenobarbital)	Concomitant use may enhance metabolism of dacarbazine by induction of microsomal enzymes; dosage adjustment may be necessary.

Toxicity/Side Effects	**Acute and/or Potentially Life-Threatening:** Anaphylaxis and hepatic toxicity (rare), including hepatic vein thrombosis and acute hepatic necrosis. **Serious:** Severe nausea and vomiting. Onset is within 1–3 hours up to 12 hours, with severity and intensity decreasing with each subsequent dose. Antiemetic prophylaxis with a serotonin antagonist in combination with dexamethasone is warranted. **Other:** Dermatologic: Alopecia, rash, photosensitivity, and pain and burning at injection site. GI: Anorexia, metallic taste, stomatitis, and diarrhea. Hematologic: Mild to moderate myelosuppression is common and dose-related. Leukopenia and thrombocytopenia may be delayed with an onset within seven days, a nadir in 21–25 days, and recovery by day 21–28. Anemia also may develop. Miscellaneous: Facial flushing, headache, nasal congestion, paresthesia, flu-like syndrome (e.g., fever, malaise, headache, sinus congestion, myalgia that last up to several days after administration), hypocalcemia (associated with high-dose therapy), blurred vision, and weakness.
Special Considerations	Protect dacarbazine solutions from light to decrease likelihood of decomposition of drug, as well as to decrease local pain and irritation at injection site. Care should be taken to avoid extravasation of drug because of risk of severe pain and tissue necrosis. In addition, diluting the drug in 100–500 ml D$_5$W or NS, slowing the infusion rate, and applying ice to the injection site may reduce the pain and discomfort associated with the administration of dacarbazine. Because of the emetogenic potential of this agent, antiemetic prophylaxis with a serotonin antagonist in combination with dexamethasone is warranted. Patients also should be instructed to wear sunscreen (SPF 15) to minimize potential for photosensitivity reaction.

Monitoring Parameters	Monitoring is recommended prior to initiation of therapy and at periodic intervals during therapy unless otherwise specified. • CBC with differential: Recommended prior to initiation of therapy, prior to each subsequent dose, and at periodic intervals during therapy. • Platelet count: Recommended prior to initiation of therapy, prior to each subsequent dose, and at periodic intervals during therapy. • Hemoglobin and/or hematocrit: Recommended prior to initiation of therapy, prior to each subsequent dose, and at periodic intervals during therapy. • Liver function tests: ALT, AST, alkaline phosphatase, total bilirubin, LDH. • Renal function tests: CrCl, actual or calculated, and/or SCr recommended prior to initiation of therapy, prior to each subsequent dose, and at periodic intervals during therapy.
Indications	Indicated in the treatment of metastatic melanoma, as well as in second-line treatment of Hodgkin's disease. Off-label uses include islet cell carcinoma, soft-tissue sarcoma, and neuroblastoma.
Dosage Adjustment Recommendations	It is recommended that the dose of dacarbazine be adjusted in the setting of renal impairment (see Appendix B). It also is recommended to adjust dose or proceed with caution in patients with hepatic impairment.
Pharmacokinetics	Slowly and incompletely absorbed after oral administration. Dacarbazine is extensively metabolized in the liver, where it is activated by hepatic microsomal enzymes to cytotoxic metabolites. Biphasic half-life with an initial half-life of 20–40 minutes and terminal half-life of five hours. Elimination occurs through the hepatobiliary route, as well as unchanged in the urine (30%–50%).
Manufacturer	Bayer Corporation Pharmaceutical Division, West Haven, CT

Dactinomycin

Other Name	Cosmegen®, actinomycin D
Classification	Antitumor antibiotic.
Mechanism	A product of *Streptomyces parvullus,* for which the mechanism may involve binding to DNA by intercalation between base pairs and inhibition of DNA-dependent RNA synthesis.
Vesicant Information	Classified as a vesicant. If extravasated, aspirate any drug in surrounding tissue, and place ice on area for 20–30 minutes every few hours for 48 hours. Elevate limb as often as possible during first 48 hours following extravasation.
Preparation and Mixture	Reconstitute with 1.1 ml sterile water for injection to yield a clear, gold-colored solution with a final concentration of 500 mcg/ml. Do not reconstitute with preservative diluent, NS, or D_5W, as precipitation may occur. May further dilute with D_5W or NS or administer into the tubing of a running IV infusion. Standard dilution for IVPB is dose per 50 ml of D_5W or NS administered over 20–30 minutes. Do not use cellulose ester mem-

brane in-line filters, as partial removal of dactinomycin from the IV solution has been reported.

Administration	May be given as a slow IVP over 10–15 minutes or as an infusion over 20–30 minutes. DO NOT administer intramuscularly or subcutaneously.
Storage and Stability	Store intact vials at room temperature, and protect from light, humidity, and excessive heat. Reconstituted and/or diluted solutions are stable at room temperature for 24 hours.
How Supplied	Cosmegen® for Injection is supplied as a yellow lyophilized powder in sterile vials containing 500 mcg of dactinomycin.
Dosage	Common dosing regimens are 10–15 mcg/kg/day (or 0.1–0.15 mg/kg/day), 400 mcg/m²/day for a maximum of five days every three to six weeks, or 0.4–2.5 mg/m² as a single dose given at intervals of one to four weeks. Usual adult dose is 500 mcg IV daily for five days.
Compatibility Information	Compatible with dacarbazine. Use of water-containing preservatives (e.g., benzyl alcohol, parabens), D_5W, or NS to reconstitute dactinomycin may result in the formation of a precipitate.
Contraindications/ Precautions	Contraindicated in patients with a known hypersensitivity to dactinomycin or any component and children under six months of age. In addition, if dactinomycin is given at or about the same time of infection with chicken pox or herpes zoster, a severe generalized disease that may result in death may occur. Risk versus benefit should be considered in patients with hepatic function impairment (lower dosages recommended), active infection, gout or a history of gout, history of uric acid nephropathy, or significant bone marrow depression.

Drug Interactions	**Agent**	**Effect**
	Doxorubicin	Concurrent or sequential use with dacarbazine may increase cardiotoxicity; recommend not exceeding 450 mg/m² total dose of doxorubicin in this setting.
	Radiation therapy	May potentiate the effects of radiation therapy causing increased skin erythema, which may be severe, and increased GI toxicity.

Toxicity/Side Effects	**Acute and/or Potentially Life-Threatening:** Anaphylactoid reaction.
	Serious: Dactinomycin is extremely corrosive. If extravasation occurs, severe damage to soft tissues will occur.
	Other: Dermatologic: Alopecia, skin eruptions (e.g., acneiform), increased pigmentation, and radiation recall (i.e., skin irritation that may lead to necrosis in previously irradiated areas). GI: Severe nausea and vomiting with onset within 2–5 hours, lasting up to 24 hours; stomatitis, anorexia, abdominal pain, esophagitis, and diarrhea. GI ulceration and hepatic toxicity, including ascites,

	hepatomegaly, hepatitis, and liver function test abnormalities, are less common. Hematologic: Myelosuppression may be dose-limiting and severe. Onset within 7 days, nadir at 14–21 days with recovery by 21–28 days. Anemia, aplastic anemia, agranulocytosis, and pancytopenia may occur. Miscellaneous: Hypocalcemia, hyperuricemia, fatigue, depression, malaise, and fever.
Special Considerations	Antiemetic prophylaxis with a serotonin antagonist in combination with dexamethasone is warranted. Care should be taken to avoid extravasation. Do not administer IM or SC.
Monitoring Parameters	Monitoring recommended at initiation of therapy and at periodic intervals during therapy unless otherwise specified. • CBC with differential: Recommended prior to initiation of therapy, prior to each subsequent dose, and at periodic intervals during therapy. • Platelet count: Recommended prior to initiation of therapy, prior to each subsequent dose, and at periodic intervals during therapy. • Hemoglobin and/or hematocrit: Recommended prior to initiation of therapy, prior to each subsequent dose, and at periodic intervals during therapy. • Liver function tests: ALT, AST, alkaline phosphatase, total bilirubin, LDH. • Uric acid.
Indications	Indicated in the treatment of Ewing's sarcoma, sarcoma botryoides, trophoblastic tumors, testicular carcinoma, Wilms' tumor, and rhabdomyosarcoma. Also used in KS, osteosarcoma, melanoma, and cancers of the endometrium and ovary.
Dosage Adjustment Recommendations	Dosage should be based on BSA in obese or edematous patients. If marked leukopenia, thrombocytopenia, diarrhea, or stomatitis occurs, therapy should be withheld until counts return to satisfactory levels and the patient has recovered.
Pharmacokinetics	Poorly absorbed after oral administration. Widely distributed in the body after IV administration, although only negligible amounts are detected in the CSF. Dactinomycin has a half-life of approximately 36 hours and is eliminated either unchanged in the urine (10%) or excreted via the feces/bile (50%).
Manufacturer	Merck & Company, Inc., West Point, PA

Daunorubicin HCl

Other Name	Cerubidine®
Classification	Anthracene; anthracycline derivative.
Mechanism	Binds to nucleic acids by intercalation, thereby interfering with DNA synthesis.
Vesicant Information	Vesicant. Care should be taken to avoid extravasation; if extravasated, apply ice immediately, and elevate limb.

Preparation and Mixture	Reconstitute daunorubicin with 4 ml sterile water to 20-mg vial to yield 5 mg/ml dose. Further dilute with 100 ml D_5W or NS to infuse over 30–45 minutes. The ready-to-use solution, on the other hand, may be immediately used in an IV infusion without the possibility of reconstitution error.
Administration	Further dilute dose in 10–15 ml NS in a syringe prior to IVP injection or infusion through a fast-flowing side arm of IV tubing. Check blood return before, during, and after infusion. Do not extravasate. Mini-bag infusion of 50 ml over 30–45 minutes.
Storage and Stability	Reconstituted solution stable at room temperature for 24 hours and refrigerated for 48 hours. Protect from light.
How Supplied	20-mg vial of powder; ready-to-use solution 5 mg/ml containing 4 ml (total of 20 mg).
Dosage	30–60 mg/m² daily for three to five days every three to four weeks.
Compatibility Information	Incompatible with heparin and heparin-containing solutions.
Contraindications/ Precautions	Hypersensitivity to daunorubicin.

Drug Interactions	**Agent**	**Effect**
	Doxorubicin	Use of daunorubicin in a patient who has previously received doxorubicin may increase risk of cardiotoxicity. Should not be used in patients who have received complete cumulative doses of an anthracycline.
	Cyclophosphamide or mediastinal radiation therapy	Concurrent use may result in increased risk of cardiotoxicity.
	Hepatotoxic drugs	Concurrent use may increase risk of hepatotoxicity.
	Trastuzumab	Concomitant use with anthracyclines may increase incidence and severity of cardiac dysfunction.

Toxicity/Side Effects	**Acute and/or Potentially Life-Threatening:** Cardiotoxicity, specifically CHF with a subsequent decrease in the left ventricular ejection fraction (LVEF), can occur with cumulative doses > 550 mg/m². Cardiac function should be monitored regularly. Incidence may increase with prior anthracycline use, preexisting cardiac disease, concomitant cyclophosphamide, or mediastinal radiotherapy and cumulative dose. Can occur months to years following therapy. Long-term monitoring and periodic assessment of cardiac function is essential. **Serious:** Severe local tissue inflammation, ulceration, and necrosis upon extravasation. Apply ice immediately, and elevate limb. **Other:** Cardiovascular: Pericarditis, myocarditis.

Dermatologic: Skin rash, urticaria, and pigmentation of nail beds.

GI: Nausea and vomiting, usually mild to moderate; occurring in 1–3 hours and lasting for 4–24 hours; diarrhea, and stomatitis.

Hematologic: Myelosuppression, predominantly neutropenia, is dose-limiting.

Miscellaneous: Alopecia, chills, elevations in serum bilirubin, AST, and alkaline phosphatase, red discoloration of urine.

Special Considerations	Check for blood return before, during, and after infusion. Avoid extravasation. Urine may be red in color one to two days after administration. Protect from light. Do not mix with heparin.
Monitoring Parameters	Monitoring is recommended prior to initiation of therapy and at periodic intervals during therapy unless otherwise specified. • CBC with differential: Recommended prior to initiation of therapy, prior to each subsequent dose, and at periodic intervals during therapy. • Platelet count: Recommended prior to initiation of therapy, prior to each subsequent dose, and at periodic intervals during therapy. • Hemoglobin and/or hematocrit: Recommended prior to initiation of therapy, prior to each subsequent dose, and at periodic intervals during therapy. • Liver function tests: ALT, AST, alkaline phosphatase, total bilirubin, LDH. • Renal function tests: CrCl, actual or calculated, and/or SCr recommended prior to initiation of therapy, prior to each subsequent dose, and at periodic intervals during therapy. • Cardiac function tests: Multiple gated acquisition (MUGA) scan or LVEF recommended at baseline in patients with risk factors and at periodic intervals throughout therapy, as well as long-term follow-up evaluations. • Site: Monitor for stinging and burning during peripheral line or implanted port infusion.
Indications	ANLL in adults (e.g., myelogenous, monocytic, erythroid), ALL in children in combination with other agents.
Dosage Adjustment Recommendations	Lifetime maximum dose of 550 mg/m² or 450 mg/m² in patients who have been treated with radiation therapy to the chest. Dose reduction in patients with impaired renal and hepatic function (see Appendices A and B).
Pharmacokinetics	Rapid distribution to major organs. Initial half-life of 45 minutes. Terminal half-life of 18.5 hours. Metabolized by the liver and excreted in bile (40%) and in urine (25%).
Manufacturer	Wyeth-Ayerst Pharmaceuticals, Philadelphia, PA

Daunorubicin, liposomal

Other Name	DaunoXome®, daunorubicin citrate
Classification	Anthracene; anthracycline derivative.
Mechanism	Aqueous solution of the citrate salt of daunorubicin encapsulated with liposomes. Inhibits DNA and RNA synthesis by intercalating between base pairs of DNA and by steric obstruction. Liposomal formulation helps to protect the entrapped daunorubicin from chemical and enzymatic deg-

	radiation, minimizes protein binding, and decreases uptake by normal tissues. Once in the tumor microenvironment, daunorubicin is released over time.
Vesicant Information	Although grade 3 and 4 local injection site inflammation has been reported, no instances of local tissue necrosis have been reported. One should take appropriate precautions to avoid extravasation.
Preparation and Mixture	Supplied as a solution containing 2 mg/ml of daunorubicin. Dilute 1:1 with 5% Dextrose Injection, USP, by transferring calculated volume from vial into a sterile infusion bag containing an equal volume of D_5W. Do not use an in-line filter for IV infusion.
Administration	IV over 60 minutes.
Storage and Stability	Store intact vials of liposomal daunorubicin under refrigeration at 2°–8°C (36°–46°F). Do not freeze. Protect from light. Diluted liposomal daunorubicin should be administered immediately. If not used immediately, diluted liposomal daunorubicin should be stored under refrigeration for a maximum of six hours.
How Supplied	Supplied as a translucent, red, liposomal dispersion in single-use vials, each containing 50 mg daunorubicin base at a concentration of 2 mg/ml.
Dosage	Usual adult dose is 40 mg/m^2 IV over 60 minutes every two weeks.
Compatibility Information	Liposomal daunorubicin should be diluted only with D_5W. Not compatible with other medications, other diluents, or bacteriostatic solutions.
Contraindications/ Precautions	Contraindicated in patients who have experienced a serious hypersensitivity reaction to liposomal daunorubicin or any of its constituents. Risk versus benefit should be considered in patients with preexisting cardiac disease (may increase risk of cardiac toxicity; monitor cardiac function), renal or hepatic function impairment (excretion may be delayed; dosage reduction recommended), existing or recent chicken pox or herpes zoster infection, or significant bone marrow depression (treatment should be withheld if granulocytes < 750 cells/mm^3).

Drug Interactions	**Agent**	**Effect**
	Cyclophosphamide	Concomitant use may increase risk of cardiotoxicity.
	Radiation therapy to mediastinum	Concomitant use may increase risk of cardiotoxicity.
	Anthracene derivatives	Prior use may increase risk of cardiotoxicity; dosage adjustment may be necessary.
	Hepatotoxic drugs	Concurrent use may increase risk of hepatotoxicity.
	Trastuzumab	Concomitant use with anthracyclines may increase incidence and severity of cardiac dysfunction.

Toxicity/Side Effects	**Acute and/or Potentially Life-Threatening:** Cardiotoxicity, specifically CHF with a subsequent decrease in the LVEF, can occur with cumulative doses > 300 mg/m^2. Cardiac function should be monitored regularly. Incidence may increase with prior anthracycline use, preexisting cardiac disease, concomitant cyclophosphamide or mediastinal radiotherapy, and cumulative dose.
	Serious: Infusion-related reaction, manifested as back pain, chest tightness, or flushing, may occur during first five minutes of infusion and is most likely related to the liposomal component of the preparation.
	Other: Cardiovascular: Chest pain, palpitations, hypertension, edema, syncope, and tachycardia. GI: Nausea and vomiting, usually mild to moderate; abdominal pain, diarrhea, dry mouth, dysphagia, constipation, and stomatitis. Hematologic: Myelosuppression, predominantly neutropenia, is dose-limiting. Neurologic: Neuropathy, fatigue, headache, depression, dizziness, and insomnia. Miscellaneous: Alopecia, dyspnea, pruritus, arthralgia, and myalgia.
Special Considerations	Liposomal daunorubicin NOT interchangeable with free daunorubicin. Cardiac function should be monitored regularly in patients receiving liposomal daunorubicin because of the potential risk for cardiotoxicity and CHF. Although local tissue necrosis has not been reported following extravasation, caution should be used when administering this agent. An infusion-related reaction may occur during the first five minutes of the infusion; symptomatic therapies should be available (e.g., diphenhydramine, corticosteroids). Liposomal daunorubicin is considered to be a mild to moderate emetogen; consider an as-needed antiemetic (e.g., prochlorperazine) for nausea and/or vomiting, which may occur.
Monitoring Parameters	Monitoring is recommended prior to initiation of therapy and at periodic intervals during therapy unless otherwise specified. • CBC with differential: Recommended prior to initiation of therapy, prior to each subsequent dose, and at periodic intervals during therapy. • Platelet count: Recommended prior to initiation of therapy, prior to each subsequent dose, and at periodic intervals during therapy. • Hemoglobin and/or hematocrit: Recommended prior to initiation of therapy, prior to each subsequent dose, and at periodic intervals during therapy. • Cardiac function tests: MUGA or LVEF recommended prior to initiation of therapy, at periodic intervals during therapy, and at total cumulative doses of 320 mg/m^2, 480 mg/m^2, and every 240 mg/m^2 thereafter. • Liver function tests: ALT, AST, alkaline phosphatase, total bilirubin, LDH. • Renal function tests: CrCl, actual or calculated, and/or SCr recommended prior to initiation of therapy, prior to each subsequent dose, and at periodic intervals during therapy. • Observation for evidence of opportunistic infection.
Indications	Liposomal daunorubicin is indicated in the treatment of advanced HIV-associated KS. Liposomal daunorubicin is being investigated in other

	settings in which daunorubicin has been established as efficacious (e.g., lymphoma, sarcomas, leukemias).
Dosage Adjustment Recommendations	Recommended to reduce dose in the setting of renal and hepatic function impairment (see Appendices A and B). In addition, blood counts should be obtained prior to each dose and therapy withheld if absolute granulocyte count is < 750 cells/mm^3.
Pharmacokinetics	The plasma pharmacokinetics of liposomal daunorubicin differ significantly from conventional daunorubicin. The small volume of distribution (confined to the vascular fluid volume) and clearance for the liposomal product appear to result in a higher daunorubicin exposure. Half-life is approximately 4.4 hours, which most likely represents a distribution half-life. Animal studies suggest that liposomal daunorubicin crosses the blood-brain barrier.
Manufacturer	Gilead Sciences, Foster City, CA (merged with NexStar Pharmaceuticals, Inc.)

Denileukin diftitox

Other Name	ONTAK®, DAB$_{389}$ IL-2
Classification	Biologic; targeted fusion molecule.
Mechanism	Denileukin is a recombinant DNA-derived cytotoxic protein composed of the amino acid sequences for diphtheria toxin fragments A and B (Met$_1$-Thr$_{387}$)-His followed by the amino acid sequences Ala$_1$-Thr$_{133}$ for interleukin-2. This fusion protein is designed to direct the cytocidal action of diphtheria toxin to IL-2 receptor expressing cells, resulting in inhibition of cellular protein synthesis and cell death. Malignant cells expressing one or more of the subunits of the IL-2 receptor are found in certain leukemias and lymphomas.
Vesicant Information	Not classified as a vesicant or an irritant.
Preparation and Mixture	Bring frozen solution to room temperature, up to 25°C (77°F). The vials may be thawed at room temperature for one to two hours or in the refrigerator at 2°–8°C (36°–46°F) for not more than 24 hours. Denileukin must not be heated. The thawed solution may have a haze visible; this should clear at room temperature and must not be used unless the solution is clear, colorless, and without visible particulate matter. The solution may be mixed by gentle swirling; do not shake. The concentration of denileukin must be at least 15 mcg/ml during all steps of the preparation process. Withdraw the calculated dose from the vial, and inject into an empty IV bag. For each 1 ml (150 mcg) of denileukin, add 9 ml of sterile saline without preservative. May prepare and dilute denileukin in plastic syringes or plastic IV bags. Do not use glass containers. Prepared solutions should be administered within six hours using a syringe pump or IV infusion. Unused portions should be discarded immediately. Do not administer through an in-line filter. Denileukin should not be refrozen.
Administration	For IV use only. Denileukin should be infused over at least 15 minutes. DO NOT administer as an IV bolus injection.

Storage and Stability	Store frozen at or below −10°C. Once solution is thawed, do not refreeze. Prepared solutions of denileukin should be administered within six hours. Unused portions should be discarded immediately.
How Supplied	Denileukin is supplied in a package of six 2-ml, single-use vials of 150 mcg/ml sterile, frozen solution.
Dosage	The recommended treatment regimen is 9 or 18 mcg/kg/day administered intravenously for five consecutive days every 21 days. The optimal duration of therapy has not been determined, although only 2% of patients who did not demonstrate at least a 25% decrease in tumor burden prior to the fourth cycle subsequently responded.
Compatibility Information	No compatibility information available; do not physically mix denileukin with other drugs.
Contraindications/ Precautions	Contraindicated for use in patients with known hypersensitivity to denileukin or any of its components (e.g., diphtheria toxin, IL-2, excipients). Patients should be monitored carefully for signs of infection because of the potential impairment in immune function of denileukin-treated patients. Risk versus benefit should be considered in patients with preexisting cardiovascular disease because of the development of a vascular leak syndrome.
Drug Interactions	No clinical drug interaction studies have been conducted.
Toxicity/Side Effects	**Acute and/or Potentially Life-Threatening:** Acute hypersensitivity-type reactions have been reported in up to two-thirds of patients during or within 24 hours of denileukin infusion; approximately half of these events occurred on the first day of dosing regardless of treatment cycle. The constellation of symptoms includes one or more of the following: hypotension (50%), back pain (30%), dyspnea (28%), vasodilation (28%), rash (25%), chest pain or tightness (24%), tachycardia, dysphagia or laryngismus, syncope, allergic reaction, or anaphylaxis. These events were severe in 2% of patients. Management includes interruption or a decrease in the rate of infusion and the administration of IV antihistamines, corticosteroids, and/or epinephrine. Resuscitative equipment should be readily available during denileukin administration. **Serious:** Vascular leak syndrome may occur and is characterized by two or more of the following: hypotension, edema, and/or hypoalbuminemia. The onset of symptoms usually is delayed, occurring within first two weeks of infusion, and may persist or worsen after denileukin treatment cessation. This syndrome is usually self-limited. Risk versus benefit should be considered before denileukin treatment in patients with preexisting cardiovascular disease. Preexisting low serum albumin levels may predispose patients to this syndrome. It is postulated, because of denileukin binding to activated lymphocytes and macrophages, that impairment of immune function occurs. Infections have been reported in 48% of patients, of whom 23% were considered severe. Patients should be monitored for signs of infection as these patients are at particular risk for cutaneous infections because of their disease. **Other:** Cardiovascular: Hypotension, vasodilation, tachycardia, thrombotic events, and hypertension.

Endocrine: Hypoalbuminemia (97%), transaminase increase (76%; occurred during first course of therapy and usually self-limited), edema (62%), hypocalcemia, weight decrease, dehydration, and hypokalemia.

GI: Nausea and vomiting (78%), anorexia (44%), diarrhea (delayed onset and prolonged), and pancreatitis (rare).

Hematologic: Anemia (24%), thrombocytopenia, lymphopenia (in up to 34%; lymphocyte counts drop during dosing period and return to normal by day 15), and leukopenia.

Neurologic: Dizziness (23%), paresthesia, nervousness, confusion, and insomnia.

Miscellaneous: Myalgia, arthralgia, rash, pruritus, sweating, hematuria, albuminuria, and hypo- or hyperthyroidism.

Special Considerations	Consider antiemetics (e.g., serotonin antagonists, prochlorperazine) prior to administration and as needed. In addition, anorexia, hypotension, anemia, confusion, rash, and nausea and/or vomiting occurred more frequently in patients older than age 65. Do not use glass containers for administration because of adsorption to glass. Do not administer as an IV bolus injection; must be infused over at least 15 minutes.
Monitoring Parameters	Monitoring is recommended prior to initiation of therapy and at periodic intervals during therapy unless otherwise specified. • Prior to the administration of denileukin, the patient's malignant cells should be tested for CD25 expression. • CBC with differential: Recommended prior to initiation of therapy and at weekly intervals during therapy. • Hemoglobin and/or hematocrit: Recommended prior to initiation of therapy, prior to each subsequent dose, and at periodic intervals during therapy. • Serum chemistry panel including albumin: Recommended prior to initiation of therapy and at weekly intervals during therapy. • Liver function tests: ALT, AST, alkaline phosphatase, total bilirubin, LDH. • Renal function tests: CrCl, actual or calculated, and/or SCr recommended prior to initiation of therapy, prior to each subsequent dose, and at periodic intervals during therapy. • Weight, edema, and blood pressure: Should be carefully monitored on an outpatient basis.
Indications	Denileukin is indicated for the treatment of patients with persistent or recurrent cutaneous T cell lymphoma whose malignant cells express the CD25 component of the IL-2 receptor. Also being studied in the treatment of non-Hodgkin's lymphoma and psoriasis.
Dosage Adjustment Recommendations	Administration of denileukin should be delayed until serum albumin levels are 3 g/dl or greater.
Pharmacokinetics	Denileukin displays 2-compartmental kinetics after first dose with a distribution phase half-life of approximately 2–5 minutes and a terminal phase half-life of 70–80 minutes. The development of antibody formation to the diphtheria toxin domains increases clearance two- to threefold.
Manufacturer	Seragen, Inc., Hopkinton, MA

Dexrazoxane

Other Names	Zinecard®, ICRF-187
Classification	Miscellaneous; cardioprotective agent; chelating agent.
Mechanism	Appears to be converted intracellularly to a ring-opened chelating agent that interferes with iron-mediated free radical generation.
Vesicant Information	Not classified as a vesicant or an irritant.
Preparation and Mixture	Add 25 or 50 ml of 0.167 molar (M/6) sodium lactate injection (provided by the manufacturer) to the 250- or 500-mg vial, respectively, to produce a solution containing 10 mg/ml. Reconstituted solutions may be further diluted with 50–100 ml of either Sodium Chloride for Injection, 0.9%, USP, or 5% Dextrose Injection, USP, to a final concentration ranging from 1.3–5 mg/ml.
Administration	Dexrazoxane solutions may be given by slow IV injection or rapid IV drip over 15–30 minutes. Dexrazoxane is administered just prior to the administration of doxorubicin. Doxorubicin must be administered within 30 minutes from the beginning of the dexrazoxane infusion. Doxorubicin should not be administered prior to dexrazoxane.
Storage and Stability	Store intact vials at controlled room temperature between 15°–30°C (59°–86°F). Reconstituted and/or diluted solutions are stable at room temperature or under refrigeration for six hours.
How Supplied	Dexrazoxane for injection is a sterile, pyrogen-free lyophilized powder available in vials containing 250 mg or 500 mg and packaged with a 25-ml or 50-ml vial, respectively, of 0.167 molar (M/6) Sodium Lactate Injection, USP.
Dosage	The recommended dosage ratio of dexrazoxane:doxorubicin is 10 parts dexrazoxane to 1 part doxorubicin (e.g., 500 mg/m² dexrazoxane for every 50 mg/m² doxorubicin) repeated with each treatment of doxorubicin. Dexrazoxane is administered just prior to the administration of doxorubicin. Doxorubicin must be administered within 30 minutes from the beginning of the dexrazoxane infusion.
Compatibility Information	Dexrazoxane may be further diluted after reconstitution with Sodium Chloride for Injection, 0.9%, USP, or 5% Dextrose Injection, USP. Dexrazoxane should not be mixed with other medications.
Contraindications/ Precautions	Should not be used with chemotherapy regimens that do not contain an anthracycline.
Drug Interactions	There was no significant change in the pharmacokinetics of doxorubicin or its predominant metabolite, doxorubinol, in the presence of dexrazoxane.
Toxicity/Side Effects	**Acute and/or Potentially Life-Threatening:** None noted. **Serious:** Severity of myelosuppression may be greater with the addition of dexrazoxane to the chemotherapy regimen. **Other:** Pain at the injection site.

Special Considerations	Dexrazoxane should be given prior to doxorubicin. Doxorubicin should be given within 30 minutes after the beginning of the dexrazoxane infusion. Dexrazoxane is indicated in patients who have received a cumulative doxorubicin dose of 300 mg/m²; some data suggest reduced efficacy of fluorouracil, cyclophosphamide, and doxorubicin chemotherapy for metastatic breast cancer when dexrazoxane was administered starting with the initiation of chemotherapy.
Monitoring Parameters	Monitoring is recommended prior to initiation of therapy and at periodic intervals during therapy unless otherwise specified. • CBC with differential: Recommended prior to initiation of therapy, prior to each subsequent dose, and at periodic intervals during therapy. • Hemoglobin and/or hematocrit: Recommended prior to initiation of therapy, prior to each subsequent dose, and at periodic intervals during therapy. • Platelet count: Recommended prior to initiation of therapy, prior to each subsequent dose, and at periodic intervals during therapy. • Cardiac function tests: Recommended at periodic intervals because dexrazoxane reduces but does not eliminate the risk of anthracycline-induced cardiotoxicity. • Liver function tests: ALT, AST, alkaline phosphatase, total bilirubin, LDH.
Indications	Indicated for reducing the incidence and severity of cardiomyopathy associated with doxorubicin administration in women with metastatic breast cancer who have received a cumulative doxorubicin dose of 300 mg/m². Used off-label to reduce the incidence and severity of cardiomyopathy associated with the anthracyclines in a variety of settings (e.g., lymphoma, sarcoma).
Dosage Adjustment Recommendations	None noted.
Pharmacokinetics	Rapidly distributed throughout the body after IV administration, the drug is not bound to plasma proteins and is metabolized in the liver, and approximately 42% of the drug is excreted unchanged in the urine. Elimination half-life is approximately two to three hours.
Manufacturer	Pharmacia & Upjohn, Peapack, NJ

Docetaxel

Other Names	Taxotere®
Classification	Antimicrotubule agent.
Mechanism	Promotes the assembly and blocks the disassembly of microtubules, which prevents cancer cell division, causing cell death.
Vesicant Information	Irritant.
Preparation and Mixture	Remove vials of docetaxel and diluent (13% weight to weight [w/w] ethanol in water) from refrigerator, and let stand at room temperature for five minutes. Add entire contents of diluent to docetaxel, which ensures a final

concentration of 10 mg/ml. Gently rotate contents for 15 seconds. Premix solution should be clear yellow to brownish-yellow; however, some foam may form at top of contents because of the polysorbate 80. Discard premix solution if not clear or contains a precipitate. Allow premix solution to stand for a few minutes to allow most of foam to dissipate. Withdraw calculated amount of premix docetaxel solution (10 mg/ml), and add to a 250-ml infusion bag or bottle of Sodium Chloride for Injection, 0.9%, USP, or 5% Dextrose Injection, USP to produce a final concentration of 0.3–0.9 mg/ml. If the dose of docetaxel to be administered is > 240 mg, use a larger volume of infusion vehicle so that the final concentration does not exceed 0.9 mg/ml. Thoroughly mix the infusion by manual rotation. Solutions must be prepared in a glass bottle, polypropylene, or polyolefin plastic bag to prevent leaching of plasticizers. Nonpolyvinylchloride (non-PVC) tubing should also be used.

Administration	Docetaxel is administered as an IV infusion over one hour.
Storage and Stability	Intact vials should be stored under refrigeration and protected from light. Vials should be stored at room temperature for five minutes before using. Premix and initial diluted solutions are stable for eight hours at either room temperature or under refrigeration. Final diluted (fully prepared) solutions are stable for four hours and should be used within four hours (including the one-hour infusion time).
How Supplied	Docetaxel is available in 20-mg and 80-mg vials as a lyophilized white or almost white powder prepackaged with the 13% (w/w) ethanol in water diluent and formulated in polysorbate 80.
Dosage	Usual adult dose is 60–100 mg/m^2 administered intravenously as a one-hour infusion every three weeks. Weekly dosing regimens also common.
Compatibility Information	Compatible with Sodium Chloride for Injection, 0.9%, USP, and 5% Dextrose Injection, USP. Solutions must be prepared in a glass bottle, polypropylene, or polyolefin plastic bag to prevent leaching of plasticizers. Non-PVC tubing also should be used.
Contraindications/ Precautions	Contraindicated in patients with a previous hypersensitivity to docetaxel or to other drugs formulated with polysorbate 80. Docetaxel should not be used in patients with neutrophil counts < 1,500 cells/mm^3. Risk versus benefit should be considered in patients with preexisting pleural effusion, active infection, a history of alcohol abuse, or significant bone marrow depression.
Drug Interactions	No formal clinical studies have been performed to evaluate drug interactions; however, in vitro studies have shown the metabolism of docetaxel may be modified by concomitant administration of drugs that inhibit, induce, or are metabolized by the cytochrome P450 3A4 enzyme system. These include cyclosporine, ketoconazole, erythromycin, terfenadine, and troleandomycin. Caution should be used when prescribing these drugs while the patient is receiving docetaxel.
Toxicity/Side Effects	**Acute and/or Potentially Life-Threatening:** Treatment-related mortality increased in patients with abnormal liver function. Severe hypersensitivity reactions characterized by hypotension and/or bronchospasm or generalized rash/erythema may occur. Discontinuation of infusion and

symptomatic treatment may be necessary. Corticosteroid prophylaxis warranted.

Serious: Severe fluid retention characterized by poorly tolerated peripheral edema, generalized edema, pleural effusion requiring urgent drainage, cardiac tamponade, or pronounced abdominal distention may occur in up to 6.5% of patients, despite corticosteroid prophylaxis.

Other:
Cardiovascular (rare): Hypotension, sinus tachycardia, heart failure, atrial flutter, unstable angina, pulmonary edema, and dysrhythmia.
Dermatologic: Rash, erythema, alopecia, nail changes, mild hyperpigmentation, and possible desquamation.
GI: Mild nausea and vomiting, stomatitis, and diarrhea.
Liver function tests: Increased bilirubin, ALT, AST, and alkaline phosphatase.
Hematologic: Myelosuppression is dose-limiting; neutropenia (nadir within eight days and median duration of seven days), thrombocytopenia, and anemia.
Neurologic: Asthenia (severe in 14.9% of cases), myalgia, arthralgia, and paresthesia.
Miscellaneous: Fever, dyspnea, fluid retention, fluid-associated weight gain, and infusion site reactions (e.g., hyperpigmentation, inflammation, phlebitis, swelling of vein).

Special Considerations	To reduce the incidence and severity of fluid retention and hypersensitivity reactions, all patients should be premedicated with oral corticosteroids (e.g., dexamethasone 8 mg twice daily for three to five days) beginning one day prior to initiation of docetaxel. Close monitoring of patient for hypersensitivity and fluid retention is warranted. Docetaxel is mildly emetogenic; is consider prescribing an as-needed antiemetic (e.g., prochlorperazine).
Monitoring Parameters	Monitoring is recommended prior to initiation of therapy and at periodic intervals during therapy unless otherwise specified. • CBC with differential: Recommended prior to initiation of therapy, prior to each subsequent dose, and at periodic intervals during therapy. • Hemoglobin and/or hematocrit: Recommended prior to initiation of therapy, prior to each subsequent dose, and at periodic intervals during therapy. • Platelet count: Recommended prior to initiation of therapy, prior to each subsequent dose, and at periodic intervals during therapy. • Liver function tests: ALT, AST, alkaline phosphatase, total bilirubin, LDH. • Vital signs: During and after infusion; monitor for signs/symptoms of hypersensitivity.
Indications	Docetaxel is FDA-indicated in the treatment of patients with locally advanced or metastatic breast cancer after failure of prior chemotherapy, as well as in the treatment of patients with non-small cell lung cancer that does not respond to cisplatin-based chemotherapy. Also used in variety of other settings, including ovarian cancer.
Dosage Adjustment Recommendations	Docetaxel is not recommended for patients with hepatic impairment, especially moderate to severe impairment, because of the increased risk of severe toxicity (see Appendix A). If bilirubin is greater than the upper

limits of normal, or the ALT/AST > 1.5 times the upper limits of normal concomitant with alkaline phosphatase > 2.5 times upper limits of normal, docetaxel should not be administered. If docetaxel considered essential for a patient with hepatic impairment, significant dose reduction is necessary. Docetaxel administration should be delayed if neutrophil count is < 1,500 cells/mm^3 and/or platelet count is < 100,000 cells/mm^3. In addition, a reduction in each subsequent dose is recommended for patients with severe neutropenia (< 500 cells/mm^3) for more than seven days, febrile neutropenia, severe infection, severe peripheral neuropathy, or severe or cumulative cutaneous reactions. For patients originally receiving 100 mg/m^2, a dose reduction to 75 mg/m^2 is appropriate. If complications persist or recur, dosage should be further reduced to 55 mg/m^2. Lastly, patients who originally receive 60 mg/m^2 and who do not develop the above may tolerate higher doses.

Pharmacokinetics	Exhibits a triphasic decline in plasma concentrations and is highly bound to plasma proteins. Undergoes oxidative metabolism by the liver with isoenzymes of the cytochrome P450 3A4 system involved. Following metabolism, docetaxel is eliminated in the urine (6%) and the feces (75%) with most of the drug eliminated within the first 48 hours.
Manufacturer	Rhône-Poulenc Rorer Pharmaceuticals Inc., Collegeville, PA

Doxorubicin HCl

Other Names	Adriamycin®, Rubex®
Classification	Anthracene; anthracycline derivative.
Mechanism	The anthracyclines have several modes of action but seem to share at least one common cytotoxic mechanism with other antitumor antibiotics: intercalation between base pairs in the DNA double helix. The anthracycline portion of the molecule appears to intercalate between stacked nucleotide pairs in the DNA helix, causing inhibition of DNA and RNA synthesis. Doxorubicin can be cytotoxic in all phases of the cell-cycle although maximally cytotoxic in S phase. Also inhibits the enzyme topoisomerase II, as well as causes generation of free radicals.
Vesicant Information	Vesicant; local skin and deep-tissue damage will occur at the site of inadvertent extravasation. Apply ice immediately, and elevate limb. One promising antidote is dimethyl sulfoxide 1.5 ml applied every six hours for 14 days.
Preparation and Mixture	Lyophilized drug may be reconstituted with sterile water for injection, D$_5$W, NS, and most other common IV solutions. For IVP doses, reconstitution with either D$_5$W or NS is advised to ensure isotonicity of the resultant solution.
Administration	Short IVP infusions and IV bolus injections are common methods for administration. A slow IVP over several minutes offers several advantages. First, serious extravasations can be minimized by using slow IVP over one to two minutes with constant check on blood return. Second, injection also may be infused via a side port of a running IV line. Do not infuse doxorubicin HCl

near previous venipuncture. Remember that doxorubicin causes severe tissue damage if extravasation occurs. Start a fresh peripheral IV site to infuse doxorubicin HCl. All prolonged infusions must be given through a tunneled central venous catheter or port on a volumetric infusion pump.

Storage and Stability	Manufacturers generally report at least two-year stability for intact vials of lyophilized powder when stored at room temperature and away from direct light. The commercial solution formulations must be stored under refrigeration. One manufacturer includes methylparaben as a solubility enhancer and as an antimicrobial to facilitate multidosing from a single vial.
How Supplied	IV use only; 10-, 20-, 50-, 100-, 150-, and 200-mg vials; liquid or lyophilized form.
Dosage	Numerous drug administration schedules have been reported for doxorubicin HCl. As a single agent, doses of 60–75 mg/m^2 have been used, repeated no more than every three weeks. For patients with normal cardiac function, it is recommended not to exceed 550 mg/m^2 maximum cumulative lifetime dose of doxorubicin HCl to minimize risk of cardiac toxicity. In patients with risk factors (e.g., elderly, mediastinal irradiation, preexisting heart disease, concurrent cyclophosphamide use), it is recommended not to exceed a cumulative lifetime dose of 400 mg/m^2. The total dose limit also must consider the doses of any other anthracyclines or DNA-intercalating compounds the patient has received in the past.
Compatibility Information	The reader is referred to other resources on admixture for detailed information.
Contraindications/ Precautions	Elderly patients with cardiac history; hypersensitivity to doxorubicin; pregnancy and lactation.

Drug Interactions	**Agent**	**Effect on Doxorubicin**
	Amphotericin B	Reduced resistance.
	Caffeine	Blocked cytotoxicity.
	Cyclosporine	Modulation of doxorubicin resistance.
	Gentamicin	Antagonized bacterial activity.
	Allopurinol	Antitumor effects.
	Cimetidine	Decreased clearance, increased plasma exposure.
	Warfarin	Lack of pharmacokinetic or antitumor interaction.
	Insulin	Enhanced antitumor effects.
	Interferon alfa	Cytotoxic synergy.

Doxorubicin can be radiosensitizing and radiomimetic. In other words, doxorubicin can cause reactivation of soft tissue reactions in areas previously irradiated, referred to as "radiation recall."

Toxicity/Side Effects	**Acute and/or Potentially Life-Threatening:** Cardiotoxicity, specifically CHF with a subsequent decrease in the LVEF, can occur with cumulative doses > 450–550 mg/m^2. Cardiac function should be monitored regularly. Incidence may increase with prior anthracycline use, preexisting cardiac disease, concomitant cyclophosphamide or mediastinal radiotherapy, and cumulative dose. Can occur months to years following therapy. Long-term monitoring and periodic assessment of cardiac function are essential. **Serious:** Severe local tissue inflammation, ulceration, and necrosis upon extravasation. Apply ice immediately, and elevate limb. **Other:** Cardiovascular: Pericarditis, myocarditis. Dermatologic: Alopecia, skin rash, urticaria, pigmentation of nail beds, venous flare phenomena (noted with erythematous streaking along the vein used for doxorubicin infusion, urticaria, and pruritus; symptoms usually abate with treatment of IV antihistamines and glucocorticosteroids) and radiation recall (redness, warmth, erythema, and dermatitis in radiation port; occurs five to seven days after doxorubicin administration; topical corticosteroids and topical cooling indicated). GI: Nausea and vomiting, usually mild to moderate in moderate doses and highly emetogenic with high-dose doxorubicin ($\geq$ 60 mg/m^2); occurring in 1–3 hours and lasting for 4–24 hours; diarrhea, esophagitis, anorexia, necrosis of the colon, and stomatitis. Hematologic: The dose-limiting side effect of doxorubicin is bone marrow suppression. Leukopenia (nadir of 10–14 days) is common in up to 60%–80% of patients. Hematologic recovery is usually resolved within one week of the nadir. Miscellaneous: Facial flushing, hyperuricemia, and red discoloration of urine.
Special Considerations	Impaired immune system, myelosuppression. Avoid inhalation when mixing drug. Limit lifetime cumulative dose to 550 mg/m^2; 400 mg/m^2 for patients with risk factors for increased cardiac toxicity.
Monitoring Parameters	Monitoring is recommended prior to initiation of therapy and at periodic intervals during therapy unless otherwise specified. • CBC with differential: Recommended prior to initiation of therapy, prior to each subsequent dose, and at periodic intervals during therapy. • Hemoglobin and/or hematocrit: Recommended prior to initiation of therapy, prior to each subsequent dose, and at periodic intervals during therapy. • Platelet count: Recommended prior to initiation of therapy, prior to each subsequent dose, and at periodic intervals during therapy. • Cardiac function tests: MUGA or LVEF recommended at baseline in patients with risk factors and at periodic intervals throughout therapy, as well as long-term evaluations. • Liver function tests: ALT, AST, alkaline phosphatase, total bilirubin, LDH.
Indications	FDA-approved for a wide spectrum of antitumor activity in solid tumors and hematologic cancers (e.g., sarcomas, adenocarcinomas, melanomas, leukemias, lymphomas).

Dosage Adjustment Recommendations	Dose reduced in patients with impaired hepatobiliary function (see Appendix A).
Pharmacokinetics	The drug is rapidly distributed in body tissues with 75% bound to plasma proteins, especially albumin. There is significant distribution of doxorubicin into human breast milk. Terminal elimination half-life of 30–40 hours and the incomplete (50%) total recovery of drug in urine, bile, and feces. Organs and tissues with high-dose concentrations include liver, lymph nodes, muscles, bone marrow, fat, and skin. The conjugated metabolites are excreted in the bile and feces.
Manufacturer	Adriamycin®, Pharmacia & UpJohn, Peapack, NJ; Rubex®, Bristol-Myers Squibb Oncology /Immunology Division, Princeton, NJ

Doxorubicin, liposomal

Other Names	Doxil®, doxorubicin hydrochloride liposome
Classification	Anthracene; anthracycline derivative.
Mechanism	Liposomal doxorubicin incorporates a polyethylene glycol derivative around a liposomal-coated core of doxorubicin (called Stealth® [Alza Pharmaceuticals, Mountain View, CA] technology). Doxorubicin binds to nucleic acids by intercalation with base pairs of DNA interfering with DNA synthesis, inhibits the enzyme topoisomerase II, and causes the production of free radicals that cleave DNA and cell membranes.
Vesicant Information	Considered an irritant. Precautions should be taken to avoid extravasation. If any signs or symptoms of extravasation occur, immediately terminate infusion. Ice may be applied over the site of extravasation for 30–60 minutes to help to alleviate the local reaction. If significant reaction, consider application of ice at intervals of 15 minutes for 24 hours. Elevate and rest extremity for 24–48 hours. Application of heat or sodium bicarbonate can be harmful and is contraindicated.
Preparation and Mixture	Liposomal doxorubicin, up to a maximum of 90 mg, must be diluted in 250 ml of 5% Dextrose Injection, USP. Do not administer as a bolus injection or an undiluted solution. Do not use if precipitate is present. Do not use with in-line filters.
Administration	Administer as an IV infusion over 30 minutes. Do not administer as an IM or SC injection.
Storage and Stability	Refrigerate unopened vials at 2°–8°C (36°–46°F). Avoid freezing. Diluted liposomal doxorubicin should be stored under refrigeration and administered within 24 hours.
How Supplied	Supplied as a sterile, red, translucent liposomal dispersion in 10-ml glass, single-use vials containing 20 mg doxorubicin hydrochloride at a concentration of 2 mg/ml.
Dosage	The recommended dose for AIDS-associated KS is 20 mg/m^2 IV over 30 minutes every three weeks; for ovarian cancer, 50 mg/m^2 IV over 30 minutes every four weeks. In other settings, dosages range from 40–80 mg/m^2 IV every three to four weeks.

Compatibility Information	Do not mix with other drugs. Do not use any other diluent other than 5% Dextrose Injection, USP. Do not use any bacteriostatic agent, such as benzyl alcohol.
Contraindications/ Precautions	Contraindicated in patients with a history of hypersensitivity to conventional doxorubicin or to the components of the liposomal product. Risk versus benefit should be considered in patients with existing bone marrow depression, history of cardiovascular disease, or existing or recent chicken pox or herpes zoster infection, or patients with hepatic function impairment.
Drug Interactions	No formal drug interaction studies have been conducted with liposomal doxorubicin; however, may interact with drugs known to interact with conventional doxorubicin.

Agent	Effect
Trastuzumab	Concomitant use with anthracyclines may increase incidence and severity of cardiac dysfunction.

| Toxicity/Side Effects | **Acute and/or Potentially Life-Threatening:** An acute infusion-related reaction consisting of SOB, chills, facial swelling, and low blood pressure may occur during the initial few minutes of the first infusion and usually resolves with the cessation of the infusion. Cardiotoxicity (e.g., cardiomyopathy, fast or irregular heartbeat, SOB, left ventricular failure) has been reported; however, experience with liposomal doxorubicin is limited. Therefore, warnings related to the use of conventional doxorubicin should be observed.

Serious: Palmar-plantar erythrodysesthesia, characterized by ulceration, erythema, and desquamation of the hands and feet with pain and inflammation, may occur. Usually mild and most commonly occurs after six to eight weeks of therapy, although reported incidence < 5%. In severe cases, management consists of holding treatment until resolution and resuming therapy with longer intervals between doses.

Other:
Dermatologic: Pigmentation of nail beds, alopecia, allergic reaction (e.g., rash, chills, fever, itching), injection site pain or reactions, and radiation erythema and recall.
GI: Nausea (dose-related; mild to moderate in most regimens), vomiting, constipation, diarrhea, and stomatitis.
Hematologic: Anemia, neutropenia (dose-limiting; onset in 7 days, nadir by day 10–14, and recovery by day 21–28), and thrombocytopenia; myelosuppression may occur in up to 80% of patients.
Miscellaneous: Dyspnea, hyperglycemia, dizziness, back pain, and headache. |
|---|---|
| Special Considerations | Liposomal doxorubicin IS NOT interchangeable with free doxorubicin. Cardiac function should be monitored regularly in patients receiving liposomal doxorubicin because of the potential risk for cardiotoxicity and CHF. An infusion-related reaction may occur during the first five minutes of the infusion; symptomatic therapies should be available (e.g., diphenhydramine, |

corticosteroids). Although considered an irritant, caution should be taken to prevent extravasation. If any signs or symptoms of extravasation occur, immediately terminate infusion. Ice may be applied over the site of extravasation for 30–60 minutes to help to alleviate the local reaction. Liposomal doxorubicin considered to be a mild to moderate emetogen; consider an as-needed antiemetic (e.g., prochlorperazine) for nausea and/or vomiting.

Monitoring Parameters	Monitoring is recommended prior to initiation of therapy and at periodic intervals during therapy unless otherwise specified. • CBC with differential: Recommended prior to initiation of therapy, prior to each subsequent dose, and at periodic intervals during therapy. • Platelet count: Recommended prior to initiation of therapy, prior to each subsequent dose, and at periodic intervals during therapy. • Hemoglobin and/or hematocrit: Recommended prior to initiation of therapy, prior to each subsequent dose, and at periodic intervals during therapy. • Liver function tests: ALT, AST, alkaline phosphatase, total bilirubin. • Cardiac function tests: MUGA or LVEF recommended prior to initiation of therapy and at periodic intervals during therapy. • Renal function tests: CrCl, actual or calculated, and/or SCr recommended prior to initiation of therapy, prior to each subsequent dose, and at periodic intervals during therapy.
Indications	Liposomal doxorubicin is indicated in the treatment of advanced AIDS-associated KS in patients who have progressed or are intolerant to primary therapies and in the treatment of metastatic carcinoma of the ovary in patients with disease that is refractory to both paclitaxel- and platinum-based chemotherapy. In addition, investigated in other settings in which doxorubicin has been established as efficacious (e.g., sarcomas, breast cancer, early-stage ovarian cancer).
Dosage Adjustment Recommendations	Dosage adjustments recommended in hepatic and renal impairment (see Appendices A and B). In addition, the dose of liposomal doxorubicin should be adjusted based on ANC and platelet count (ANC 500–999 and/or platelet count 25,000–49,000, wait until neutrophil count > 1,000 and platelet count > 50,000, then redose at 25% dose reduction; if ANC < 500 and/or platelet count < 25,000, wait until neutrophil count > 1,000 and platelet count > 50,000, then redose at 50% dose reduction). Dose reductions also recommended for grade of stomatitis (grade 1: no dose reduction necessary; grade 2: wait one week and if symptoms improve, redose at 100%; grade 3: wait one week and if symptoms improve, redose at 25% dose reduction; grade 4: wait one week and if symptoms improve, redose at 50% dose reduction).
Pharmacokinetics	Liposome encapsulation is thought to enhance the accumulation of doxorubicin in tumors and KS lesions. Steady-state volume of distribution confined mostly to vascular fluid volume with 70% of drug bound to plasma proteins. Metabolism takes place in both the liver and the plasma to active and inactive metabolites.
Manufacturer	Alza Pharmaceuticals, Mountain View, CA

Epirubicin

Other Names	Ellence®
Classification	Anthracene; anthracycline derivative.
Mechanism	Epirubicin intercalates DNA, which triggers DNA cleavage by topoisomerase II. It also inhibits DNA helicase activity, ultimately interfering with replication and transcription.
Vesicant Information	Epirubicin is classified as a vesicant. Severe local tissue necrosis will occur if epirubicin extravasates during administration. Do not administer epirubicin by SC or IM route.
Preparation and Mixture	Epirubicin is provided as a preservative-free, ready-to-use solution in two single-use vial sizes.
Administration	May only be administered IV. Should be administered into the tubing of a freely flowing IV infusion (0.9% sodium chloride or 5% glucose solution) over three to five minutes. This technique is intended to minimize the risk of thrombosis or perivenous extravasation, which could lead to severe cellulitis, vesication, or tissue necrosis. A direct push injection is not recommended because of the risk of extravasation, which may occur even in the presence of adequate blood return on needle aspiration.
Storage and Stability	Vials should be stored under refrigeration between 2°–8°C (36°–46°F) and protected from light. Do not freeze. Epirubicin should be used within 24 hours of the first penetration of the rubber stopper.
How Supplied	Available in 25-ml (50-mg) and 100-ml (200-mg) preservative-free, single-use vials containing 2 mg epirubicin per ml.
Dosage	The recommended starting dose of epirubicin is 100 mg/m^2 IV on day 1 of a three-week cycle or 60 mg/m^2 IV on days 1 and 8 of a four-week cycle as a component of adjuvant combination chemotherapy. It is recommended to administer a fluoroquinolone or trimethoprim-sulfamethoxazole as prophylaxis with epirubicin 120 mg/m^2.
Compatibility Information	Compatible with 5% Dextrose Injection, USP, Sodium Chloride for Injection, 0.9%, USP, or sterile water for injection.
Contraindications/ Precautions	Patients with a baseline neutrophil count < 1,500 cells/mm^3; severe myocardial insufficiency or recent myocardial infarction; previous treatment with anthracyclines at maximum cumulative doses; hypersensitivity to epirubicin, other anthracyclines, or anthracenediones; or severe hepatic dysfunction should not receive epirubicin.
Drug Interactions	Concomitant use of epirubicin with other agents that can cause heart failure (e.g., calcium channel blockers) requires close monitoring of cardiac function throughout treatment. Because epirubicin is extensively metabolized by the liver, changes in hepatic function induced by concomitant therapies may affect epirubicin metabolism, pharmacokinetics, therapeutic efficacy, and/or toxicity. Cimetidine increases the AUC of epirubicin by 50%.

Toxicity/Side Effects	**Acute and/or Potentially Life-Threatening:** Life-threatening CHF, the most severe form of anthracycline-induced cardiomyopathy, is dependent on the cumulative dose of epirubicin. The risk of developing CHF increases rapidly with increasing total cumulative doses of epirubicin in excess of 900 mg/m^2; this cumulative dose should only be exceeded with extreme caution. Delayed cardiotoxicity usually develops late in the course of therapy or within two to three months after completion of treatment.

Serious:

Cardiac function: Anthracyclines (e.g., epirubicin) can induce an early (acute) or late (delayed) onset cardiac toxicity. Early cardiac toxicity of epirubicin consists mainly of sinus tachycardia and/or ECG abnormalities, such as nonspecific ST-T wave changes, but tachyarrhythmias, including premature ventricular contractions and ventricular tachycardia, bradycardia, and atrioventricular and bundle-branch block, also have been reported. Delayed cardiac toxicity results from a characteristic cardiomyopathy that is manifested by reduced LVEF and/or signs and symptoms of CHF (e.g., tachycardia, dyspnea, pulmonary edema, dependent edema, hepatomegaly, ascites, pleural effusion, gallop rhythm).

Hematologic: Dose-dependent, reversible leukopenia and neutropenia are the most common acute dose-limiting toxicities of epirubicin. The WBC nadir is usually reached 10–14 days from initiation of treatment. WBC and neutrophil counts generally return to normal values by day 21 after drug administration. Severe thrombocytopenia and anemia also may occur.

Tumor lysis syndrome: Hyperuricemia and other metabolic abnormalities may occur with epirubicin treatment. While not generally a problem in patients with breast cancer, tumor lysis syndrome may occur.

Secondary leukemia: The occurrence of secondary AML has been reported in patients treated with anthracyclines and is more common when such drugs are given in combination with DNA-damaging antineoplastic agents, when patients have been heavily pretreated with cytotoxic drugs, or when doses of the anthracyclines have been escalated. The risk of secondary AML with epirubicin is approximately 0.2% at three years and 0.8% at five years.

Other:

Dermatologic: Reversible alopecia occurs frequently, with hair regrowth occurring within two to three months after treatment discontinuation. Flushes, skin and nail hyperpigmentation, photosensitivity, and hypersensitivity to irradiated skin (i.e., radiation-recall reaction) may occur. Urticaria and anaphylaxis have been reported in patients treated with epirubicin; signs and symptoms of these reactions may vary from skin rash and pruritus to fever, chills, and shock.

GI: Mucositis may occur and is characterized by pain or a burning sensation, erythema, erosions, ulcerations, bleeding, or infection. Mucositis generally appears early after drug administration and, if severe, may progress over a few days to mucosal ulcerations; most patients recover from this adverse event by the third week of therapy. Hyperpigmentation of the oral mucosa also may occur. Nausea, vomiting, diarrhea, and abdominal pain can occur.

Special Considerations	Avoid epirubicin administration in veins over joints or in extremities with compromised venous or lymphatic drainage. A burning or stinging sensation may be indicative of perivenous infiltration (which also may occur without causing pain); immediately terminate the infusion and restart in another vein. Facial flushing, as well as local erythematous streaking along the vein, may be indicative of excessively rapid administration and may precede local phlebitis or thrombophlebitis. Administration of epirubicin after previous radiation therapy may induce an inflammatory recall reaction at the site of the irradiation. Do not administer epirubicin by SC or IM route.
Monitoring Parameters	Monitoring is recommended prior to initiation of therapy and at periodic intervals during therapy unless otherwise specified. • CBC with differential: Recommended prior to initiation of therapy, prior to each subsequent dose, and at periodic intervals during therapy. • Platelet count: Recommended prior to initiation of therapy, prior to each subsequent dose, and at periodic intervals during therapy. • Hemoglobin and/or hematocrit: Recommended prior to initiation of therapy, prior to each subsequent dose, and at periodic intervals during therapy. • Liver function tests: ALT, AST, alkaline phosphatase, total bilirubin. • Cardiac function tests: MUGA or LVEF recommended prior to initiation of therapy and at periodic intervals during therapy. • Renal function tests: CrCl, actual or calculated, and/or SCr recommended prior to initiation of therapy, prior to each subsequent dose, and at periodic intervals during therapy. • Serum uric acid, potassium, calcium, and phosphorous: Monitor immediately after initial chemotherapy administration in patients potentially susceptible to tumor lysis syndrome.
Indications	Epirubicin is indicated as a component of adjuvant therapy in patients with evidence of axillary node tumor involvement following resection of primary breast cancer.
Dosage Adjustment Recommendations	Reduce the day 1 dose of subsequent cycles to 75% of the day 1 dose in current cycle in patients experiencing during treatment cycle nadir platelet counts < 50,000/mm^3, ANC < 250/mm^3, neutropenic fever, or grades 3 or 4 nonhematologic toxicity. Day 1 chemotherapy in subsequent courses of treatment should be delayed until platelet counts are ≥ 100,000/mm^3, ANC ≥ 1,500/mm^3, and nonhematologic toxicities have recovered to ≤ grade 1. For patients receiving a divided dose of epirubicin, the day 8 dose should be 75% of day 1 if platelet counts are 75,000–100,000/mm^3 and ANC is 1,000–1,499/mm^3. If day 8 platelet counts are < 75,000/mm^3, ANC < 1,000/mm^3, or grade 3/4 nonhematologic toxicity has occurred, omit the day 8 dose. In patients with elevated serum AST or serum total bilirubin concentrations, the following dose reductions are recommended based on clinical trials: total bilirubin 1.2–3 mg/dL or AST two to four times the upper limit of normal, give 50% of recommended starting dose; total bilirubin > 3 mg/dl or AST > four times upper limit of normal, give 25% of recommended starting dose. Consider lower doses of epirubicin in patients with severe renal impairment (SCr > 5 mg/dl).

Pharmacokinetics	The plasma concentration of epirubicin declines in a triphasic manner with mean half-lives for the alpha, beta, and gamma phases of about 3 minutes, 2.5 hours, and 33 hours, respectively.
	Following IV administration, epirubicin is rapidly and widely distributed into the tissues. Binding of epirubicin to plasma proteins, predominantly albumin, is approximately 77% and is not affected by drug concentration. Epirubicin also appears to concentrate in red blood cells (RBCs); whole blood concentrations are approximately twice those of plasma. Epirubicin is extensively and rapidly metabolized by the liver and also is metabolized by other organs and cells, including RBCs. Epirubicin and its major metabolites are eliminated through biliary excretion and, to a lesser extent, by urinary excretion.
Manufacturer	Pharmacia & Upjohn, Peapack, NJ

Estramustine

Other Names	Emcyt®
Classification	Hormonal agent; antimicrotubule agent; alkylating agent.
Mechanism	Structurally, a phosphorylated combination of estradiol and mechlorethamine; however, has weak alkylating activity. Thought to bind to microtubule-associated proteins and disrupt normal cytoskeletal structure of cells by depolymerization.
Vesicant Information	Not classified as a vesicant or an irritant. Estramustine is commercially available as an oral product.
Preparation and Mixture	No preparation or admixture necessary. Estramustine is commercially available as an oral product.
Administration	Oral.
Storage and Stability	Bottles should be stored under refrigeration at 2°–8°C (36°–46° F). Protect from light. Capsules may be stored at room temperature for 24–48 hours without affecting potency.
How Supplied	Supplied as opaque white capsules, each containing estramustine phosphate sodium as the disodium salt monohydrate equivalent to 140 mg of estramustine phosphate. Packaged in bottles of 100.
Dosage	Recommended daily dose is 14 mg/kg of body weight or 600 mg/m², given in three to four divided doses. Patients should be treated for 30–90 days before determinations are made on possible benefits of therapy.
Compatibility Information	Not applicable. Estramustine is commercially available as an oral product.
Contraindications/ Precautions	Contraindicated in active thrombophlebitis or thromboembolic disorders, hypersensitivity to estramustine or any component, estradiol, or nitrogen mustard. Risk versus benefit should be considered in patients with asthma, cardiac insufficiency, coronary artery disease, epilepsy, mental depression, migraine headaches, renal or hepatic insufficiency, peptic ulcer, thrombophlebitis, thrombosis, or thromboembolic disorders.

Drug Interactions	**Agent**	**Effect**
	Milk- or calcium-containing products	Decreased/impaired absorption of estramustine.

Toxicity/Side Effects	**Acute and/or Potentially Life-Threatening:** An increased risk of thrombosis, including fatal and nonfatal myocardial infarction, is present in men receiving estrogens for prostate cancer.
	Serious: See above.
	Other:
	Cardiovascular: Edema and hypertension.
	Dermatologic: Pigment changes.
	GI: Diarrhea, nausea (usually lessens with continued therapy), mild increases in AST or LDH, flatulence, and anorexia.
	Hematologic: Mild leukopenia.
	Miscellaneous: Decreased libido, breast tenderness/enlargement, dyspnea, insomnia, lethargy, depression, leg cramps, thrombophlebitis, tinnitus, night sweats, and hypercalcemia.

Special Considerations	Take on empty stomach, one hour before or two hours after a meal. Estramustine should be swallowed with water. Milk, milk products, or calcium-rich foods or medications should not be taken simultaneously with estramustine. Do not take more or less of this medication than prescribed. Do not take missed dose. Do not double-up on doses. Consider an as-needed antiemetic (e.g., prochlorperazine) for nausea.

Monitoring Parameters	Monitoring is recommended prior to initiation of therapy and at periodic intervals during therapy unless otherwise specified.
	• CBC with differential: Recommended prior to initiation of therapy, prior to each subsequent dose, and at periodic intervals during therapy.
	• Platelet count: Recommended prior to initiation of therapy, prior to each subsequent dose, and at periodic intervals during therapy.
	• Liver function tests: ALT, AST, alkaline phosphatase, total bilirubin, LDH.

Indications	Indicated in the palliative treatment of patients with metastatic and/or progressive prostate cancer.

Dosage Adjustment Recommendations	None noted.

Pharmacokinetics	Well absorbed orally and dephosphorylated in the intestines and eventually oxidized and hydrolyzed to estramustine, estradiol, estrone, and nitrogen mustard. Half-life of 20 hours and eliminated in the feces via the bile.

Manufacturer	Pharmacia & Upjohn, Peapack, NJ

Etoposide

Other Names	VePesid®, VP-16
Classification	Antimicrotubule agent; plant alkaloid; podophyllotoxin derivative.
Mechanism	Cell-cycle specific alkaloid that inhibits DNA synthesis in the S and G_2 phases. Inhibition of DNA synthesis is promoted by the action of

topoisomerase II. This enzyme is responsible for unbinding and resealing of chromosomes during the mitotic phase. This process causes the DNA strands to be dysfunctional and break, thus not allowing the cells to enter mitotic phase, resulting in cell death.

Vesicant Information	Irritant.
Preparation and Mixture	Reconstitute with sterile water. Available in multidose vials of 100 mg/5 ml, 150 mg/7.5 ml, 500 mg/25 ml, and 1 g/50 ml. Oral etoposide should be kept refrigerated.
Administration	IV. Avoid rapid infusion; infuse over 30–60 minutes.
Storage and Stability	Store vials at room temperature and capsules at 2°–8°C (36°–46°F). Stable for 24 months. Solutions of etoposide of 0.2 mg/ml are stable for 96 hours and 0.4 mg/ml are stable for 24 hours at room temperature.
How Supplied	Supplied as 20-mg/ml in 5-ml, 10-ml, and 25-ml vials or 50-mg capsules.
Dosage	Dosage is in combination regimen. In testicular cancer, dose range is 50–100 mg/m^2/day on days 1–5 or 100 mg/m^2/day on days 1, 3, and 5. Repeated every three to four weeks. In small cell lung cancer, dose range is 35 mg/m^2/day for four days or 50 mg/m^2/day for five days. Oral dosing continuously over 21 days with one to two weeks respite. Oral dose is twice the IV dose rounded to the nearest 50 mg.
Compatibility Information	The reader is referred to other resources on admixture for detailed information.
Contraindications/Precautions	Patients with hypersensitivity or previous anaphylactic reaction. Lactation.

Drug Interactions	**Agent**	**Effect**
	Calcium antagonists	Increases cytotoxicity of etoposide in vitro.
	Carmustine	Increased incidence of hepatotoxicity with concomitant use.
	Cyclosporine	Increases cytotoxicity of etoposide.
	MTX	Increased intracellular accumulation of MTX.
	Warfarin	May elevate PT with concomitant use.

Toxicity/Side Effects	**Acute and/or Potentially Life-Threatening:** Anaphylactic-like reaction manifested by chills, fever, tachycardia, bronchospasm, dyspnea, and hypotension. Treatment is symptomatic; stop infusion, and, at the discretion of the physician, administer pressor agents, corticosteroids, antihistamines, and/or volume expanders.
	Serious: Hepatic toxicity, although uncommon, has been reported with the use of high-dose etoposide.

	Other: Cardiovascular: Hypotension (related to infusion time; give over 30–60 minutes), tachycardia. Dermatologic: Alopecia. GI: Nausea, vomiting, anorexia, diarrhea, stomatitis, and abdominal pain. Hematologic: Anemia, leukopenia, and thrombocytopenia are dose-limiting; WBC nadir on day 5–15 with recovery by day 24–28. Neurologic: Peripheral neuropathy exacerbated by prior course of vincristine. Respiratory: Bronchospasms resulting in wheezing.
Special Considerations	Hypotension, infuse slowly. Administer antihistamine and corticosteroids for wheezing. Monitor for anaphylactic reaction. Oral dose is twice the IV dose because of bioavailability. Administer the oral dose as a once daily dose if total daily dose is ≤ 400 mg or in divided doses if total daily dose > 400 mg.
Monitoring Parameters	Monitoring is recommended prior to initiation of therapy and at periodic intervals during therapy unless otherwise specified. • CBC with differential: Recommended prior to initiation of therapy, prior to each subsequent dose, and at periodic intervals during therapy. • Platelet count: Recommended prior to initiation of therapy, prior to each subsequent dose, and at periodic intervals during therapy. • Hemoglobin and/or hematocrit: Recommended prior to initiation of therapy, prior to each subsequent dose, and at periodic intervals during therapy. • Liver function tests: ALT, AST, alkaline phosphatase, total bilirubin. • PT: If on concurrent warfarin therapy, monitor frequently.
Indications	FDA-approved in the treatment of testicular and small cell lung carcinoma. Also used in the treatment of lymphomas, bladder cancer, sarcomas, Wilms' tumor, Ewing's sarcoma, prostate cancer, and KS.
Dosage Adjustment Recommendations	Dose reduction if impaired renal function or elevated bilirubin (see Appendices A and B).
Pharmacokinetics	Excreted primarily in the urine. Initial half-life is 1.5 hours with terminal half-life range of 4–11 hours. Oral capsule bioavailability is 50%.
Manufacturer	Bristol-Myers Squibb Oncology/Immunology Division, Princeton, NJ

Etoposide phosphate

Other Names	Etopophos®
Classification	Antimicrotubule; plant alkaloid; podophyllotoxin derivative.
Mechanism	Rapidly and completely converted in vivo by dephosphorylation to active moiety, etoposide.
Vesicant Information	Not categorized as a vesicant or an irritant.
Preparation and Mixture	Reconstitute vial with Sterile Water for Injection, USP, 5% Dextrose Injection, USP, Sodium Chloride for Injection, 0.9%, USP, Sterile Bacteriostatic

Water for Injection with Benzyl Alcohol, or Bacteriostatic Sodium Chloride for Injection with Benzyl Alcohol to a concentration equivalent to 20 mg/ml or 10 mg/ml etoposide (22.7 mg/ml or 11.4 mg/ml etoposide phosphate, respectively). The quantity of diluent for reconstitution is listed below.

Vial	Volume of Diluent	Final Concentration
100 mg	5 ml	20 mg/ml
	10 ml	10 mg/ml
500 mg	25 ml	20 mg/ml
	50 ml	10 mg/ml
1,000 mg	50 ml	20 mg/ml
	100 ml	10 mg/ml

Following reconstitution, etoposide phosphate may be administered without further dilution or may be further diluted to a concentration as low as 0.1 mg/ml etoposide with 5% Dextrose Injection, USP, or Sodium Chloride for Injection, 0.9%, USP.

Administration	IV infusion over 5–210 minutes.
Storage and Stability	Store intact vials under refrigeration 2°–8°C (36°–46°F) and protect from light. Reconstituted solutions are stable in glass or plastic containers under refrigeration for seven days or at room temperature for 24 hours if reconstituted with sterile water for injection, NS, or D_5W or 48 hours if reconstituted with Sterile Bacteriostatic Water for Injection with Benzyl Alcohol or Bacteriostatic Sodium Chloride for Injection with Benzyl Alcohol. Diluted solutions are stable at room temperature or under refrigeration for up to 24 hours.
How Supplied	Supplied as a sterile lyophilized powder in vials containing etoposide phosphate equivalent to 100 mg, 500 mg, or 1,000 mg etoposide.
Dosage	Dosed as etoposide equivalent.
Compatibility Information	Not available.
Contraindications/ Precautions	Contraindicated in patients with a known hypersensitivity to etoposide, etoposide phosphate or any component, as well as in IT administration of the drug. Risk versus benefit should be considered in patients with hepatic or renal function impairment (lower dosages recommended), significant bone marrow depression, or active infection.

Drug Interactions	**Agent**	**Effect**
	Calcium antagonists	Increases cytotoxicity of etoposide in vitro.
	Carmustine	Increased incidence of hepatotoxicity with concomitant use.
	Cyclosporine	Increases cytotoxicity of etoposide.
	MTX	Increased intracellular accumulation of MTX.
	Warfarin	May elevate PT with concomitant use.

Toxicity/Side Effects	See etoposide.
Special Considerations	Advantages of etoposide phosphate are rate of infusion and less fluid necessary for preparation and dilution.
Indications	See etoposide.
Dosage Adjustment Recommendations	Dosage adjustments necessary in renal and hepatic impairment (see Appendices A and B). May be prudent to follow more stringent guidelines for dosage adjustment in renal and hepatic impairment found in etoposide monograph.
Pharmacokinetics	Rapidly and completely converted to etoposide in plasma by dephosphorylation. See etoposide for further pharmacokinetic information.
Manufacturer	Bristol-Myers Squibb Oncology/Immunology Division, Princeton, NJ

Floxuridine

Other Names	FUDR®, 5-FUDR, 5-fluoro-2'-deoxyuridine
Classification	Antimetabolite agent; pyrimidine analogue.
Mechanism	Rapidly catabolized to fluorouracil. The primary effect of fluorouracil is to interfere with DNA synthesis through inhibition of thymidylate synthetase.
Vesicant Information	Not classified as a vesicant or an irritant.
Preparation and Mixture	Reconstitute with 5 ml Sterile Water for Injection, USP, to yield a solution containing 100 mg/ml. The calculated daily dose is then diluted with 5% Dextrose Injection, USP, or Sodium Chloride for Injection, 0.9%, USP, to the volume appropriate for the infusion apparatus used.
Administration	IV infusion over 15 minutes or longer or intra-arterially infused over 7–14 days.
Storage and Stability	The intact vials should be stored at room temperature 15°–30°C (59°–86°F). Reconstituted solutions are stable under refrigeration for two weeks.
How Supplied	Supplied as a sterile, nonpyogenic, lyophilized powder containing 500 mg floxuridine in a 5-ml vial.
Dosage	Recommended dosage schedules of floxuridine by continuous arterial infusion is 0.1–0.6 mg/kg/day usually for periods of 14–21 days, with a rest period of two weeks between cycles. Therapy is continued until toxicity or response occurs. Dosages of 0.4–0.6 mg/kg/day usually required for hepatic artery infusions (HAI) because of hepatic metabolism. A common regimen for HAI is 4–6 mg/m²/day as a continuous infusion for two weeks followed by a two-week rest period. Lower floxuridine (0.2–0.3 mg/kg/day) doses may be utilized when in combination with leucovorin.
Compatibility Information	Concentrations of floxuridine of 2.5–12 mg/ml in bacteriostatic 0.9% sodium chloride with heparin (200 units/ml), leucovorin, and dexamethasone

is chemically stable for two weeks in an implantable infusion device for HAI therapy. Floxuridine (1–4 mg/ml) and leucovorin (0.03–0.96 mg/ml) are stable in plastic containers for 48 hours at room and refrigerated temperatures.

Contraindications/ Precautions	Patients with poor nutritional status, depressed bone marrow function, or potentially serious infections should not receive floxuridine. Risk versus benefit should be considered in patients with renal or hepatic impairment (lower dosage recommended), history of hepatitis, previous cytotoxic therapy with alkylating agents or prior high-dose pelvic irradiation (lower dosage recommended), or recent or existing chicken pox or herpes zoster infection.
Drug Interactions	**Agent** **Effect** Radiation therapy Additive bone marrow depression. Cytotoxic chemotherapy Additive bone marrow depression.
Toxicity/Side Effects	**Acute and/or Potentially Life-Threatening:** Related to procedural complications of regional artery infusion and include arterial aneurysm, thrombosis, embolism and ischemia, hepatic necrosis and abscess formation, bleeding, and infection. **Serious:** Gastroenteritis, GI ulceration, hepatotoxicity, or intra- and extrahepatic sclerosis. **Other:** Dermatologic: Alopecia, dermatitis, rash or itching, and scaling or redness of hands or feet. GI: Nausea and vomiting, glossitis, and stomatitis. Hematologic: Anemia, thrombocytopenia, and neutropenia. Miscellaneous: Fever, weakness, malaise, and lethargy.
Special Considerations	It is recommended to place patients on H_2-antagonist therapy (e.g., ranitidine, famotidine) to reduce possibility of peptic ulcer. Although nausea and vomiting not severe, patients may require an as-needed antiemetic (e.g., prochlorperazine).
Monitoring	Monitoring recommended prior to initiation of therapy and at periodic intervals during therapy unless otherwise specified. • CBC with differential: Recommended prior to initiation of therapy, prior to each subsequent dose, and at periodic intervals during therapy. • Platelet count: Recommended prior to initiation of therapy, prior to each subsequent dose, and at periodic intervals during therapy. • Hemoglobin and/or hematocrit: Recommended prior to initiation of therapy, prior to each subsequent dose, and at periodic intervals during therapy. • Liver function tests: ALT, AST, alkaline phosphatase, total bilirubin, LDH. • Renal function tests: CrCl, actual or calculated, and/or SCr recommended prior to initiation of therapy, prior to each subsequent dose, and at periodic intervals during therapy. • Examination of patient's mouth for ulceration.

Indications	Indicated in the palliative management of GI adenocarcinoma metastatic to the liver. May also be utilized in the local management of other tumor types metastatic to the liver or in the treatment of primary liver cancer. In addition, infusional therapy has been utilized in cancers of the ovary, bladder, head and neck, and kidney, as well as in the treatment of acute lymphocytic and nonlymphocytic leukemias.
Dosage Adjustment Recommendations	Therapy should be withheld for patients experiencing severe diarrhea, esophagopharyngitis, GI ulceration or bleeding, hemorrhage from any site, marked thrombocytopenia, marked neutropenia, stomatitis, or intractable vomiting. Therapy may be reinstituted at a lower dose when toxicity has subsided. In addition, dosage adjustments are warranted in patients with renal or hepatic impairment (see Appendices A and B). Hold the floxuridine dose for any impairment greater than stated.
Pharmacokinetics	Metabolized in the liver with a half-life of 0.3–0.6 hours.
Manufacturer	Roche Laboratories, Nutley, NJ

Fludarabine phosphate

Other Names	Fludara®
Classification	Antimetabolite; nucleotide analogue of the antiviral agent adenine arabinoside.
Mechanism	Inhibits DNA synthesis by inhibiting DNA polymerase and ribonucleotide reductase.
Vesicant Information	Not classified as a vesicant or an irritant.
Preparation and Mixture	Reconstitute 50-mg vial with 2 ml of sterile water for injection. Solution is clear and contains 25 mg/ml of fludarabine. Further dilution for infusion should be in 100–125 ml of D_5W or NS. Reconstituted solution can be stored for up to eight hours at room temperature or refrigerated.
Administration	Short-term IV infusion, usually over 30 minutes.
Storage and Stability	Intact vial to be stored under refrigeration (2°–8°C; 36°–46°F) or for up to eight hours at room temperature (22°–25°C; 72°–77°F).
How Supplied	Each 6-ml vial contains 50 mg lyophilized drug as a sterile white powder.
Dosage	Usual dosage of fludarabine is 18–30 mg/m²/day for five days. Infuse over 30 minutes daily. The standard recommended dosage for CLL therapy: 25mg/m²/day for five days; repeated every 28–35 days for three cycles.
Compatibility Information	The reader is referred to other resources on admixture for detailed information.
Contraindications/ Precautions	Contraindicated in patients with hypersensitivity to the drug. Lactation. Anaphylaxis; coma and death in very high doses.
Drug Interactions	Use cautiously when administering concomitantly with other myelosuppressive agents. Pentostatin increases pulmonary toxicity and may prove lethal.

Toxicity/Side Effects	**Acute and/or Potentially Life-Threatening:** Life-threatening and sometimes fatal autoimmune hemolytic anemia.
	Serious: Interstitial pneumonitis with infiltrates and effusions, hemoptysis, hypoxia, dyspnea, and cough. Tumor lysis syndrome also may occur with bulky disease. Renal failure may occur; use cautiously in patients with preexisting renal insufficiency.
	Other: Dermatologic: Rash, pruritus, and alopecia. GI: Mild nausea and vomiting, diarrhea, constipation, and stomatitis. Genitourinary: Urinary retention, hematuria, dysuria, and proteinuria. Hematologic: Dose-limiting side effects are granulocytopenia and thrombocytopenia. Neurologic: Fatigue, weakness, paresthesia, headache, depression, agitation, neuropathy, and confusion. Miscellaneous: Chills, fever, and myalgia.
Special Considerations	Use cautiously in patients with renal insufficiency. Toxicity effects are dose-dependent. Increased toxicity risk in geriatric population related to renal insufficiency. Consider IV gammaglobulin to decrease infections in patients with CLL.
Monitoring Parameters	Monitoring is recommended prior to initiation of therapy and at periodic intervals during therapy unless otherwise specified. • CBC with differential: Recommended prior to initiation of therapy, prior to each subsequent dose, and at periodic intervals during therapy. • Platelet count: Recommended prior to initiation of therapy, prior to each subsequent dose, and at periodic intervals during therapy. • Hemoglobin and/or hematocrit: Recommended prior to initiation of therapy, prior to each subsequent dose, and at periodic intervals during therapy. • Liver function tests: ALT, AST, alkaline phosphatase, total bilirubin, LDH. • Renal function tests: CrCl, actual or calculated, and/or SCr recommended prior to initiation of therapy, prior to each subsequent dose, and at periodic intervals during therapy. • Stool cultures: If persistent diarrhea to rule out infectious etiology.
Indications	FDA-approved in the treatment of CLL. Off-label uses include mycosis fungoides, non-Hodgkin's lymphoma, multiple myeloma, melanoma, pancreatic adenocarcinoma, and hairy-cell leukemia.
Dosage Adjustment Recommendations	Reduce dose for renal impairment (see Appendix B).
Pharmacokinetics	Eliminated via kidneys. Half-life is 10 hours.
Manufacturer	Berlex Laboratories, Richmond, CA

Fluorouracil

Other Names	5-fluorouracil, 5-FU, Efudex®, Adrucil®, Fluoroplex®
Classification	Antimetabolite; fluorinated pyrimidine.

Mechanism	Cell-cycle specific in S phase. Inhibition of RNA formation and DNA synthesis through decrease in sufficient thymine, resulting in cell death.
Vesicant Information	Not classified as a vesicant or an irritant.
Preparation and Mixture	Reconstitution not required. Store at room temperature. Light-sensitive. Further dilution in NS or D_5W for infusion. Inspect doses for precipitate; if solution does not clear with agitation or warming to 40°C, discard.
Administration	IV. IVP via side arm of fast-flowing compatible fluids. Continuous infusion over 12–24 hours (per protocol) in NS or D_5W. Check blood return throughout long-term infusion. Topical: skin preparation, apply using powder-free gloves.
Storage and Stability	Protect from light. Store at 15°–30°C (59°–86°F).
How Supplied	Supplied as 50 mg/ml in 10 ml, 20 ml, 50 ml, and 100 ml. Available topically as 1% (30-g) and 5% (25-g) topical cream and 1% (30-ml), 2% (10-ml), and 5% (10-ml) topical solution.
Dosage	Numerous regimens used and include 12 mg/kg/day (400–500 mg/m²/day) for four to five days either as single daily IV injection or four-day continuous infusion, 370 mg/m²/day for five days, and 600 mg/m² weekly for six weeks. Manufacturer recommends that no standard dose should exceed 800 mg/day, although higher doses (up to 2 g/day) are routinely administered via continuous infusion.
Compatibility Information	The reader is referred to other resources on admixture for detailed information.
Contraindications/ Precautions	IT administration should be avoided. Hypersensitivity to fluorouracil, myelosuppression.

Drug Interactions	Agent	Effect
	Leucovorin calcium	Synergistic; increase toxicity of fluorouracil; must be given prior to or concomitantly with fluorouracil.
	Allopurinol	Allopurinol inhibits thymidine phosphorylase; antitumor effect unaltered but decreases toxicity of fluorouracil.
	MTX	Mutually antagonistic; schedule-dependent; administer fluorouracil after MTX.

Toxicity/Side Effects	**Acute and/or Potentially Life-Threatening:** GI adverse events are route- and schedule-dependent. Continuous-infusion fluorouracil can be associated with severe diarrhea and mucositis. The infusion should be discontinued if intractable diarrhea or severe mucositis develops. Subsequent therapy should be dose modified.
	Serious: Angina, hypotension, ECG changes, myocardial ischemia, and arrhythmias; similar to ischemic changes. Usually occurs within first two days of therapy and may be treated symptomatically with nitroglycerin

and calcium channel blockade. Thought to be caused by coronary vasospasm induced by fluorouracil.

Other:

Dermatologic: Hand-foot syndrome, photosensitivity, alopecia, hyperpigmentation, especially along venous circulation, nail color changes with possible loss of nails, and skin rash.

GI: Mild to moderate nausea, vomiting, anorexia, heartburn, proctitis, and esophagitis.

Neurologic: Confusion, headache, disorientation, acute cerebellar ataxia, lethargy, and weakness.

Ocular: Photophobia, visual changes, conjunctivitis, and increased tearing.

Special Considerations	Patient should avoid excessive exposure to the sun while on therapy. Do not use occlusive dressing over topical agent because of inflammation of normal skin.
Monitoring Parameters	Monitoring is recommended prior to initiation of therapy and at periodic intervals during therapy unless otherwise specified. • CBC with differential: Recommended prior to initiation of therapy, prior to each subsequent dose, and at periodic intervals during therapy. • Platelet count: Recommended prior to initiation of therapy, prior to each subsequent dose, and at periodic intervals during therapy. • Hemoglobin and/or hematocrit: Recommended prior to initiation of therapy, prior to each subsequent dose, and at periodic intervals during therapy. • Liver function tests: ALT, AST, alkaline phosphatase, total bilirubin, LDH. • Renal function tests: CrCl, actual or calculated, and/or SCr recommended prior to initiation of therapy, prior to each subsequent dose, and at periodic intervals during therapy. • Examination of patient's mouth for ulceration. • Stool cultures: If persistent diarrhea to rule out infectious etiology.
Indications	FDA-approved uses: Colon, rectum, breast, stomach, and pancreatic carcinoma, head and neck cancer, actinic keratosis. Off-label use: esophageal carcinoma.
Dosage Adjustment Recommendations	Dose reduction should be considered in patients with impaired renal or liver function (see Appendices A and B), significant myelosuppression, severe diarrhea and/or mucositis and poor nutrition. Reduce dose by 25%–33% when given in a regimen with leucovorin calcium.
Pharmacokinetics	Metabolized by the liver. Half-life is 8–20 minutes; terminal half-life is 20 hours. Excreted by the kidneys in the urine and the lungs as carbon dioxide. Crosses the blood-brain barrier.
Manufacturer	Efudex®, ICN Pharmaceuticals, Inc., Costa Mesa, CA; Fluoroplex®, Allergan Inc., Irvine, CA

Gemcitabine

Other Names	Gemzar®, gemcitabine hydrochloride
Classification	Antimetabolite; pyrimidine analogue.
Mechanism	Intracellular conversion to two active metabolites: gemcitabine diphosphate, which inhibits the enzyme responsible for catalyzing synthesis of deoxynucleoside triphosphates required for DNA synthesis, and gemcitabine triphosphate, which competes with endogenous deoxynucleoside triphosphates for incorporation into DNA with subsequent inhibition of DNA synthesis. Cell-cycle specific for the S phase and G_1/S phase boundary.
Vesicant Information	Not classified as a vesicant or an irritant.
Preparation and Mixture	Reconstitute with 5 ml or 25 ml Sodium Chloride for Injection, 0.9%, USP, (without preservative) to the 200-mg or 1-g vial, respectively, yielding a clear, colorless to light straw-colored solution with a concentration of 38 mg/ml. This solution may be administered as prepared or further diluted with Sodium Chloride for Injection, 0.9%, USP, to a concentration as low as 0.1 mg/ml.
Administration	IV infusion over 30 minutes.
Storage and Stability	Store intact vials at room temperature 20°–25°C (68°–77°F). Reconstituted and/or diluted solutions stable at room temperature for up to 24 hours. Do not refrigerate.
How Supplied	Supplied as a white, lyophilized powder in single-use vials containing 200 mg (10-ml vial size) or 1 g (50-ml vial size) of gemcitabine.
Dosage	FDA-approved regimen for pancreatic cancer is 1,000 mg/m² intravenously over 30 minutes once weekly for up to seven weeks (or until toxicity necessitates reducing or holding a dose), followed by a one-week rest period. Subsequent cycles consist of weekly infusions for three weeks followed by a one-week rest period. Two schedules have been investigated in the treatment of non-small cell lung cancer: Gemcitabine 1,000 mg/m² over 30 minutes on days 1, 8, and 15 of each 28-day cycle with cisplatin dosed at 100 mg/m² on day 1 administered after the gemcitabine infusion and gemcitabine 1,250 mg/m² over 30 minutes on days 1 and 8 of each 21-day cycle with cisplatin dosed at 100 mg/m² on day 1 administered after the gemcitabine infusion. Other regimens utilize gemcitabine 1,000 mg/m² as a weekly infusion for three weeks followed by a one-week rest period. Dosage adjustments are recommended based on hematologic and nonhematologic toxicities. A dosage increase to 1,250 mg/m² is recommended for patients who have completed the first cycle of therapy, provided that the ANC and platelet nadirs exceed 1,500 and 100,000 cells per cubic millimeter, respectively, and if no greater than grade 1 nonhematologic toxicity has occurred. Patients who tolerate subsequent cycle at 1,250 mg/m² may have the dose increased to 1,500 mg/m² for subsequent cycles, provided they meet the same criteria (ANC and platelet nadirs > 1,500 and 100,000 and no greater than grade 1 nonhematologic toxicity).

Compatibility Information	The compatibility of gemcitabine with other drugs has not been studied. No incompatibilities have been observed with infusion bottles, PVC bags, or administration sets.
Contraindications/ Precautions	Contraindicated in patients with a known hypersensitivity to the drug. Risk versus benefit should be considered in patients with existing bone marrow depression, infection, or hepatic or renal function impairment (dose reduction may be necessary).
Drug Interactions	No confirmed drug interactions have been reported.
Toxicity/Side Effects	Prolongation of infusion times > 60 minutes or dosing more frequently than weekly has shown to increase toxicity.
	Acute and/or Potentially Life-Threatening: Hemolytic uremic syndrome, although rare, has been reported. Renal failure may not be reversible with discontinuation of therapy, and dialysis may be required. Bronchospasm and anaphylactoid reactions also have been reported.
	Serious: Cardiovascular events, such as myocardial infarction, cerebrovascular accident, arrhythmia, and hypertension have occurred. Many of these patients had a prior history of cardiovascular disease.
	Other: Dermatologic: Rash (occurs in up to 30%; macular or finely granular maculopapular pruritic eruption of mild to moderate severity involving the trunk and extremities) and alopecia. GI: Nausea and vomiting (mild to moderate, occurring in up to two-thirds of patients), diarrhea, constipation, and stomatitis. Hematologic: Myelosuppression is dose-limiting; anemia, thrombocytopenia, and neutropenia. Gemcitabine therapy may be dose-modified or suspended based on degree of hematologic toxicity. Miscellaneous: Fever (40%), paresthesia, dyspnea, elevated liver enzymes and bilirubin, edema (generalized and peripheral), and flu-like syndrome (e.g., fever, asthenia, headache, cough, chills, myalgia).
Special Considerations	Gemcitabine is a mild to moderate emetogen; antiemetic prophylaxis (e.g., prochlorperazine) recommended. Toxicities associated with gemcitabine may occur more frequently and be more severe if administered more frequently than once weekly or if infused over a time period longer than 60 minutes. Do not refrigerate reconstituted or diluted solutions, as crystallization may occur.
Monitoring Parameters	Monitoring is recommended prior to initiation of therapy and at periodic intervals during therapy unless otherwise specified. • CBC with differential: Recommended prior to initiation of therapy, prior to each subsequent dose, and at periodic intervals during therapy. • Platelet count: Recommended prior to initiation of therapy, prior to each subsequent dose, and at periodic intervals during therapy. • Hemoglobin and/or hematocrit: Recommended prior to initiation of therapy, prior to each subsequent dose, and at periodic intervals during therapy.

- Renal function tests: CrCl, actual or calculated, and/or SCr recommended prior to initiation of therapy, prior to each subsequent dose, and at periodic intervals during therapy.
- Liver function tests: ALT, AST, alkaline phosphatase, total bilirubin, LDH.

Indications	Indicated as first-line treatment for patients with locally advanced (nonresectable stage II or stage III) or metastatic (stage IV) adenocarcinoma of the pancreas. Also indicated for patients previously treated with fluorouracil. Gemcitabine also is indicated in combination with cisplatin for the first-line treatment of patients with inoperable, locally advanced (stage IIIA or IIIB) or metastatic (stage IV) non-small cell lung cancer. Off-label uses of gemcitabine are numerous and include breast and bladder cancer.
Dosage Adjustment Recommendations	Patients receiving gemcitabine should be monitored prior to each dose with a CBC with differential and platelet count. If marrow suppression is detected, the dose of gemcitabine should be modified according to the following guidelines.

ANC	Platelet count	% of full dose
$\geq 1,000$	and $\geq 100,000$	100
500–999	or 50,000–99,000	75
< 500	or < 50,000	Hold

	In addition, gemcitabine should be used with caution in patients with renal or hepatic function impairment. Dose modification is recommended, although no guidelines are available.
Pharmacokinetics	The duration of infusion and gender of the patient significantly affect the volume of distribution and elimination of gemcitabine; undergoes intracellular metabolism to produce two active metabolites. Renally eliminated as the inactive uracil metabolite and unchanged drug.
Manufacturer	Eli Lilly and Company, Indianapolis, IN

Hydroxyurea

Other Names	Hydrea®
Classification	Miscellaneous.
Mechanism	Exact mechanism unknown; thought to interfere with DNA synthesis by inhibiting ribonucleoside diphosphate reductase, preventing conversion of ribonucleotides to deoxyribonucleotides; cell-cycle specific for the S phase and may hold other cells in G_1 phase.
Vesicant Information	Not a vesicant or an irritant. Hydroxyurea is commercially available as an oral product.
Preparation and Mixture	No preparation or admixture necessary. Hydroxyurea is commercially available as an oral product.
Administration	Oral.

Storage and Stability	Store capsules in a tight container at room temperature; avoid excess heat.
How Supplied	Supplied as 500-mg capsules in bottles of 100. The capsules are imprinted with the following: 830.
Dosage	All dosages should be based on ideal or actual body weight, whichever is less. Dose should be titrated to patient response and WBC count. Usual adult dose ranges from 10–30 mg/kg/day or 500–3,000 mg/day. Intermittent dosing for solid tumors is 60–80 mg/kg as a single dose every third day.
Compatibility Information	Not applicable. Hydroxyurea is commercially available as an oral product.
Contraindications/ Precautions	Contraindicated in patients with marked bone marrow depression (e.g., leukopenia [< 2,500 WBCs]), thrombocytopenia (< 100,000 platelets), or severe anemia). Risk versus benefit should be considered in patients with gout or a history of gout, infection, history of uric acid nephropathy, or renal function impairment (dosage reduction recommended).

Drug Interactions	**Agent**	**Effect**
	Cytarabine	Modulates metabolism and cytotoxicity of cytarabine; reduced cytarabine dose recommended.
	Fluorouracil	Increased potential for neurotoxicity with concomitant therapy.
	Zidovudine, didanosine, zalcitabine	Increased effect of antiretroviral with concomitant therapy.

Toxicity/Side Effects	**Acute and/or Potentially Life-Threatening:** None noted.
	Serious: Neurotoxicity (e.g., confusion, convulsions, dizziness, headache, hallucinations), although rare, has been reported.
	Other:
	Dermatologic: Hyperpigmentation, erythema of hands and face, dry skin, alopecia, and maculopapular rash.
	GI: Mild to moderate nausea and vomiting, diarrhea, constipation, stomatitis, and anorexia.
	Hematologic: Myelosuppression is dose-limiting; leukopenia (rapid decline and recovery), thrombocytopenia, and anemia.
	Miscellaneous: Drowsiness, abnormal liver enzymes, impairment of renal tubule function (elevation of SCr and blood urea nitrogen [BUN]), hyperuricemia, dysuria, and fever.
Special Considerations	Dosage should be adjusted to meet individual requirements, based on clinical response and toxicity. Dosed on ideal or actual body weight, whichever is less. Capsules may be opened and contents emptied into glass of water if taken immediately for patients who are unable to swallow the capsules. Do not take missed dose or double-up on doses. Mild to moderate

	nausea and vomiting may occur; consider an as-needed antiemetic (e.g., prochlorperazine).
Monitoring Parameters	Monitoring is recommended prior to initiation of therapy and at periodic intervals during therapy unless otherwise specified. • CBC with differential: Recommended prior to initiation of therapy, prior to each subsequent dose, and at periodic intervals during therapy. • Platelet count: Recommended prior to initiation of therapy, prior to each subsequent dose, and at periodic intervals during therapy. • Hemoglobin and/or hematocrit: Recommended prior to initiation of therapy, prior to each subsequent dose, and at periodic intervals during therapy. • Liver function tests: ALT, AST, alkaline phosphatase, total bilirubin, LDH. • Renal function tests: CrCl, actual or calculated, and/or SCr recommended prior to initiation of therapy, prior to each subsequent dose, and at periodic intervals during therapy. • Uric acid.
Indications	Indicated in the treatment of melanoma, resistant CML, and recurrent, metastatic, or inoperable carcinoma of the ovary. Used off-label in a variety of benign and malignant hematologic disorders. In addition, used concomitantly with irradiation therapy for local control of primary squamous cell carcinomas of the head and neck.
Dosage Adjustment Recommendations	Recommended to adjust dose in renal function impairment (see Appendix B). Dosage adjustments also are recommended for toxicity, although no guidelines are available. Also, lower doses are recommended for the elderly.
Pharmacokinetics	Readily absorbed from GI tract. Widely distributed in the body. Half-life of three to four hours. Reaches peak plasma concentrations within two hours. Eliminated through renal excretion and respiratory excretion.
Manufacturer	Bristol-Myers Squibb Oncology/Immunology Division, Princeton, NJ

Idarubicin

Other Names	Idamycin®, Idamycin PFS®, idarubicin hydrochloride
Classification	Anthracene; anthracycline derivative.
Mechanism	DNA-intercalating analogue of daunorubicin, which has an inhibitory effect on nucleic acid synthesis and interacts with the enzyme topoisomerase II.
Vesicant Information	Classified as a vesicant. If extravasation occurs, apply ice immediately for 30–60 minutes, then alternate off/on every 15 minutes for 24 hours. Elevate and rest extremity for 48 hours. Application of heat or sodium bicarbonate can be harmful and is contraindicated.
Preparation and Mixture	Calculated dose of Idamycin PFS should be drawn up into a syringe and administered slowly into the tubing of a free-flowing IV infusion of Sodium Chloride for Injection, 0.9%, USP or 5% Dextrose Injection, USP. Idamycin lyophilized powder is reconstituted by adding 5 ml or 10 ml, respectively, of Sodium Chloride for Injection, 0.9%, USP, to the 5- or 10-

	ml vial, producing a solution of 1 mg/ml of idarubicin. May be further diluted in 50–100 ml D$_5$W or NS and administered as an IV infusion.
Administration	IVP (slowly over 10–15 minutes into free-flowing IV infusion) or IV infusion (over 15 minutes).
Storage and Stability	Store intact vials of lyophilized powder at room temperature and protect from light. Store Idamycin PFS under refrigeration and protect from light. Reconstituted powder stable for 72 hours at room temperature and seven days under refrigeration. With further dilution, product is stable for four weeks under refrigeration.
How Supplied	Supplied as a lyophilized powder (Idamycin) in single-use vials containing 5 and 10 mg idarubicin or as a sterile, red-orange, preservative-free solution (Idamycin PFS) in single-use vials containing 5 and 10 mg idarubicin.
Dosage	Most common regimen in leukemia induction is 8–12 mg/m^2/day for three days in combination with cytarabine. The usual dosage regimen for consolidation therapy is 10–12 mg/m^2/day for two days.
Compatibility Information	Do not dilute with bacteriostatic solutions. Incompatible with fluorouracil, heparin, etoposide, hydrocortisone, vincristine, MTX, and dexamethasone.
Contraindications/ Precautions	Contraindicated in patients with history of hypersensitivity to idarubicin, daunorubicin, or any component. Risk versus benefit should be considered in patients with infection, heart disease (increased risk of cardiotoxicity), impaired renal or hepatic function (dosage reduction is recommended), gout or a history of gout, or history of uric acid nephropathy.
Drug Interactions	No formal drug interaction studies have been performed.

Agent	Effect
Anthracyclines (daunorubicin and doxorubicin)	Use of idarubicin in a patient who has previously received an anthracycline increases risk of cardiotoxicity.
Radiation therapy to mediastinum	Concomitant use may increase risk of cardiotoxicity.
Trastuzumab	Concomitant use with anthracyclines may increase incidence and severity of cardiac dysfunction.

Toxicity/Side Effects	**Acute and/or Potentially Life-Threatening:** Myocardial toxicity as manifested by potentially fatal CHF, acute life-threatening arrhythmias, or other cardiomyopathies may occur. CHF with a subsequent irreversible decrease in the LVEF can occur with cumulative doses > 137.5 mg/m^2. Cardiac function should be monitored regularly. Incidence may increase with prior anthracycline use, preexisting cardiac disease, concomitant cyclophosphamide or mediastinal radiotherapy, and cumulative dose.
	Serious: Tissue necrosis caused by extravasation; tumor lysis syndrome with subsequent hyperuricemia, uric acid nephropathy, and renal failure

	(preventative measures such as hydration and urinary alkalinization are warranted in certain settings). **Other:** Dermatologic: Rash, alopecia, urticaria, and erythematous streaking along the vein. GI: Nausea, vomiting, constipation, diarrhea, and stomatitis. Hematologic: Myelosuppression is dose-limiting; anemia, severe leukopenia (nadir 8–14 days; recovery 21 days), and severe thrombocytopenia (nadir 10–15 days; recovery 21 days). Neurologic: Headache, fever, peripheral neuropathy, and seizures. Miscellaneous: Pain at injection site, reddish urine, post-irradiation recall, and elevation in liver enzymes.
Special Considerations	Avoid extravasation; severe local tissue necrosis has been reported. Idarubicin is considered to cause a moderately high amount of emetogenicity; prophylactic antiemetics are recommended (e.g., serotonin antagonist in combination with dexamethasone). May cause reddish discoloration of urine. Local erythematous streaking along vein may indicate too rapid infusion rate.
Monitoring Parameters	Monitoring is recommended prior to initiation of therapy and at periodic intervals during therapy unless otherwise specified. • CBC with differential: Recommended prior to initiation of therapy, prior to each subsequent dose, and at periodic intervals during therapy. • Platelet count: Recommended prior to initiation of therapy, prior to each subsequent dose, and at periodic intervals during therapy. • Hemoglobin and/or hematocrit: Recommended prior to initiation of therapy, prior to each subsequent dose, and at periodic intervals during therapy. • Cardiac function. • Liver function tests: ALT, AST, alkaline phosphatase, total bilirubin, LDH. • Renal function tests: CrCl, actual or calculated, and/or SCr recommended prior to initiation of therapy, prior to each subsequent dose, and at periodic intervals during therapy. • Uric acid. • Examination of patient's mouth for oral ulceration.
Indications	Indicated in the treatment of AML in adults in combination with other antileukemic agents. Also used in ALL in children.
Dosage Adjustment	Dosage adjustments recommended in renal and hepatic impairment (see Appendices A and B).
Pharmacokinetics	Large volume of distribution because of extensive tissue binding and CSF distribution; half-life is 12–27 hours; time to peak plasma concentration is within two to four hours after administration; eliminated in the urine and bile.
Manufacturer	Pharmacia & Upjohn Company, Peapack, NJ

Ifosfamide

Other Names	Ifex®
Classification	Alkylating agent; nitrogen mustard derivative.
Mechanism	Metabolized by the liver to active metabolites, ifosfamide mustard, and acrolein, which alkylate or bind to intracellular molecular structures, including nucleic acids. Cytotoxicity primarily because of cross-linking strands of DNA and RNA, as well as inhibition of protein synthesis.
Vesicant Information	Not classified as a vesicant or an irritant.
Preparation and Mixture	Reconstitute the 1-g and 3-g vials with 20 ml or 60 ml, respectively, of Sterile Water for Injection, USP, or Bacteriostatic Water for Injection, USP (benzyl alcohol or parabens preserved). Final concentration of resulting solution is 50 mg/ml. May be further diluted to a concentration of 0.6 mg/ml–20 mg/ml with the following fluids: 5% Dextrose Injection, USP, Sodium Chloride for Injection, 0.9%, USP, lactated Ringer's Injection, USP, or Sterile Water for Injection, USP.
Administration	IV infusion (30 minutes to 24-hour continuous infusion) or slow IVP in minimum of 75 ml saline.
Storage and Stability	Store intact vials at room temperature. Reconstituted and/or diluted solutions stable for 24 hours under refrigeration per the manufacturer. Other sources give the reconstituted and/or diluted solutions a seven-day expiration at room temperature and a six-week expiration if stored under refrigeration.
How Supplied	Supplied as a white crystalline powder in single-use vials containing 1 g and 3 g ifosfamide and packaged in combination with mesna (uroprotectant).
Dosage	Standard regimens include 1,200–2,000 mg/m²/day for five days or 2,000–2,600 mg/m²/day for three days (days 1–3 or days 1, 3, and 5) administered as a 30-minute infusion up to a 24-hour continuous infusion repeated every three to four weeks. Alternatively, may be dosed as 3.6 g/m² intravenously over four hours for two consecutive days in combination regimens. With high-dose therapy, maximum tolerated doses appear to be 16 g/m²/cycle.
Compatibility Information	Compatible with mesna in NS up to nine days stored at room temperature.
Contraindications/ Precautions	Contraindicated in patients with a previous hypersensitivity; continued use contraindicated in patients with severely depressed bone marrow function. Risk versus benefit should be considered in patients with infection, including existing or recent chicken pox or herpes zoster, or in patients with hepatic or renal function impairment (dosage adjustment recommended).

Drug Interactions	Agent	Effect
	Cytochrome P450 enzyme inducers (e.g., phenytoin, phenobarbital, chloral hydrate)	Concomitant administration may induce the activation of ifosfamide, which may affect the activity and/or toxicity of ifosfamide.

Toxicity/Side Effects	**Acute and/or Potentially Life-Threatening:** CNS effects or encephalopathy, consisting of agitation, confusion, somnolence, hallucinations, unusual tiredness, dizziness, depressive psychosis, seizures, or coma. Fatalities have been reported. Occurs more frequently with one-day infusions (versus five-day), in patients with impaired renal function and/or hypoalbuminemia, and with concomitant use of drugs with sedative properties (e.g., opiates, benzodiazepines, phenothiazines).
	Serious: Urotoxicity, including hemorrhagic cystitis, dysuria, and urinary frequency, may occur within hours of administration to weeks after administration and thought to be caused by metabolite, acrolein. Ifosfamide must be administered with a uroprotective agent (e.g., mesna). Usually resolves within days after discontinuation of ifosfamide but may persist and has been fatal. Incidence is reduced by fractionation of dose, adequate hydration, and administration of mesna. Nephrotoxicity, most likely related to renal tubular damage, also has been reported and is manifested by an increase in BUN and/or SCr. Acute renal failure and metabolic acidosis have been reported.
	Other: Dermatologic: Alopecia, nail changes, skin hyperpigmentation, and dermatitis. May interfere with normal wound healing. GI: Nausea and vomiting has occurred in up to 58% of patients and is dose- and schedule-related (more common with bolus dosing and more significant with higher doses), anorexia, stomatitis, diarrhea, constipation, and elevation in liver enzymes. Hematologic: Mild to moderate myelosuppression as a single agent (leukopenia most common, thrombocytopenia and anemia less frequent); moderate to severe myelosuppression when used in combination or with high-dose therapies. Miscellaneous: SIADH, immunosuppression, sterility, possible second malignancy, nasal congestion, cardiotoxicity, pulmonary toxicity, and polyneuropathy.

Special Considerations	To prevent bladder toxicity, adequate hydration (oral or IV, at least two liters/day) and uroprotection with mesna must accompany ifosfamide administration. If microscopic hematuria is present, subsequent administration of ifosfamide should be withheld until complete resolution. Further administration should be given with more vigorous hydration and uroprotection. Ifosfamide is moderately to highly emetogenic, depending on dose and schedule; antiemetic prophylaxis consisting of a serotonin antagonist in combination with dexamethasone is warranted. Antiemetics, as well as other drugs with sedative properties, may increase risk of CNS toxicity.

Monitoring Parameters	Monitoring is recommended prior to initiation of therapy and at periodic intervals during therapy unless otherwise specified.

- CBC with differential: Recommended prior to initiation of therapy, prior to each subsequent dose, and at periodic intervals during therapy.
- Platelet count: Recommended prior to initiation of therapy, prior to each subsequent dose, and at periodic intervals during therapy.
- Hemoglobin and/or hematocrit: Recommended prior to initiation of therapy, prior to each subsequent dose, and at periodic intervals during therapy.
- Renal function tests: CrCl, actual or calculated, and/or SCr recommended prior to initiation of therapy, prior to each subsequent dose, and at periodic intervals during therapy.
- Liver function tests: ALT, AST, alkaline phosphatase, total bilirubin, LDH.
- Urinalysis for microscopic hematuria: Recommended prior to each dose.

Indications	FDA-approved as the third-line treatment in combination with other chemotherapeutics for germ cell testicular cancer. Also may be used in the treatment of sarcomas, lymphomas, leukemias, and cancers of the head and neck, cervix, uterus, ovary, endometrium, breast, and pancreas.
Dosage Adjustment Recommendations	Recommended to reduce dose in the setting of renal function impairment (see Appendix B). Studies to establish optimum dose in the setting of hepatic impairment have not been conducted. Recommend withholding/discontinuing treatment with ifosfamide until toxicity resolution for both CNS toxicity and urotoxicity.
Pharmacokinetics	Dose-dependent. Limited amount crosses blood-brain barrier. Half-life of seven hours for lower doses (up to 2.4 g/m^2/day) and biphasic for higher doses. Requires biotransformation in the liver to active metabolite; 15%–50% excreted unchanged in urine.
Manufacturer	Bristol-Myers Squibb Oncology/Immunology Division, Princeton, NJ.

Imatinib mesylate

Other Names	Gleevec®
Classification	Miscellaneous; tyrosine kinase inhibitor.
Mechanism	Inhibits the bcr-abl tyrosine kinase, thus inhibiting proliferation, and induces apoptosis in bcr-abl positive cell lines. In addition, in vitro studies demonstrate inhibition of the receptor tyrosine kinases for platelet-derived growth factor, stem cell factor, and c-kit.
Vesicant Information	Not classified as a vesicant or an irritant. Imatinib mesylate is commercially available as an oral product.
Preparation and Mixture	No preparation or admixture necessary. Imatinib mesylate is commercially available as an oral product.
Administration	Oral.
Storage and Stability	Store at 25°C (77° F).

How Supplied	Supplied as hard, orange to grayish opaque gelatin capsules containing 100 mg of imatinib free base and imprinted in red ink with the following: NVR SI. Packaged in bottles of 120 capsules.
Dosage	Dosing for chronic phase CML is 400 mg/day and 600 mg/day for patients in accelerated phase or blast crisis. Dosage should be administered orally, once daily with a meal or large glass of water. Treatment is continued for as long as the patient is deriving a benefit. In the absence of severe adverse drug reactions, patients whose disease is progressing, patients who have failed to achieve an adequate hematologic response after three months of treatment or loss of a previously achieved hematologic response may be increased to 600 mg/day and 800 mg/day for chronic phase CML and blast or accelerated phase CML, respectively.
Compatibility Information	Not applicable. Imatinib mesylate is commercially available as an oral product.
Contraindications/ Precautions	Imatinib mesylate is contraindicated in patients with hypersensitivity to imatinib or to any other component of Gleevec. Women of childbearing potential should be advised to avoid becoming pregnant (Pregnancy Category D). In addition, significant fluid retention and edema as well as hepatotoxicity have been reported. Risk versus benefit should be considered in patients with underlying impaired liver function.

Drug Interactions	**Agent**	**Effect**
	Inhibitors of the P450 isoenzyme system (e.g., ketoconazole, itraconazole, erythromycin, clarithromycin)	May increase imatinib plasma concentrations.
	Inducers of the P450 isoenzyme system (e.g., phenobarbital, phenytoin, carbamazepine, rifampin)	May decrease imatinib plasma concentration.
	Simvastatin	Increase in mean C and AUC of simvastatin by imatinib. Caution should be used with other CYP3A4 substrates such as cyclosporine, pimozide, dihydropyridine calcium channel blockers, and certain HMG-CoA reductase inhibitors.
	Warfarin	Interaction possible; patients who require anticoagulation should receive low-molecular-weight or standard heparin.

Toxicity/Side Effects	**Acute and/or Potentially Life-Threatening:** In clinical trials, one patient died with pleural effusion, congestive heart failure, and renal failure.
	Serious: Often associated with edema and occasionally serious fluid retention. Weigh and monitor patients regularly. Severe fluid retention (pleural and pericardial effusion, pulmonary edema, and/or ascites) is

reported in 1%–2% of patients. In addition, severe superficial edema has been reported.

Other:

Dermatologic: Skin rash, pruritus, and petechiae.

Gastrointestinal: Nausea, vomiting, abdominal pain, diarrhea, anorexia, nasopharyngitis, dyspepsia, and constipation.

Hematologic: Neutropenia and thrombocytopenia; both more common with higher doses. Median duration of a neutropenic and thrombocytopenic episode ranges from two to three weeks and three to four weeks, respectively.

Miscellaneous: Myalgia, arthralgia, fever, fatigue, hepatotoxicity (can be severe and needs regular monitoring), muscle cramps, hemorrhage, musculoskeletal pain, epistaxis, weakness, cough, night sweats, and headache.

Special Considerations	Women of childbearing potential should be advised to avoid becoming pregnant. An unexpected rapid weight gain should be carefully investigated to rule out fluid retention. The probability of edema and severe fluid retention was increased with higher doses and age greater than 65. Diuretics, interruption of therapy, and other supportive care measures need to be considered. Imatinib therapy has been associated with GI irritation. Patient should be instructed to take capsules with food or large glass of water. Take missed dose as soon as remembered; contact physician if not remembered until prior to next dose.
Monitoring Parameters	Monitoring is recommended prior to initiation of therapy and at periodic intervals during therapy unless otherwise specified. • CBC with differential (should perform weekly for the first month of therapy, biweekly for the second month, and periodically thereafter as clinically indicated [e.g., every two to three months]). • Liver function tests (transaminases, bilirubin, and alkaline phosphatase; monitored before initiation of treatment and monthly or as clinically indicated thereafter). • Renal function (SCr, BUN). • Monitor weight and other signs/symptoms of fluid retention. An unexpected rapid increase in weight should be investigated. Diuretics, interruption of imatinib therapy, and other supportive care measures may be needed. • Pregnancy testing (baseline prior to initiation of therapy and as clinically pertinent thereafter).
Indications	Indicated for the treatment of patients with CML in blast crisis, accelerated phase, or chronic phase after failure to interferon alpha therapy.
Dosage Adjustment	If a severe nonhematologic toxicity develops, imatinib therapy should be withheld until the toxicity has resolved. This includes significant fluid retention. Thereafter, treatment can be resumed as appropriate depending on the initial severity of the toxicity. If the bilirubin increases to greater than 3 times the upper limit of normal (ULN) or transaminases greater than 5 times ULN, imatinib therapy should be withheld until bilirubin returns to less than

1.5 times ULN and transaminases to less than 2.5 times ULN. Reinstitute therapy at a reduced daily dose (e.g., if receiving 400 mg/day reduce to 300 mg daily and if receiving 600 mg/day reduce to 400 mg daily). Dosage reductions for hematologic toxicity also are warranted. If receiving 400 mg/day for the treatment of chronic phase CML and the patient's ANC falls below $1,000/mm^3$ and/or platelets fall below $50,000/mm^3$, stop imatinib therapy until ANC increases to at least $1,500/mm^3$ and platelets increase to at least $75,000/mm^3$. Imatinib therapy should be reinstituted at 400 mg/day. If recurrence of this hematologic toxicity occurs, withhold therapy as above and re-institute with a dose reduction to 300 mg/day. In the treatment of accelerated phase CML or blast crisis, if ANC falls below $500/mm^3$ and/or platelets fall below $10,000/mm^3$ after receiving the drug for at least one month, determine if cytopenia is related to leukemia (marrow aspirate or biopsy). If unrelated to leukemia, reduce dose to 400 mg/day. If cytopenia persists for two weeks, further reduce to 300 mg/day. If cytopenia persists despite dose reductions after four weeks, stop imatinib therapy until ANC is at least $1,000/mm^3$ and platelets at least $20,000/mm^3$. Therapy should then be resumed at 300 mg/day.

Pharmacokinetics	Well absorbed after oral administration with mean bioavailability of 98%. Protein bound, mostly to albumin. Half-life of imatinib and its major active metabolite are approximately 18 and 40 hours, respectively.
Manufacturer	Novartis Pharma AG, Basle, Switzerland; distributed by Novartis Pharmaceutical Corporation, East Hanover, NJ

Irinotecan

Other Names	Camptosar®, CPT-11, camptothecin-11
Classification	Miscellaneous; topoisomerase 1 inhibitor.
Mechanism	Irinotecan and its active metabolite, SN-38, inhibit topoisomerase 1 by binding reversibly to the enzyme, which is essential to DNA religation and replication.
Vesicant Information	Considered an irritant; thrombophlebitis has been reported. Should extravasation occur, flush site with sterile water and apply ice.
Preparation and Mixture	Doses should be diluted in Sodium Chloride for Injection, 0.9%, USP, or 5% Dextrose Injection, USP, to a final concentration of 0.12–1.1 mg/ml. Because of acidic pH of irinotecan, 500 ml of D_5W preferred diluent.
Administration	Administer as IV infusion over 90 minutes.
Storage and Stability	Store intact vials at room temperature, 15°–30°C (59°–86°F), and protect from light. The diluted solution is chemically and physically stable at room temperature and in ambient fluorescent lighting for 24 hours. Solutions prepared with D_5W are stable for 48 hours if protected from light and stored under refrigeration. Because of possible microbial contamination during dilution, it is advisable that solutions diluted in D_5W are used within 24 hours if stored under refrigeration and solutions prepared with

either D$_5$W or NS are used within six hours if stored at room temperature. Do not freeze. Do not store solutions prepared with NS under refrigeration because of the development of particulates.

How Supplied	Supplied as single dose in amber-colored glass vials containing 2 ml or 5 ml of irinotecan at a concentration of 20 mg/ml.
Dosage	Recommended starting dose as a single agent is 125 mg/m^2 IV over 90 minutes once weekly for four weeks followed by a two-week rest period. Cycles are repeated in six-week intervals (four weeks on therapy, two weeks rest). Subsequent doses may be adjusted to as high as 150 mg/m^2 or to as low as 50 mg/m^2 in 25–50 mg/m^2 increments based on the individual patient's tolerance of treatment (see dosage adjustment recommendations). Investigationally, irinotecan has been administered as a single agent at 300–350 mg/m^2 every 21 days, as well as in combination with other chemotherapeutic agents (e.g., flourouracil, leucovorin, docetaxel, cisplatin).
Compatibility Information	Other drugs should not be added to the infusion solution.
Contraindications/ Precautions	Contraindicated in patients with a known hypersensitivity to the drug. Risk versus benefit should be considered in patients with preexisting or treatment-related bone marrow depression (delay, omission, and/or reduction of dose may be necessary), hepatic function impairment (dose reduction warranted), existing or recent infection, or pulmonary disease or impairment.

Drug Interactions	**Agent**	**Effect**
	Dexamethasone	Concomitant use may result in hyperglycemia, especially in patients with history of diabetes or glucose intolerance; may increase incidence of lymphocytopenia.
	Diuretics	Concomitant use may increase severity of dehydration associated with irinotecan-induced diarrhea or vomiting.
	Laxatives	Concurrent use with irinotecan may increase risk of severe diarrhea.
	Pelvic/abdominal irradiation	Prior pelvic/abdominal irradiation increases risk of severe irinotecan-induced myelosuppression.

Toxicity/Side Effects	**Acute and/or Potentially Life-Threatening:** Early or acute onset diarrhea (i.e., occurring during or within 24 hours of administration) is cholinergic in nature and may be severe but usually is transient. May be preceded by complaints of diaphoresis and abdominal cramping. Administration of 0.25–1 mg of IV atropine should be considered for treatment of diaphoresis, abdominal cramping, and/or early diarrhea unless medically contraindicated. Late onset diarrhea occurring more than 24 hours after administration is a common and dose-limiting toxicity, occurring in > 80% of patients. May be severe and prolonged enough to cause life-threatening

dehydration and/or electrolyte disturbances. Median time to onset is 11 days. Median duration is three to seven days. Prompt initiation of loperamide therapy is recommended. One recommended loperamide dosing regimen is 4 mg at onset of diarrhea followed by 2 mg every two hours until diarrhea has subsided for at least 12 hours (note: this dosing regimen exceeds the usual dosage recommendation). During the night, the patient may take 4 mg every four hours. Syndrome consisting of fever, dyspnea, and a reticulonodular pattern on chest radiograph occurred in some patients with preexisting lung tumors or nonmalignant pulmonary disease in early clinical trials; causality to irinotecan has not been established.

Serious: Neutropenia is a common and dose-limiting toxicity with the incidence of severe (grade 3 or 4) neutropenia occurring in 26.3% of patients in clinical trials. Patients who have received prior pelvic or abdominal radiation therapy have a significantly increased incidence of grade 3 or 4 neutropenia.

Other:
Dermatologic: Alopecia and rash.
GI: Nausea, vomiting, anorexia, constipation, flatulence, dyspepsia, stomatitis, and transient elevations in liver enzymes.
Hematologic: Neutropenia, thrombocytopenia, and anemia.
Neurologic: Insomnia, dizziness, headache, and fever.
Miscellaneous: Vasodilation/flushing, coughing, rhinitis, and weakness.

Special Considerations	Prompt administration of atropine for early onset diarrhea and loperamide for late onset diarrhea is encouraged. Prophylactic administration of loperamide is not recommended. Encourage adequate oral repletion if diarrhea or vomiting occurs. Patient should be instructed to have loperamide readily available and to notify physician immediately if diarrhea develops. Irinotecan has moderate to moderately high emetogenic potential; prophylactic dexamethasone with or without a serotonin antagonist is recommended. In addition, an as-needed antiemetic should be prescribed (e.g., prochlorperazine).
Monitoring Parameters	Monitoring is recommended prior to initiation of therapy and at periodic intervals during therapy unless otherwise specified. • CBC with differential: Recommended prior to initiation of therapy, prior to each subsequent dose, and at periodic intervals during therapy. • Platelet count: Recommended prior to initiation of therapy, prior to each subsequent dose, and at periodic intervals during therapy. • Hemoglobin and/or hematocrit: Recommended prior to initiation of therapy, prior to each subsequent dose, and at periodic intervals during therapy. • Liver function tests: ALT, AST, alkaline phosphatase, total bilirubin, LDH.
Indications	Indicated for the treatment of patients with metastatic carcinoma of the colon or rectum whose disease has recurred or progressed following fluorouracil-based therapy. Studied investigationally in gastric, esophageal, and pancreatic cancers.
Dosage Adjustment Recommendations	A new course of therapy should not begin until the granulocyte count has recovered to $\geq 1,500 /mm^3$, the platelet count has recovered to

$\geq 100,000$ /mm^3, and treatment-related diarrhea has fully resolved. Depending on tolerability, the patient's dose should be adjusted in 25–50 mg/m^2 increments; recommended weekly doses range from 50–150 mg/m^2. Treatment should be delayed one to two weeks to allow for recovery from treatment-related toxicities. If the patient has not recovered after a two-week delay, consideration should be given to discontinue irinotecan. The following table serves as a guideline for dosage adjustment; all dose modifications are based on worst preceding toxicity based on manufacturer's guidelines.

NCI Toxicity Grade	During a Course/ Cycle of Therapy	Adjustment for Next Cycle (After Adequate Recovery) Compared to Previous Cycle
No toxicity	Maintain dose level.	Increase 25 mg/m^2 up to maximum of 150 mg/m^2.
Hematologic toxicity (neutropenia, thrombocytopenia, and anemia)		
1	Maintain dose level.	Maintain dose level.
2	Decrease 25 mg/m^2.	Maintain dose level.
3	Omit dose, then decrease 25 mg/m^2 when resolved to $\leq$ grade 2.	Decrease 25 mg/m^2.
4	Omit dose, then decrease 50 mg/m^2 when resolved to $\leq$ grade 2.	Decrease 50 mg/m^2.
Neutropenic fever (grade 4 neutropenia and $\geq$ grade 2 fever)		
	Omit dose, then decrease 50 mg/m^2 when resolved.	Decrease 50 mg/m^2.
Diarrhea		
1 (2–3 more stools/ day than pretx)	Maintain dose level.	Maintain dose level.
2 (4–6 more stools/ day than pretx)	Decrease 25 mg/m^2.	Maintain dose level if only grade 2 toxicity.
3 (7–9 more stools/ day than pretx)	Omit dose, then decrease 25 mg/m^2 when resolved to $\leq$ grade 2	Decrease 25 mg/m^2 if only grade 3 toxicity.
4 ($\geq$ more stools/ day than pretx)	Omit dose, then decrease 50mg/m^2 when resolved to $\leq$ grade 2.	Decrease 50 mg/m^2.
Other nonhematologic toxicities		
1	Maintain dose level.	Maintain dose level.
2	Decrease 25 mg/m^2.	Decrease 25 mg/m^2.
3	Omit dose, then decrease 25 mg/m^2 when resolved to $\leq$ grade 2.	Decrease 50 mg/m^2.
4	Omit dose, then decrease 50 mg/m^2 when resolved to $\leq$ grade 2.	Decrease 50 mg/m^2.

	The use of irinotecan in patients with significant hepatic impairment has not been established and should be used with extreme caution. A reduction in the dose should be considered. Patients with mild to modest elevations in total serum bilirubin levels (1–2 mg/dl) had a significantly greater likelihood of experiencing first-course grade 3 or 4 neutropenia than patients with bilirubin levels < 1 mg/dl.
Pharmacokinetics	Irinotecan rapidly undergoes metabolic conversion to the active metabolite SN-38. SN-38 thought to be significantly more potent than parent compound. Both irinotecan and SN-38 undergo reversible, pH-dependent conversion between their two forms (active lactone form and inactive hydroxyacid form). Both irinotecan and SN-38 are protein-bound, 30%–68% and 95%, respectively, with terminal half-lives of approximately 10 hours. Irinotecan is eliminated via biliary and urinary excretion and conversion to SN-38. SN-38 is eliminated via glucuronidation and biliary excretion.
Manufacturer	Pharmacia & Upjohn Company, Peapack, NJ

Leucovorin

Other Names	Wellcovorin®, folinic acid, calcium leucovorin, citrovorum factor, leucovorin calcium
Classification	Folic acid antagonist.
Mechanism	Reduced form of folic acid; thus, does not require reduction by dihydrofolate reductase and is not affected by dihydrofolate reductase inhibitors (e.g., MTX). This allows for purine and thymidine synthesis and, thus, DNA, RNA, and protein synthesis to occur. Leucovorin competes for the same transport system into the cell as MTX and, if given at appropriate time intervals, rescues bone marrow and GI cells from MTX toxicity. Leucovorin also serves as a biomodulator of fluorouracil by providing high concentrations of folate cofactor, which allows FdUMP (active metabolite of fluorouracil) to bind more efficiently to thymidylate synthetase, making it unavailable for DNA synthesis, thus killing more cancer cells.
Vesicant Information	Not classified as a vesicant or an irritant.
Preparation and Mixture	Reconstitute 100-mg vial and 350-mg vial with 10 ml and 17 ml of Bacteriostatic Water for Injection, USP, with benzyl alcohol or Sterile Water for Injection, USP, yielding a concentration of 10 mg/ml or 20 mg/ml of leucovorin calcium, respectively. Leucovorin may be further diluted in 5% Dextrose Injection, USP, Sodium Chloride for Injection, USP, or lactated Ringer's solution. Standard dilutions are 50–100 mg leucovorin in 50 ml D_5W (minimum volume is 50 ml). Because of the benzyl alcohol contained in Bacteriostatic Water for Injection, USP, doses > 10 mg/m² are to be reconstituted with Sterile Water for Injection, USP, and used immediately. Leucovorin calcium for injection does not contain preservatives.
Administration	Leucovorin may be administered as an IM or IV injection or given orally as tablets or solution. The IV rate of administration should not exceed 160 mg/minute because of the calcium content of the product. In addition,

oral administration of doses > 25 mg is not recommended because of saturable oral absorption. DO NOT administer leucovorin intrathecally.

Storage and Stability	Store leucovorin for injection dry powder and reconstituted solutions at room temperature 15°–30°C (59°–86°F), and protect from light. Solutions reconstituted with Bacteriostatic Water for Injection, USP, with benzyl alcohol are stable for seven days. Solutions reconstituted with Sterile Water for Injection, USP, are to be used immediately. Solutions reconstituted with Bacteriostatic Water for Injection, USP, and further diluted with NS or D_5W are stable for 14 days at room temperature in Becton Dickinson polypropylene syringes at a concentration of 10 mg/ml or in PVC bags at a concentration of 1–10 mg/ml. Leucovorin tablets should be stored at room temperature and protected from light.
How Supplied	Wellcovorin brand of leucovorin calcium is supplied as vials containing 100 mg. Immunex supplies a 350-mg vial of leucovorin calcium, and generic companies supply 50- and 100-mg vials of leucovorin calcium. Oral leucovorin is supplied in 5-, 10-, 15-, and 25-mg tablets as well as a 60-ml oral solution containing 1 mg/ml leucovorin calcium.
Dosage	Leucovorin rescue after high-dose MTX (12–15 g/m^2) therapy: 10 mg/m^2 (or approximately 15 mg) orally every six hours for 10 doses. Begin within 24–42 hours of MTX administration, and continue until serum MTX concentration less than 5×10^{-8} molar. In the presence of severe GI toxicity (e.g., nausea, vomiting, mucositis), leucovorin should be administered parenterally. Leucovorin dose should be adjusted to SCr levels and serum MTX concentrations (see dosage adjustment recommendations).
	Leucovorin synergy with fluorouracil for colorectal cancer: most commonly used regimens include 20 mg/m^2 leucovorin IV followed by fluorouracil at 425 mg/m^2 or leucovorin 200 mg/m^2 slow IVP over minimum of three minutes followed by 370 mg/m^2 fluorouracil. Both regimens are administered daily for five days and repeated at four-week intervals.
	Oral and IV leucovorin also is used, although not FDA-approved, after IT MTX as well as after MTX immunosuppression in the allogeneic HCT setting.
Compatibility Information	Incompatible with fluorouracil; precipitation will occur if these agents are combined in the same IV solution.
Contraindications/ Precautions	Leucovorin is contraindicated in the treatment of pernicious and other megaloblastic anemias.

Drug Interactions

Agent	Effect
Anticonvulsants (e.g., barbiturates, hydantoin, primidone)	Large doses of leucovorin may counteract the anticonvulsant effects and increase the frequency of seizures.
Fluorouracil	Concomitant use may enhance the therapeutic and toxic effects of fluorouracil (may be considered a therapeutic advantage).
Sulfamethoxazole and trimethoprim	Concomitant use may lead to antibiotic therapeutic failures in the treatment of *Pneumocystis carinii* infections; trimethoprim is a folic acid antagonist.

Toxicity/Side Effects	Allergic sensitization, including anaphylactoid reactions and urticaria, has been reported following the administration of both oral and parenteral forms of leucovorin. No other adverse events have been attributed to leucovorin.
Special Considerations	In the setting of high-dose MTX, adequate hydration (at least 3l/day), urinary alkalinization, and leucovorin administration are necessary to prevent excessive MTX toxicity, including the renal toxicity associated with MTX and its metabolites. Daily monitoring of the SCr, plasma or serum MTX concentration, and urinary pH are essential. Administration of leucovorin should be consecutive rather than concomitant with MTX administration, as to not interfere with the antineoplastic effects of MTX. Oral leucovorin may be taken with or without regard to meals. Take as directed at evenly spaced intervals throughout day and night. Take missed scheduled dose as soon as remembered. Do not double-up doses. Consult physician for clarification on missed dose or if vomiting occurs immediately after oral administration.
Monitoring Parameters	Monitoring is recommended prior to initiation of therapy and at periodic intervals during therapy unless otherwise specified. • CrCl determination, measured or calculated: Recommended prior to the initiation of high-dose MTX to help to determine MTX dose adjustment if necessary and aid in identifying patients with delayed MTX clearance. • SCr: Recommended prior to and every 24 hours after intermediate and high-dose MTX administration to detect developing renal function impairment; an increase of > 50%–100% above baseline at 24 hours usually is associated with significant renal toxicity. • Plasma or serum MTX concentrations: Recommended at 12- to 24-hour intervals until concentration (less than) 5×10^{-8} molar; determines dose and duration of leucovorin therapy needed to maintain rescue. • Urinary pH: Monitor prior to administration of MTX and every six hours throughout leucovorin rescue; recommend pH of > 7 prior to MTX administration and continued until serum MTX concentration < 5×10^{-8} molar to minimize risk of MTX nephropathy.
Indications	Indicated as rescue after high-dose MTX therapy in the treatment of osteosarcoma. In addition, leucovorin rescue is used in the treatment and prophylaxis of MTX toxicity in a number of different settings (e.g., high-dose MTX used in the treatment of gastric cancer, sarcomas, CNS lymphoma, and non-Hodgkin's lymphoma), treatment and prophylaxis of pyrimethamine and trimethoprim toxicity, and antidotal therapy for overdoses associated with MTX or other folic acid antagonists. Also indicated for use in combination with fluorouracil to prolong survival in the palliative treatment of patients with advanced colorectal cancer.
Dosage Adjustment Recommendations	Leucovorin rescue dose and duration depends on serum or plasma MTX concentrations and SCr. The following are guidelines for leucovorin dosage and administration (based on manufacturer's guidelines).

Clinical Situation	Laboratory Findings	Leucovorin Dosage and Duration Recommendation
Normal MTX elimination	Serum MTX concentration of approximately 10 micromolar at 24 hours, 1 micromolar at 48 hours, and < 0.2 micromolar at 72 hours after administration	10 mg/m^2 or 15 mg oral, IM, or IV every six hours for 10 doses (starting at 24 hours after MTX administration).
Delayed late MTX elimination	Serum MTX concentration > 0.2 micromolar at 72 hours and > 0.05 micromolar at 96 hours after administration.	Continue leucovorin 10 mg/m^2 or 15 mg every six hours until serum MTX concentration < 0.05 micromolar.
Delayed early MTX elimination	Serum MTX concentration ≥ 50 micromolar at 24 hours or 5 micromolar at 48 hours after administration OR a 100% or greater increase in SCr level at 24 hours after administration.	Leucovorin 150 mg IV every three hours until serum MTX concentration < 1 micromolar, then 15 mg IV every three hours until serum MTX concentration < 0.05 micromolar.

In addition to these dosing guidelines, other published guidelines and dosing nomograms are available.

Pharmacokinetics	Well absorbed orally with decreases in absorption with doses > 25 mg. Onset of activity within five minutes for IV administration and within 30 minutes for oral administration. Rapidly converted to active metabolite (5-methyl-tetrahydrofolate) in the intestinal mucosa and by the liver. Half-life is 15 minutes for parent drug and 35 minutes for active metabolite. Primarily eliminated in the urine (80%–90%) with small amounts excreted in feces.
Manufacturer	Wellcovorin®, Glaxo Wellcome, Inc., Research Triangle Park, NC; Leucovorin Calcium for Injection, Immunex Corporation, Seattle, WA

Levamisole

Other Names	Ergamisol®, levamisole hydrochloride
Classification	Biochemical modulator; immune modulator.
Mechanism	Not clearly understood. Activity with fluorouracil in the treatment of colorectal cancer thought to be caused by biochemical modulation of fluorouracil and independent of levamisole's immunomodulatory effects.
Vesicant Information	Not classified as a vesicant or an irritant. Levamisole is available commercially as an oral product.

Preparation and Mixture	No preparation or admixture necessary. Levamisole is available commercially as an oral product.
Administration	Oral.
Storage and Stability	Store at room temperature below 40°C (104°F), preferably between 15°–30°C (59°–86°F). Protect from moisture.
How Supplied	Supplied as white, coated tablets containing the equivalent of 50-mg levamisole base in blister packages of 36 tablets and imprinted with the following: Janssen and L/50.
Dosage	Regimen for the adjuvant treatment of colorectal cancer is 50 mg orally every eight hours for three days, repeated every two weeks for one year (begin no earlier than seven days and no later than 30 days after surgery). Levamisole is given concomitantly with fluorouracil 450 mg/m² IV daily for five days, followed by 450 mg/m² one per week beginning 28 days after initiation of the five-day course and continued for a total treatment of one year.
Compatibility Information	Not applicable. Levamisole is available commercially as an oral product.
Contraindications/ Precautions	Contraindicated in patients with a known hypersensitivity to the product. Risk versus benefit should be considered in patients with preexisting bone marrow depression, infection, and seizure disorder.

Drug Interactions	**Agent**	**Effect**
	Alcohol	Disulfiram-like reaction may occur with concomitant administration.
	Phenytoin	Concomitant use may increase serum levels and toxicity of phenytoin; monitoring of serum phenytoin levels recommended.
	Warfarin	Concomitant use may cause prolongation of PT; monitoring of PT with corresponding adjustment in warfarin dose recommended.

Toxicity/Side Effects	**Acute and/or Potentially Life-Threatening:** Agranulocytosis, sometimes fatal; onset frequently accompanied by flu-like syndrome (e.g., fever, chills), although flu-like syndrome may occur without the occurrence of agranulocytosis. Increased incidence associated with higher than recommended doses. In addition, an encephalopathy-like syndrome with demyelination has been reported. Onset of symptoms and clinical presentation varied and include coma, confusion, lethargy, memory loss, muscle weakness, paresthesia, seizures, and speech disturbances. Therapy with levamisole and fluorouracil should be discontinued immediately. Most patients generally recover or improve with drug discontinuation; however, in some cases, recovery or improvement has not occurred, and deaths have been reported. Although rare, a life-threatening exfoliative dermatitis has been reported.
	Serious: Allergic-type reaction manifested by a flu-like syndrome, which can occur outside the setting of agranulocytosis (see above), may occur;

onset usually within hours of drug administration; may be mild and transient or severe and progressive.

Other:
Dermatologic: Rash, pruritus, urticaria, and alopecia.
Cardiovascular: Edema and chest pain.
GI: Nausea, vomiting, diarrhea, stomatitis, anorexia, abdominal pain, flatulence, constipation, taste perversion, and dyspepsia.
Hematologic: Leukopenia, thrombocytopenia, granulocytopenia, and anemia.
Neurologic: Fever, paresthesia, headache, fatigue, dizziness, somnolence, depression, anxiety, nervousness, and insomnia.
Miscellaneous: Rigors, arthralgia, myalgia, hepatotoxicity, altered sense of smell, infection, abnormal tearing, blurred vision, and conjunctivitis.

Special Considerations	Discuss with patient the importance of not taking more or less of medication than prescribed. Do not double doses and do not take a missed dose. Consult physician if vomiting occurs shortly after levamisole administration.
Monitoring Parameters	Monitoring is recommended prior to initiation of therapy and at periodic intervals during therapy unless otherwise specified. • CBC with differential: Recommended prior to initiation of therapy, prior to each subsequent dose, and at periodic intervals during therapy; also recommended prior to each dose of fluorouracil. • Platelet count: Recommended prior to initiation of therapy, prior to each subsequent dose, and at periodic intervals during therapy. • Hemoglobin and/or hematocrit: Recommended prior to initiation of therapy, prior to each subsequent dose, and at periodic intervals during therapy. • Liver function tests: ALT, AST, alkaline phosphatase, total bilirubin, LDH.
Indications	Levamisole is indicated as adjuvant treatment in combination with fluorouracil after surgical resection in patients with Dukes' stage C colon cancer.
Dosage Adjustment Recommendations	Patients with cirrhosis should be monitored closely for adverse effects. Dose reduction or discontinuation of levamisole may be warranted if adverse effects are noted. Discontinue levamisole if WBC < 2,500/mm³ for more than 10 days, despite deferring fluorouracil therapy. In addition, both levamisole and fluorouracil therapy should be deferred if platelet count is not adequate (> 100,000/mm³).
Pharmacokinetics	Rapidly absorbed from GI tract. Undergoes extensive hepatic biotransformation. Half-life of three to four hours (metabolites 16 hours). Undergoes both renal (70%) and fecal elimination.
Manufacturer	Janssen Pharmaceutica Inc., Titusville, NJ

Lomustine

Other Names	CCNU, CeeNU®
Classification	Alkylating agent.

Mechanism	Inhibits DNA and RNA synthesis. Cell-cycle nonspecific.
Vesicant Information	Not classified as a vesicant or an irritant. CCNU is commercially available as an oral product.
Preparation and Mixture	Supplied as capsules. Dispense only one dose at a time. Handle with gloves.
Administration	Oral on an empty stomach, preferably at bedtime. Schedule administration every six to eight weeks. Dispense to the nearest 10 mg.
Storage and Stability	Avoid exposure to excess heat (> 40°C; > 104°F). Unopened manufacturer-sealed container is stable for two years.
How Supplied	Oral capsules available in a six-pack containing 10 mg, 30 mg, or 100 mg of CCNU.
Dosage	Dosed as a single agent at 100–130 mg/m² every six weeks; 100 mg/m² when given in the setting of compromised bone marrow function. Subsequent doses readjusted after initial treatment based on nadir platelet and leukocyte counts. If nadir leukocyte count 2,000–2,900/m³, platelets 25,000–74,999/m³: administer 75% of prior dose; if leukocytes < 2,000/m³, platelets < 25,000/m³: administer 50% of prior dose.
Compatibility Information	Avoid over-the-counter preparations with CCNU.
Contraindications/ Precautions	Hypersensitivity to CCNU. Prolonged myelosuppression. Pregnant or lactating patient.

Drug Interactions	**Agent**	**Effect**
	Radioactive dyes	CCNU causes a transient increase in liver function tests.
	Cimetidine	May potentiate myelotoxicity of CCNU.
	Phenobarbital	May decrease the effectiveness of CCNU.

Toxicity/Side Effects

Acute and/or Potentially Life-Threatening: Pulmonary toxicity of CCNU, although rare, can be dose-limiting and life-threatening and has been reported to occur six months to up to years after treatment. Patients present with SOB, tachypnea, and nonproductive cough. Usually characterized as interstitial pneumonia and fibrosis, which may be progressive and fatal. Patients who receive ≥ 1,100 mg/m² are at higher risk, although other factors (e.g., past history of lung disease, smoking, prior mediastinal irradiation, concurrent administration of other agents associated with pulmonary toxicity) may play a role. Pulmonary function tests should be obtained at baseline and repeated during treatment. Patients with a baseline below 70% of predicted FVC or DLCO are particularly at risk.

Serious: Renal toxicity, progressive azotemia, and renal failure, although rare, have been reported; usually associated with high cumulative doses and prolonged therapy.

Other:
Dermatologic: Alopecia.

GI: Moderate to severe nausea and vomiting (occurs within three to six hours of administration and usually lasts for 24 hours), stomatitis, and reversible elevation of liver enzymes.

Hematologic: Delayed, dose-related, and cumulative myelosuppression; occurs four to six weeks after administration and may be prolonged lasting for one to two weeks. Nadir platelets at day 26–34; nadir WBC at day 41–46. Refractory anemia and acute leukemia also have been reported.

Neurologic: Lethargy, ataxia, and disorientation.

Special Considerations	Do not drink alcohol while taking CCNU. Pulmonary fibrosis with accumulated dose > 1,100 mg/m². Hold dose until WBC > 4,000/mm³ and platelet count > 100,000/mm³. Bone marrow recovery takes six to eight weeks. Avoid accidental overdose by dispensing one treatment at a time. Highly emetogenic; premedicate with a serotonin antagonist in combination with dexamethasone.
Monitoring Parameters	Monitoring is recommended prior to initiation of therapy and at periodic intervals during therapy unless otherwise specified. • CBC with differential: Recommended prior to initiation of therapy, prior to each subsequent dose, and at periodic intervals during therapy. • Platelet count: Recommended prior to initiation of therapy, prior to each subsequent dose, and at periodic intervals during therapy. • Hemoglobin and/or hematocrit: Recommended prior to initiation of therapy, prior to each subsequent dose, and at periodic intervals during therapy. • Liver function tests: ALT, AST, alkaline phosphatase, total bilirubin, LDH. • Renal function tests: CrCl, actual or calculated, and/or SCr recommended prior to initiation of therapy, prior to each subsequent dose, and at periodic intervals during therapy. • Pulmonary function tests: Recommended prior to therapy and at frequent intervals thereafter. • Blood pressure: During administration.
Indications	Approved as a single agent used in combination with other modalities or in combination with other myelosuppressives in primary or metastatic brain tumors, as well as in the secondary treatment of Hodgkin's disease.
Dosage Adjustment Recommendations	Subsequent doses readjusted after initial treatment based on nadir platelet and leukocyte counts. If nadir leukocyte count 2,000–2,900/mm³, platelets 25,000–74,999/mm³: administer 75% of prior dose; if leukocytes < 2,000/mm³, platelets < 25,000/mm³: administer 50% of prior dose. Consider lower doses (100 mg/m²) when dosing in combination with other myelosuppressive agents.
Pharmacokinetics	Cross-resistance exists between lomustine and carmustine. Rapidly absorbed from the GI tract. Oral bioavailability 60%–90%. Lipid-soluble and one of the few agents that crosses the blood-brain barrier. Seventy-five percent excreted in the urine within four days. Peak plasma level: one to six

	hours. Largely excreted via the kidneys and a small amount in the lungs and feces. Plasma half-life of six hours.
Manufacturer	Bristol-Myers Squibb Oncology/Immunology Division, Princeton, NJ

Mechlorethamine

Other Names	Mustargen®, nitrogen mustard, mustine, mechlorethamine hydrochloride, HN_2
Classification	Alkylating agent; nitrogen mustard derivative.
Mechanism	Bifunctional alkylating agent that inhibits DNA and RNA synthesis via formation of carbonium ions; intra- and interstrand cross-linking of DNA causing miscoding, breakage, and failure of replication.
Vesicant Information	Classified as a vesicant. Mechlorethamine produces pain, swelling, and thrombophlebitis of vein immediately upon extravasation and is known to cause severe and prolonged skin ulceration and tissue necrosis. Administer drug through the rubber or plastic tubing of a free-flowing IV to reduce the possibility of a severe local reaction. Treatment of mechlorethamine extravasation should begin immediately. Apply ice and elevate limb immediately and as much as possible for first 48 hours following extravasation.
Preparation and Mixture	Using a sterile 10-ml syringe, inject 10 ml of Sterile Water for Injection, USP, or Sodium Chloride for Injection, 0.9%, USP, into a vial of mechlorethamine. With the needle and syringe still in the rubber stopper, shake the vial several times to dissolve the drug completely. The resultant solution contains 1 mg of mechlorethamine hydrochloride per 1 ml. Final concentration of drug to be administered not to exceed 1 mg/ml. Do not use if solution is discolored or if droplets of water are visible within the vial prior to reconstitution. Solution is highly unstable and should be used within one hour of reconstitution/dilution. May be diluted in up to 100 ml Sodium Chloride for Injection, 0.9%, USP, for intracavitary use.
Administration	Administer as a slow IVP through a free-flowing IV over one to three minutes. Venous patency should be confirmed by flushing the vein with a small volume of D_5W or NS prior to drug administration. May also be used topically and for intracavitary or intrapericardial administration.
Storage and Stability	Store intact vials at room temperature and protect from light and humidity. Reconstituted and diluted solutions are highly unstable and decompose on standing and, therefore, should be used within one hour of preparation.
How Supplied	Supplied as a light yellow-brown crystalline powder as mechlorethamine hydrochloride in vials of 10 mg.
Dosage	IV dosage regimens include 6 mg/m² on days 1 and 8 of a 28-day cycle in combination with other chemotherapeutics; single-agent regimens

include 0.4 mg/kg or 12–16 mg/m^2 for one dose repeated at four- to six-week intervals or divided doses of 0.1 mg/kg/day for four successive daily doses repeated at four- to six-week intervals. Intrapericardial and intracavitary administration utilizes doses of 0.2 mg/kg and 0.4 mg/kg, respectively. Topical administration of mechlorethamine has been used in the treatment of cutaneous lesions of mycosis fungoides. A skin test should be performed to detect sensitivity and possible irritation.

Compatibility Information	Compatible with NS and sterile water for injection. Data available on compatibility with amifostine, fludarabine, granisetron, ondansetron, and vinorelbine; refer to manufacturer or other literature sources for specific information. Mechlorethamine is incompatible with other antineoplastic agents because of instability.
Contraindications/ Precautions	Contraindicated in the presence of known infectious diseases and in patients who have had previous anaphylactic reactions to the drug. Risk versus benefit should be considered in patients with preexisting bone marrow depression and in patients with a history of gout or urate renal stones. Caution also should be used in patients who have had previous cytotoxic drug therapy or radiation therapy (dosage reduction recommended).
Drug Interactions	No known drug interactions, although mechlorethamine may raise the concentration of uric acid in the blood, and dosage of antigout medications may need to be adjusted to control hyperuricemia and gout.
Toxicity/Side Effects	**Acute and/or Potentially Life Threatening:** Acute nausea and vomiting occurs in majority of patients; highly emetogenic (> 90%); onset within 30 minutes to three hours; duration two to eight hours. Premedication with a serotonin antagonist in combination with dexamethasone required. Patients with refractory nausea and/or vomiting may require the addition of other antiemetics and/or sedatives (e.g., prochlorperazine, benzodiazepines, barbiturates). **Serious:** Leukopenia and thrombocytopenia may be severe; onset in four to seven days; nadir in 14 days; recovery by day 21–28. **Other:** Dermatologic: Rash and alopecia. Endocrine: Delayed menses, oligomenorrhea, temporary or permanent amenorrhea, impaired spermatogenesis, azoospermia, and hyperuricemia. GI: Diarrhea, anorexia, and metallic taste. Neurologic: Fever, vertigo, and peripheral neuropathy. Miscellaneous: Weakness, tinnitus, ototoxicity, thrombophlebitis, hepatotoxicity, hypersensitivity, and secondary malignancies.
Special Considerations	Highly emetogenic (> 90%); premedication with a serotonin antagonist in combination with dexamethasone required. Patients with refractory nausea and/or vomiting may require the addition of other antiemetics and/or sedatives (e.g., prochlorperazine, benzodiazepines, barbiturates). Avoid extravasation; administer mechlorethamine through a free-flowing IV line; verify patency of vein prior to administration.

Monitoring Parameters	Monitoring is recommended prior to initiation of therapy and at periodic intervals during therapy unless otherwise specified. • CBC with differential: Recommended prior to initiation of therapy, prior to each subsequent dose, and at periodic intervals during therapy. • Platelet count: Recommended prior to initiation of therapy, prior to each subsequent dose, and at periodic intervals during therapy. • Hemoglobin and/or hematocrit: Recommended prior to initiation of therapy, prior to each subsequent dose, and at periodic intervals during therapy. • Liver function tests: ALT, AST, alkaline phosphatase, total bilirubin, LDH. • Serum uric acid. • Audiometric testing.
Indications	IV mechlorethamine is indicated for the treatment of Hodgkin's disease (stages III and IV), lymphosarcoma, CML or CLL, polycythemia vera, mycosis fungoides, and bronchogenic carcinoma. Administered intrapleurally, intraperitoneally, or intrapericardially in the palliative treatment of metastatic carcinoma resulting in effusion.
Dosage Adjustment Recommendations	It is recommended that total dosage in patients who have received prior cytotoxic chemotherapy or radiotherapy should not exceed 0.2–0.3 mg/kg. Mechlorethamine therapy should be withdrawn if leukocyte or platelet count falls markedly. Therapy may be resumed at a lower dosage when leukocyte and platelet count returns to satisfactory level.
Pharmacokinetics	After IV administration, drug undergoes rapid chemical transformation, rapidly deactivated in body fluids and tissues. Effect occurs within minutes with unchanged drug undetectable within a few minutes. Apparent elimination is renal although less than 0.01% as unchanged drug.
Manufacturer	Merck & Co, Inc., West Point, PA

Melphalan

Other Names	Alkeran®, L-PAM, phenylalanine mustard
Classification	Alkylating agent; nitrogen mustard derivative.
Mechanism	Bifunctional alkylating agent; cytotoxicity primarily because of cross-linking of strands of DNA and RNA, as well as inhibition of protein synthesis.
Vesicant Information	Not classified as a vesicant or an irritant.
Preparation and Mixture	Melphalan for injection is reconstituted by rapidly injecting 10 ml of supplied diluent into vial of lyophilized powder. Immediately shake vigorously until solution is clear. Resultant concentration is 5 mg/ml. Immediately dilute reconstituted solution with Sodium Chloride for Injection, 0.9%, USP, to a concentration no greater than 0.45 mg/ml. Because of the instability of the solutions, the time between reconstitution/dilution and administration should be kept to a minimum. Prepared fresh solution is stable for one hour after dilution and must be administered within that time period.

Administration	Melphalan is administered orally on an empty stomach or intravenously over 15 minutes.
Storage and Stability	Both oral tablets and injectable powder should be stored at room temperature and protected from light. Reconstituted solution stable for 90 minutes; diluted solution stable for approximately 60 minutes. Must be prepared fresh; solution is stable for one hour after dilution and must be administered within that time period. Do not refrigerate solution; precipitation may occur. Oral tablets should be stored in a dry place and dispensed in a glass container.
How Supplied	Supplied orally as a white, scored tablet containing 2 mg melphalan in bottles of 50 and with the following: ALKERAN and A2A. Melphalan for injection supplied as a single-use clear glass vial of freeze-dried melphalan hydrochloride equivalent to 50 mg melphalan and one 10-ml clear glass vial of sterile diluent.
Dosage	Most common regimens for oral melphalan include 0.15 mg/kg/day for seven days followed by a rest period of at least three weeks, after which a maintenance dose of 0.05 mg/kg/day is instituted when leukocyte and platelet counts are recovering; 0.1–0.25 mg/kg/day for two to three weeks or 0.25 mg/kg/day for four to five days followed by a rest period of two to four weeks, then maintenance dose of 2–4 mg a day when leukocyte and platelet counts are recovering; 0.25 mg/kg/day or 7 mg/m^2/day for five days every five to six weeks adjusted to produce mild leukopenia and thrombocytopenia; and 0.2 mg/kg/day for five days repeated every four to five weeks if blood counts return to normal. Intravenously, melphalan is dosed at 16 mg/m^2 at two-week intervals for four doses then at four-week intervals after recovery from toxicity; dosage adjustments made based on nadir blood cell counts. High-dose therapies also used in the HCT setting.
Compatibility Information	Melphalan 0.1 mg/ml is incompatible for y-site administration with the following drugs: amphotericin B, chlorpromazine, daunorubicin, idarubicin, lorazepam, methylprednisolone, vinorelbine, and prochlorperazine.
Contraindications/ Precautions	Contraindicated in patients who have demonstrated prior resistance to the product as well as in patients who have experienced a hypersensitivity to the product. Risk versus benefit should be considered in patients with preexisting bone marrow depression, existing or recent chicken pox or herpes zoster infection, history of gout or urate renal stones, renal function impairment (dosage adjustment recommended), and in patients who have received previous cytotoxic drug therapy or radiation therapy within three to four weeks.

Drug Interactions

Agent	Effect
Carmustine	IV melphalan may be synergistic with carmustine in causing pulmonary toxicity.
Cimetidine (and possibly other H$_2$ antagonists)	Reduction of gastric pH reported to decrease absorption and bioavailability of melphalan by up to 30%.
Cyclosporine	Concomitant use may increase risk of nephrotoxicity.

Toxicity/Side Effects	**Acute and/or Potentially Life-Threatening:** Anaphylaxis, although rare, has been reported with the IV formulation of melphalan. This reaction usually occurs after multiple courses of therapy. The infusion should be terminated followed by symptomatic treatment (e.g., volume expanders, pressor agents, corticosteroids, antihistamines). **Serious:** Myelosuppression, which occurs within two to three weeks of initiation of therapy, may be severe. Leukocyte and platelet nadir usually occur within three to five weeks and return to normal within four to eight weeks. Irreversible bone marrow failure has been reported. Cumulative myelosuppression may occur with repeated dosing. **Other:** Dermatologic: Alopecia, vesiculation of skin, pruritus, and rash. Endocrine: SIADH, sterility, and amenorrhea. GI: Mild nausea and vomiting, diarrhea, and stomatitis. Hematologic: Anemia, agranulocytosis, and hemolytic anemia. Miscellaneous: Vasculitis, bladder irritation, hemorrhagic cystitis, hypersensitivity (skin rash and itching), pulmonary fibrosis, interstitial pneumonitis, and the development of second malignancies.
Special Considerations	Reconstituted and diluted solutions of IV melphalan are highly unstable; administration should occur within one hour of dilution. Do not refrigerate solution, as precipitation may occur. Take oral melphalan on an empty stomach. Do not take more medication than prescribed. Do not double doses or take a missed dose. Melphalan causes mild nausea and vomiting; consider prescribing an as-needed antiemetic (e.g., prochlorperazine).
Monitoring Parameters	Monitoring is recommended prior to initiation of therapy and at periodic intervals during therapy unless otherwise specified. • CBC with differential: Recommended prior to initiation of therapy, prior to each subsequent dose, and at periodic intervals during therapy. • Platelet count: Recommended prior to initiation of therapy, prior to each subsequent dose, and at periodic intervals during therapy. • Hemoglobin and/or hematocrit: Recommended prior to initiation of therapy, prior to each subsequent dose, and at periodic intervals during therapy. • Renal function tests: CrCl, actual or calculated, and/or SCr recommended prior to initiation of therapy, prior to each subsequent dose, and at periodic intervals during therapy. • Serum uric acid.
Indications	IV melphalan is indicated in the palliative treatment of patients with multiple myeloma for which oral therapy is not appropriate. Oral melphalan is indicated in the palliative treatment of multiple myeloma and in the palliative treatment of unresectable epithelial carcinoma of the ovary. Also used in the treatment of breast cancer, malignant melanoma, Waldenstrom's macroglobulinemia, and Hodgkin's disease.
Dosage Adjustment Recommendations	Dosage adjustment is necessary for melphalan in patients with renal function impairment (see Appendix B). Thrombocytopenia and/or leukopenia are indications to withhold further therapy until the blood counts have sufficiently recovered (WBC 2,000–3,000 cells/mm^3; platelet count

	>100,000 cells/mm^3). Dose adjustment on the basis of blood counts at the nadir and day of treatment should be considered.
Pharmacokinetics	Absorption of the oral product is incomplete and variable; food interferes with absorption; bioavailability also unpredictable. Significant protein binding (60%–90%); 30% is irreversibly bound to plasma proteins. Half-life of approximately 90 minutes and eliminated from plasma primarily by chemical hydrolysis. Renal and nonrenal mechanisms play a minor role in elimination.
Manufacturer	Glaxo Wellcome Inc., Research Triangle Park, NC

Mercaptopurine

Other Names	Purinethol®, 6-mercaptopurine, 6-MP
Classification	Antimetabolite; purine analogue.
Mechanism	Purine antagonist that, once converted to monophosphate nucleotide in the cell, inhibits de novo protein synthesis by competing with endogenous ribotides; halts RNA synthesis. Cell-cycle S phase specific.
Vesicant Information	Not classified as a vesicant or an irritant. Mercaptopurine is available commercially as an oral product.
Preparation and Mixture	No preparation or admixture necessary. Mercaptopurine is available commercially as an oral product.
Administration	Oral.
Storage and Stability	Store at room temperature in a dry place.
How Supplied	Supplied as a pale-yellow to buff scored tablet containing 50 mg of mercaptopurine in bottles of 25 and imprinted with the following: PURINETHOL and 04A.
Dosage	Common induction dosing regimen is 2.5 mg/kg/day in single daily dose rounded to the nearest 25 mg. If there is no clinical improvement or leukocyte depression after four weeks, an increase in dosage to 5 mg/kg/day may be attempted. Maintenance dosing of 1.5–2.5 mg/kg/day or 80–100 mg/m^2/day once complete hematologic remission is obtained.
Compatibility Information	Not applicable. Mercaptopurine is available commercially as an oral product.
Contraindications/ Precautions	Contraindicated in patients without a diagnosis of ALL or in patients whose disease has demonstrated prior resistance to this drug. Risk versus benefit should be considered in patients with preexisting bone marrow depression, renal and/or hepatic impairment, existing or recent chicken pox or herpes zoster infection, or history of gout or urate renal stones or in patients who have had previous cytotoxic therapy or radiation therapy (dosage reduction is recommended).

Drug Interactions	**Agent**	**Effect**
	Allopurinol	Increases levels of mercaptopurine through inhibition of xanthine oxidase; reduce dose of mercaptopurine by up to 75% when both drugs are used concomitantly.
	Doxorubicin	Synergistic hepatic toxicity.
	Warfarin	Mercaptopurine inhibits the anticoagulant effect of warfarin; monitor PT and adjust warfarin dose accordingly.

Toxicity/Side Effects

Acute and/or Potentially Life-Threatening: Hepatotoxicity, which includes features of intrahepatic cholestasis and parenchymal cell necrosis, has been reported. A small number of deaths have been attributed to hepatic necrosis. May occur with any dosage but seems to occur more frequently when doses of 2.5 mg/kg are exceeded. Monitoring of serum transaminase levels, alkaline phosphatase, and bilirubin levels may allow early detection of hepatotoxicity. The onset of clinical jaundice, hepatomegaly, or anorexia with tenderness in the right hypochondrium are immediate indications for withholding further mercaptopurine therapy until exact etiology is identified.

Serious: Myelosuppression is most frequent side effect, which may be serious. Leukopenia, thrombocytopenia, and anemia are unavoidable in the induction phase for acute leukemia if remission is to be successful. Severe hematologic toxicity may require supportive therapies (e.g., platelet and RBC transfusions, antibiotics).

Other:
Dermatologic: Rash, hyperpigmentation, and dry, scaling skin.
GI: Nausea, vomiting, diarrhea, stomatitis, anorexia, stomach pain, glossitis, and tarry stools.
Miscellaneous: Drug fever, headache, weakness, renal toxicity, hyperuricemia, and eosinophilia.

Special Considerations

Do not take mercaptopurine with meals. Review with patient the importance of ample fluid intake, not taking more medication than prescribed, not doubling doses, and not taking missed dose. Although nausea and vomiting are mild, consider prescribing an as-needed antiemetic (e.g., phenothiazine).

Monitoring Parameters

Monitoring is recommended prior to initiation of therapy and at periodic intervals during therapy unless otherwise specified.
- CBC with differential: Recommended prior to initiation of therapy, prior to each subsequent dose, and at periodic intervals during therapy.
- Platelet count: Recommended prior to initiation of therapy, prior to each subsequent dose, and at periodic intervals during therapy.
- Hemoglobin and/or hematocrit: Recommended prior to initiation of therapy, prior to each subsequent dose, and at periodic intervals during therapy.

- Renal function tests: CrCl, actual or calculated, and/or SCr recommended prior to initiation of therapy, prior to each subsequent dose, and at periodic intervals during therapy.
- Liver function tests: ALT, AST, alkaline phosphatase, total bilirubin, LDH.
- Serum uric acid.

Indications	Mercaptopurine is indicated for remission induction and maintenance therapy of ALL. The response of this agent depends on the particular subclassification of ALL and the age of the patient (pediatric versus adult). Also used in the treatment of ANLL and non-Hodgkin's lymphoma.
Dosage Adjustment Recommendations	Dosage adjustment in renal and hepatic impairment recommended but no specific guidelines are available. In addition, mercaptopurine may have a delayed action and should be discontinued at the first sign of an abnormally large or rapid fall in leukocyte or platelet count. If subsequently the leukocyte or platelet count remains constant for two to three days or rises, treatment may be resumed.
Pharmacokinetics	Variable and incomplete absorption (16%–50%); crosses blood-brain barrier but not in appreciable amounts; 30% protein binding. Undergoes first-pass metabolism in GI mucosa and liver; degradation primarily by xanthine oxidase. Exhibits triphasic half-life and undergoes renal elimination (7%–39% as unchanged drug).
Manufacturer	Glaxo Wellcome Inc., Research Triangle Park, NC

Mesna

Other Names	Mesnex®
Classification	Uroprotectant.
Mechanism	Following IV administration, mesna is rapidly oxidized to mesna disulfide (dimesna), which remains in the intravascular compartment and is rapidly eliminated by the kidneys. In the kidney, mesna disulfide is reduced to the free thiol compound mesna, which binds with and detoxifies acrolein and other urotoxic metabolites of ifosfamide and cyclophosphamide.
Vesicant Information	Not classified as a vesicant or an irritant.
Preparation and Mixture	Mesna injection is prepared for IV administration by adding any of the following fluids to obtain a final concentration of 20 mg/ml: 5% Dextrose Injection, USP, 5% Dextrose and 0.2% Sodium Chloride for Injection, USP, 5% Dextrose and 0.33% Sodium Chloride for Injection, USP, 5% Dextrose and 0.45% Sodium Chloride for Injection, USP, Sodium Chloride for Injection, 0.9%, USP, or lactated Ringer's solution. For oral administration, the injection may be diluted in a 1:1, 1:2, 1:10, or 1:100 concentration in carbonated beverages (e.g., cola, ginger ale), juices (e.g., orange, apple), or whole milk (e.g., white, chocolate).
Administration	IV infusion over 15–30 minutes or per protocol. Injectable mesna also may be given for oral administration.

Storage and Stability	Store intact vials at controlled room temperature. Diluted solutions are physically and chemically stable at room temperature for 24 hours. Mesna drawn up in polypropylene syringes is stable for nine days at room temperature or under refrigeration. Diluted solutions for oral administration are stable for 24 hours if stored under refrigeration.
How Supplied	Supplied as 100 mg/ml in 200-mg single dose ampules and 1-g multidose vials.
Dosage	Most common regimen for mesna uroprotection is 20% w/w of the ifosfamide or cyclophosphamide dose administered intravenously 15 minutes before each ifosfamide/cyclophosphamide administration and four and eight hours after each dose of ifosfamide/cyclophosphamide. Total daily dose of mesna is equal to 60% of the total dose of the ifosfamide/ cyclophosphamide. For high-dose ifosfamide regimens, may consider dosing mesna 20% w/w of ifosfamide dose administered intravenously 15 minutes before ifosfamide administration and then at three-hour intervals after ifosfamide dose for three to six total doses; total daily dose of mesna equal to 80%–140% of the total dose of ifosfamide. Oral administration is twice the IV dose (because of limited oral bioavailability) and thus dosed at 40% w/w of the ifosfamide/cyclophosphamide dose utilizing the same four-hour interval schedule. Of note, IV mesna is the administration method of choice for the first dose before the ifosfamide/ cyclophosphamide administration; oral mesna is not recommended for the first dose. For continuous infusion mesna dosing regimens, mesna doses at least equal to those of ifosfamide or cyclophosphamide have been used.
Compatibility Information	Compatible with ifosfamide, cyclophosphamide, etoposide, potassium chloride, and bleomycin. Incompatible with carboplatin and cisplatin.
Contraindications/ Precautions	Contraindicated in patients with a known hypersensitivity to mesna or other thiol compounds.
Drug Interactions	No known drug interactions; three reported cases of increased INR in patients receiving concomitant ifosfamide/mesna and warfarin. Protime and INR should be monitored closely, as adjustments in warfarin dosage may be necessary. In addition, in vitro and in vivo animal tumor models have shown that mesna does not have any effect on the antitumor efficacy of concomitantly administered cytotoxic agents.
Toxicity/Side Effects	**Acute and/or Potentially Life-Threatening:** Allergic reactions to high-dose oral mesna have been reported in patients with autoimmune disorders. The symptoms ranged from mild hypersensitivity to systemic anaphylactic reactions. **Serious:** None noted. **Other:** GI: Nausea, vomiting, diarrhea, bad taste in mouth, and soft stools. Miscellaneous: Hypotension, malaise, headache, limb pain, rash, and itching.

Special Considerations	To maintain adequate mesna concentrations in the urinary bladder during the course of elimination of the urotoxic metabolites of ifosfamide/cyclophosphamide, repeat doses of mesna are required. Because of the disagreeable sulfur odor, mesna injection should be diluted in carbonated beverages, juices, or whole milk prior to oral ingestion. Vomiting within one hour of oral mesna ingestion should be reported to the physician; repeat dose of IV mesna should be considered.
Monitoring Parameters	Examination of urine for microscopic hematuria recommended prior to the administration of each dose of ifosfamide or cyclophosphamide.
Indications	Mesna has been shown to be effective as a prophylactic agent in reducing the incidence of ifosfamide-induced hemorrhagic cystitis.
Dosage Adjustment Recommendations	Mesna is dosed on a w/w basis of the ifosfamide or cyclophosphamide dose. When the dosage of either chemotherapeutic drug is adjusted (increased or decreased), the mesna dose should be modified accordingly.
Pharmacokinetics	Peak plasma levels occur two to three hours after administration; half-life of the parent drug approximately 0.36 hours, half-life of the mesna disulfide metabolite approximately 1.17 hours. Both mesna and mesna disulfide are excreted primarily in the urine; maximum excretion occurring at one hour after IV administration and two to three hours after oral administration.
Manufacturer	Bristol-Myers Squibb Oncology/Immunology Division, Princeton, NJ

Methotrexate

Other Names	Amethopterin, Mexate®, Folex®, Rheumatrex®
Classification	Antimetabolite; folic acid antagonist.
Mechanism	Cell-cycle S phase specific. Inhibits enzyme dihydrofolate reductase, which results in inhibition of DNA, RNA, and protein synthesis.
Vesicant Information	No extravasation necrosis reported.
Preparation and Mixture	Reconstitute the lyophylized powder with sterile water, Sodium Chloride for Injection, USP, or D_5W for injection to a final concentration of $\leq$ 25mg/ml for 20-mg and 50-mg vials and 50 mg/ml for the 1-g vial. Use preservative-free solution (e.g., lactated Ringer's, Elliott's B solution) for IT preparation.
Administration	Oral and parenteral (IV, IM, IT).
Storage and Stability	Store intact vials at room temperature and protect from light. Reconstituted solutions stable for seven days at room temperature. Further diluted solutions stable for 24 hours at room temperature.
How Supplied	Available as powder for injection in 20-mg and 1-g vials; isotonic liquid, preservative-free in 50-mg 100-mg, 200-mg, and 250-mg vials; isotonic liquid containing preservative in 50-mg and 250-mg vials.

Dosage	Dosage is determined by type of malignant disease to be treated. Conventional dose: 15–20 mg/m^2 orally twice weekly, 30–50 mg/m^2 orally or intravenously weekly, 15 mg/day for five days orally or intramuscularly every two to three weeks; intermediate dose: 50–150 mg/m^2 IVP every two to three weeks, 240 mg/m^2 IV infusion every four to seven days (with leucovorin rescue), 0.5–1g/m^2 IV infusion every two to three weeks (with leucovorin rescue); high dose: 1–12 g/m^2 IV infusion every one to three weeks (with leucovorin rescue); IT: (12 mg/m^2 or 12–15 mg in two- to five-day intervals). Usual oral doses: 10–25 mg/week; weekly dose not to exceed 50 mg.
Compatibility Information	Not compatible with fluorouracil, prednisolone sodium phosphate, and cytarabine (interferes with MTX absorption when in IV admixture).
Contraindications/ Precautions	Contraindicated in patients with a known hypersensitivity to MTX or any component. Use with caution in patients with impaired renal and liver function and preexisting profound bone marrow suppression.

Drug Interactions	**Agent**	**Effect**
	Nonsteroidal anti-inflammatory drugs (NSAIDs) and aspirin	Increase MTX effect/toxicity because of decreased renal excretion.
	Probenecid	Increase MTX effect produced by decreased renal clearance.
	Ethanol	Increase hepatotoxicity; can result in coma.
	Aminoglycosides, cyclosporine	Increase potential for nephrotoxicity.
	Procarbazine	Increase potential for nephrotoxicity.
	Phenytoin, sulfonamides, and tetracyclines	Increase effect/toxicity of MTX by displacing MTX off of plasma proteins.
	Folic acid preparations	Decrease MTX effectiveness.

Toxicity/Side Effects	**Acute and/or Potentially Life-Threatening:** Arachnoiditis manifested as a severe headache, nuchal rigidity, vomiting, and fever may occur with IT administration. In addition, a subacute toxicity may develop in the second or third week of IT therapy, consisting of motor paralysis of extremities, cranial nerve palsy, seizures, or coma. Demyelinating encephalopathy also can occur months to years after therapy. Pneumonitis associated with fever, cough, and interstitial pulmonary infiltrates; withhold MTX until symptoms resolve.
	Serious: Renal failure, azotemia, and nephropathy. Manifested by an abrupt rise in SCr and BUN and decreased urine output. Mostly associated with high-dose therapy. Prevent with aggressive IV hydration, urine alkalinization, and leucovorin rescue.
	Other:
	Dermatologic: Rash, urticaria, photosensitivity, radiation recall, alopecia, reddening of the skin, depigmentation or hyperpigmentation of the skin, and pruritus.

GI: Nausea and vomiting (emetic potential increases with increasing doses), diarrhea, anorexia, mucositis, ulcerative stomatitis (dose-limiting), and hepatic dysfunction.

Hematologic: Myelosuppression (e.g., thrombocytopenia, granulocytopenia) is dose-limiting; occurs five to seven days after therapy and usually resolves in two weeks.

Neurologic: Dizziness, headache, confusion, and drowsiness.

Miscellaneous: Hyperuricemia, cystitis, blurred vision, and arthralgia.

Special Considerations	Use cautiously in patients with impaired renal and hepatic function (see dosage adjustment recommendations). Leucovorin rescue needed with intermediate and high-dose MTX therapy (> 100 mg/m^2). Leucovorin can enhance the therapeutic effect of MTX by controlling the toxicity. Limit exposure to sunlight. Aggressive IV hydration and alkalinization of urine necessary with higher dose therapy (> 100 mg/m^2); monitor urine pH and output prior to and during administration.
Monitoring Parameters	Monitoring is recommended prior to initiation of therapy and at periodic intervals during therapy unless otherwise specified. • CBC with differential: Recommended prior to initiation of therapy, prior to each subsequent dose, and at periodic intervals during therapy. • Platelet count: Recommended prior to initiation of therapy, prior to each subsequent dose, and at periodic intervals during therapy. • Hemoglobin and/or hematocrit: Recommended prior to initiation of therapy, prior to each subsequent dose, and at periodic intervals during therapy. • Liver function tests: ALT, AST, alkaline phosphatase, total bilirubin, LDH. • CrCl determination (measured or calculated): Recommended prior to the initiation of high-dose MTX to help to determine MTX dose adjustment if necessary and aid in identifying patients with delayed MTX clearance. • SCr: Recommended prior to and every 24 hours after MTX administration to detect developing renal function impairment; an increase of > 50%–100% above baseline at 24 hours usually is associated with severe renal toxicity. • Plasma or serum MTX concentrations after high-dose therapy: Recommended at 12- to 24-hour intervals until concentration below 5×10^{-8} molar; determines dose and duration of leucovorin therapy needed to maintain rescue. • Urinary pH: Monitor prior to administration of high-dose MTX and every six hours throughout leucovorin rescue; recommend pH of > 7 prior to MTX administration and continued until serum MTX concentration < 5×10^{-8} molar to minimize risk of MTX nephropathy. • Pulmonary function tests (e.g., DLCO): Periodic evaluations if patient is symptomatic or has risk factors. • Chest x-ray: Monitor at periodic intervals in a patient at risk for pulmonary toxicity or symptomatic, particularly if not monitoring pulmonary function by DLCO. • Examination of patient's mouth for ulceration. • Stool cultures: If persistent diarrhea to rule out infectious etiology.

Indications	FDA-approved uses include ALL, meningeal leukemia, lung and breast cancer, head and neck cancer, mycosis fungoides, non-Hodgkin's lymphoma, choriocarcinoma, and osteogenic sarcoma. Off-label uses in bladder cancer and post-transplant immunosuppression.
Dosage Adjustment Recommendations	Dosage adjustments recommended in hepatic and renal dysfunction (see Appendices A and B). After higher-dose MTX therapy (>100 mg/m^2), dose of leucovorin rescue is determined by MTX serum levels (see leucovorin).
Pharmacokinetics	Oral bioavailability good. Elimination 80%–90% kidneys. Initial half-life of two to three hours; terminal half-life of 8–10 hours.
Manufacturer	Rheumatrex®, Lederle Laboratories, Pearl River, NY; Folex®, Adria Laboratories, Kalamazoo, MI; Mexate®, Bristol-Myers-Squibb Oncology/Immunology Division, Princeton, NJ

Mitomycin

Other Names	Mutamycin®, mitomycin-C
Classification	Alkylating agent; antitumor antibiotic.
Mechanism	Antibiotic produced from *Streptomyces caespitosus*. Inhibits DNA synthesis. Most active during late G$_1$ and early S phases.
Vesicant Information	Vesicant; may cause severe tissue irritation and progress to cellulitis, ulceration, and sloughing of skin. Topical dimethyl sulfoxide possible antidote.
Preparation and Mixture	Reconstitute 5-mg vial with 10 ml sterile water; 20-mg vial with 40 ml of sterile water. Set at room temperature until completely dissolved. To prepare for infusion, inject calculated dose in 100–150 ml NS, or D$_5$W.
Administration	IV or intra-arterial administration. Single agent or in combination. For infusions of 100–150 ml, infuse over 30–60 minutes or through side arm of running IV fluids. To treat bladder papillomas, instill 20–60 mg (1 mg/ml) directly into the bladder.
Storage and Stability	A purple, flocculent lyophilized powder. Reconstituted solution stable for one week at room temperature and two weeks if refrigerated.
How Supplied	5-mg, 20-mg, and 40-mg powder vial.
Dosage	Usual dose is 10–20 mg/m^2 IV as a single agent every six to eight weeks. When combined with other agents, dose at 10 mg/m^2 every six to eight weeks. HCT doses of 40–50 mg/m^2. Intra-arterial infusion dosed at 50 mg/m^2 x 1. Intravesicular instillations for bladder cancer are dosed at 20–40 mg/dose.
Compatibility Information	Compatible with NS and D$_5$W for infusion.
Contraindications/ Precautions	Contraindicated in patients with platelet count < 75,000/mm^3, leukocyte count < 3,000/mm^3, or SCr > 1.7 mg/dl or hypersensitivity to mitomycin or any component. Breast-feeding not recommended.

Drug Interactions	**Agent**	**Effect**
	Vinca alkaloids	Concomitant infusions of vincristine or vinblastine can cause severe bronchospasms and SOB.
	Doxorubicin	May enhance cardiac toxicity.

Toxicity/Side Effects

Acute and/or Potentially Life-Threatening: Acute nausea and vomiting, usually mild to moderate, seen in up to 100% of patients; occurs within one to two hours and may persist for three hours to four days after therapy. Hemolytic uremic syndrome, although uncommon (< 10%), may occur and is fatal in up to 50%. Manifests as microangiopathic hemolytic anemia, thrombocytopenia, and renal failure. Patients receiving doses > 60 mg or 50 mg/m^2 (HCT dosing) at higher risk. Interstitial pneumonitis or pulmonary fibrosis has been reported in up to 7% of patients. Manifests as dry cough and progressive dyspnea; often responsive to steroids. Cardiac failure in patients treated with doses > 30 mg/m^2.

Serious: Cumulative and dose-related (related to both total dose and schedule) myelosuppression. Moderate and severe effects on WBC and platelets, respectively. Onset and nadir three to four weeks after therapy with recovery at day 42–56. Should not be dosed earlier than every six to eight weeks.

Other:
Dermatologic: Pruritus, rash, alopecia, and discolored fingernails (purple).
GI: Stomatitis, elevated liver enzymes, diarrhea, and anorexia.
Neurologic: Malaise, fever, and peripheral neuropathy.
Miscellaneous: Thrombophlebitis and permanent sterility.

Special Considerations

Extravasation precaution; solution is purple in color; myelosuppression may be cumulative; if spill occurs, treat with 5% sodium hypochlorite or 1% potassium permanganate. Do not exceed cumulative doses of > 50 mg/m^2.

Monitoring Parameters

Monitoring is recommended prior to initiation of therapy and at periodic intervals during therapy unless otherwise specified.
- CBC with differential: Recommended prior to initiation of therapy, prior to each subsequent dose, and at periodic intervals during therapy.
- Platelet count: Recommended prior to initiation of therapy, prior to each subsequent dose, and at periodic intervals during therapy.
- Hemoglobin and/or hematocrit: Recommended prior to initiation of therapy, prior to each subsequent dose, and at periodic intervals during therapy.
- Liver function tests: ALT, AST, alkaline phosphatase, total bilirubin, LDH.
- Pulmonary function tests (e.g., DLCO): Periodic evaluations if patient symptomatic or has risk factors.
- Chest x-ray: Monitor at periodic intervals in a patient at risk for pulmonary toxicity or symptomatic, particularly if not monitoring pulmonary function by DLCO.
- Renal function tests: CrCl, actual or calculated, and/or SCr recommended prior to initiation of therapy, prior to each subsequent dose, and at periodic intervals during therapy.

Indications	FDA-approved for the use in pancreatic and gastric carcinoma. Off-label uses include breast, colorectal, lung, head and neck, and cervical carcinoma and CML.
Dosage Adjustment Recommendations	Dose reduction necessary for renal impairment (see Appendix B) as well as per leukocyte and platelet nadir; leukocyte nadir of 2,000–2,999/mm^3, platelet nadir of 25,000–74,999/mm^3: dose at 70% of prior dose; leukocyte nadir < 2,000/mm^3, platelets < 25,000/mm^3: dose at 50% of prior dose.
Pharmacokinetics	Metabolized primarily by the liver with 10% of unchanged drug eliminated renally. Initial half-life of 5–15 minutes with terminal half-life of 50 minutes. Does not cross the blood-brain barrier. Drug concentrates in lung, kidneys, tongue, muscle, and heart tissue.
Manufacturer	Bristol-Myers Squibb Oncology/Immunology Division, Princeton, NJ

Mitoxantrone hydrochloride

Other Names	Novantrone®
Classification	Anthracenedione.
Mechanism	Activity in late S phase but not cell-cycle specific. Inhibits DNA and RNA synthesis.
Vesicant Information	The reports are mixed as to whether mitoxantrone is a vesicant or nonvesicant. Administer with caution as if a vesicant.
Preparation and Mixture	Compatible with D$_5$W, NS, and lactated Ringer's solution. Dilute in at least 50 ml of solution.
Administration	Intermittent infusion or continuous infusion. Use caution when infusing; avoid extravasation. Infuse in 50 ml solution over 5–10 minutes. IVP over three to five minutes through a side arm flowing compatible IV solution. DO NOT administer IV bolus over less than three minutes.
Storage and Stability	Store intact vials at room temperature or under refrigeration. No preservatives. Chemically stable for years at room temperature, refrigerated, or frozen. Stable for up to two weeks when mixed in D$_5$W or lactated Ringer's solutions at room temperature.
How Supplied	Sterile vial solution. 10, 12.5, or 15 ml of a 2-mg/ml solution; yielding 20-mg, 25-mg, and 30-mg doses.
Dosage	For ANLL: 12 mg/m^2 daily for three days (total dose 36 mg/m^2) as a single agent.
Compatibility Information	Incompatible with heparin-containing solutions. Compatible with hydrocortisone at 2 mg/ml times 24 hours, ondansetron, and cytarabine.
Contraindications/ Precautions	Contraindicated in patients with a known hypersensitivity. Risk versus benefit should be considered in patients with preexisting myelosuppression or breast-feeding women. No IT use.

Drug Interactions	Concomitant use of cytarabine may yield enhanced toxic effects of mitoxantrone.
Toxicity/Side Effects	**Acute and/or Potentially Life-Threatening:** CHF, although incidence much less than with other anthracyclines. Predisposing factors include prior anthracycline use, history of cardiovascular disease, and mediastinal irradiation. Risk of developing cardiotoxicity is < 3% if cumulative dose < 100–120 mg/m² in patients with risk factors or < 160 mg/m² in patients with no predisposing factors. **Serious:** Seizures, tumor lysis syndrome in ANLL patients, and renal failure. **Other:** Dermatologic: Alopecia, pruritus, and skin desquamation. GI: Nausea and vomiting (moderately emetogenic), GI bleeding, stomatitis, diarrhea, and abdominal pain. Genitourinary: Blue-green discoloration of urine. Hematologic: Mildly myelosuppressive; granulocytopenia, and thrombocytopenia (onset 9–10 days, nadir 14 days, recovery 21 days). Neurologic: Headache and fever. Miscellaneous: SOB, cough, conjunctivitis, and phlebitis.
Special Considerations	Patient will have blue-green urine 24–48 hours after infusion. Occasionally blue color in sclera. Precipitate may form when refrigerated; will redissolve when warmed to room temperature. Cumulative cardiac toxicity reported, especially in patients who have received prior anthracycline agents.
Monitoring Parameters	Monitoring is recommended prior to initiation of therapy and at periodic intervals during therapy unless otherwise specified. • CBC with differential: Recommended prior to initiation of therapy, prior to each subsequent dose, and at periodic intervals during therapy. • Platelet count: Recommended prior to initiation of therapy, prior to each subsequent dose, and at periodic intervals during therapy. • Hemoglobin and/or hematocrit: Recommended prior to initiation of therapy, prior to each subsequent dose, and at periodic intervals during therapy. • Liver function tests: ALT, AST, alkaline phosphatase, total bilirubin, LDH. • Renal function tests: CrCl, actual or calculated, and/or SCr recommended prior to initiation of each dose, and at periodic intervals during therapy if at risk for tumor-lysis syndrome. • Cardiac function tests: MUGA or LVEF recommended as baseline in patients with risk factors and at periodic intervals throughout therapy, as well as long-term follow-up evaluations. • Site inspection: For stinging and burning during peripheral line or implanted port infusion.
Indications	FDA-approved for the treatment of AML or APL, as well as acute erythroid leukemia. Off-label uses include non-Hodgkin's lymphoma and hepatic and breast cancer.
Dosage Adjustment Recommendations	Caution in patients with marrow suppression; start with low initial dose (12 mg/m²). Dose reduce or withhold if severe marrow suppression.

Pharmacokinetics	Concentrates in the liver, kidney, thyroid, heart, RBCs, and pleural fluid. Metabolized by the liver. Half-life of five days. Excretion primarily biliary/fecal with 11% of unchanged drug excreted renally.
Manufacturer	Immunex Corporation, Seattle, WA

Paclitaxel

Other Names	Taxol®
Classification	Antimicrotubule; yew tree derivative.
Mechanism	Stabilizes microtubules, thereby inhibiting the microtubular reorganization necessary for mitotic division and other cellular function.
Vesicant Information	Irritant.
Preparation and Mixture	Use non-PVC administration sets. Prepare in glass, polyolefin, or polypropylene containers to prevent leaching of di-(2-ethylhexyl) phthalate (DEHP), found in PVC sets. Dilute in NS, D_5W, D_5NS.
Administration	IV. Infuse through a 0.22-micron filter with non-PVC tubing. Premedicate with H_2 blocker, diphenhydramine, and corticosteroid. Infusion may be over 3–96 hours. Intraperitoneal use of 175 mg/m^2 reported in studies.
Storage and Stability	Reconstituted solution stable at temperature between 2°–25°C (36°–77°F) for 27 hours.
How Supplied	Available in 30-mg/5-ml, 100-mg/16.7-ml, and 300-mg/50-ml multidose vials.
Dosage	Common dosing regimens include 135 mg/m^2 IV over 3 or 24 hours or 175 mg/m^2 IV over 3 hours. Weekly dosing regimens also common.
Compatibility Information	Compatible with IV fluids of NS, D_5W, D_5NS, and D_5 Ringer's lactate.
Contraindications/ Precautions	Patients with known sensitivity or reaction to paclitaxel or any component (Cremophor®, Basf Aktiengesellschaft, Ludwigshafen, Germany).
Drug Interactions	**Agent** / **Effect** Cisplatin — Myelosuppression more profound when cisplatin given prior to paclitaxel. Ketoconazole — Possible inhibition of metabolism.
Toxicity/Side Effects	**Acute and/or Potentially Life-Threatening:** Hypersensitivity reactions, including life-threatening anaphylaxis, bronchospasm, dyspnea, edema, urticaria, chills, and fever, have been reported. Patients should be kept under observation for one hour after administration of the drug and resuscitation equipment and other agents necessary to treat anaphylaxis (e.g., antihistamines, oxygen, epinephrine, IV steroids) should be available.

Serious: Significant peripheral neuropathies may develop; dose-dependent and incidence increases with increasing cumulative doses. Dose reduction necessary if neuropathy is severe.

Other:
Cardiovascular: Hypotension, bradycardia, arrhythmias, and abnormal ECG.
Dermatologic: Alopecia, skin redness, pain at the injection site, and flushing.
GI: Mild nausea and vomiting, diarrhea, elevated liver function tests, and mucositis.
Hematologic: Myelosuppression is dose- and schedule-dependent (greater incidence with longer infusion times); significant neutropenia (nadir 7–10 days, recovery by day 21) and anemia reported; thrombocytopenia less common.
Neurologic: Ataxia, arthralgia, and myalgia.
Miscellaneous: Phlebitis.

Special Considerations	Premedicate with corticosteroids (dexamethasone 20 mg po or IV 12 and 6 hours prior to each dose), H$_2$ antagonists (famotidine 20 mg IV 30–60 minutes prior to each dose), and H$_1$ antagonists (diphenhydramine 50 mg IV 30–60 minutes prior to each dose) to minimize or prevent hypersensitivity reactions.
Monitoring Parameters	Monitoring is recommended prior to initiation of therapy and at periodic intervals during therapy unless otherwise specified. • CBC with differential: Recommended prior to initiation of therapy, prior to each subsequent dose, and at periodic intervals during therapy. • Platelet count: Recommended prior to initiation of therapy, prior to each subsequent dose, and at periodic intervals during therapy. • Hemoglobin and/or hematocrit: Recommended prior to initiation of therapy, prior to each subsequent dose, and at periodic intervals during therapy. • Liver function tests: ALT, AST, alkaline phosphatase, total bilirubin, LDH. • Renal function tests: CrCl, actual or calculated, and/or SCr recommended prior to initiation of each dose. • Cardiac function tests: MUGA or LVEF recommended as baseline and periodically in patients with significant cardiac risk factors. • Vital signs: Monitoring recommended prior to, during, and immediately after each drug administration.
Indications	FDA-approved uses include the first-line treatment in combination with cisplatin of patients with advanced ovarian carcinoma, metastatic breast cancer that has failed standard anthracycline therapy and in the first-line treatment in combination with cisplatin of non-small cell lung cancer in patients who are not candidates for potentially curative surgery and/or radiotherapy. In addition, paclitaxel is approved for adjuvant treatment of node-positive breast cancer administered sequentially to standard doxorubicin-containing combination chemotherapy. Paclitaxel also is indicated as second-line treatment of AIDS-related KS. Off-label uses include the treatment of melanoma, gastric cancer, and acute leukemia.

Dosage Adjustment Recommendations	Dose reduction of 20% recommended for severe neutropenia and peripheral neuropathy. Dose reductions also recommended in the setting of hepatic impairment (see Appendix A).
Pharmacokinetics	Limited penetration into CSF, 97.5% bound to plasma proteins. Metabolized and excreted via the liver and biliary tract. Terminal half-life of 6–48 hours.
Manufacturer	Bristol-Myers Squibb Oncology/Immunology Division, Princeton, NJ

Pegaspargase

Other Names	Oncaspar®, PEG-L-asparaginase
Classification	Miscellaneous.
Mechanism	Modified version of the enzyme L-asparaginase. The enzyme L-asparaginase is modified by covalently conjugating units of monomethoxypolyethylene glycol (PEG) to the enzyme, thereby rendering the modified product less antigenic and extending the plasma half-life, allowing for lower doses and less frequent administration. L-asparaginase is an enzyme that deaminates asparagine to aspartic acid and ammonia, thereby depriving tumor cells of the amino acid for protein synthesis.
Vesicant Information	Not classified as a vesicant or an irritant, although local injection site hypersensitivity has been reported.
Preparation and Mixture	When administered intravenously, pegaspargase may be diluted in 100 ml Sodium Chloride for Injection, 0.9%, USP, or 5% Dextrose Injection, USP, into a free-flowing IV line.
Administration	The manufacturer recommends pegaspargase be administered by the IM route if possible; however, may be administered intramuscularly as an IV infusion over one to two hours. When pegaspargase is administered, no more than 2 ml should be injected at a single site.
Storage and Stability	Store intact vials under refrigeration; do not freeze. Freezing destroys activity, which cannot be detected visually. Do not use if cloudy or if precipitate is present. Do not use if stored at room temperature for greater than 48 hours. Use only one dose per vial; do not re-enter the vial. Discard any unused portion. Diluted IV solutions are stable at room temperature for 48 hours. Do not filter solution.
How Supplied	Supplied as a 5-ml single-use vial containing 750 IU/ml of pegaspargase in a clear, colorless, phosphate buffered solution.
Dosage	Pegaspargase administered IM or IV is dosed at 2,500 IU/m^2 every 14 days as a component of a combination chemotherapy regimen or as a single agent.
Compatibility Information	No compatibility information available.
Contraindications/ Precautions	Contraindicated in patients with pancreatitis or a history of pancreatitis, patients who have had significant hemorrhagic events associated with prior L-asparaginase therapy, or in patients who have had serious allergic

reactions (e.g., generalized urticaria, bronchospasm, laryngeal edema, hypotension) or other unacceptable toxicity to pegaspargase therapy. Risk versus benefit should be considered in patients with a history of bleeding disorders, existing or recent chicken pox or herpes zoster infection, diabetes mellitus, or hepatic function impairment or in patients receiving anticoagulant therapy.

Drug Interactions	**Agent**	**Effect**
	Anticoagulant therapy (e.g., aspirin, NSAIDs, dipyridamole, warfarin, heparin)	Increase risk of bleeding complications because of imbalances of coagulation factors in patients receiving pegaspargase.
	MTX	Pegaspargase antagonizes the effects of MTX when administered before MTX.

Toxicity/Side Effects

Acute and/or Potentially Life-Threatening: Hypersensitivity reactions, including life-threatening anaphylaxis, bronchospasm, dyspnea, edema, urticaria, chills, and fever, have been reported. Reactions may be acute or delayed and are especially likely in patients with known hypersensitivity to other forms of L-asparaginase. Patients should be kept under observation for one hour after the administration of the drug, and resuscitation equipment and other agents necessary to treat anaphylaxis (e.g., antihistamines, oxygen, epinephrine, IV steroids) should be available. Coagulation disorders leading to clinical hemorrhage (e.g., disseminated intravascular coagulation, hypofibrinogenemia, prolonged PTs, prolonged partial thromboplastin times [PPTs], decreased antithrombin III) or thrombosis also may occur, which may be fatal. Pancreatitis, sometimes fulminant and fatal, has occurred.

Serious: A variety of liver function abnormalities have been reported, including elevations in AST, ALT, and bilirubin; jaundice, ascites, and hypoalbuminemia have occurred clinically. Usually reversible with drug discontinuation but has been severe, leading to liver failure. Neurologically, status epilepticus, temporal lobe seizures, coma, severe confusion, disorientation, and paresthesia have occurred. These effects usually have reversed spontaneously after treatment discontinuation. Renal dysfunction and renal failure also have been reported.

Other:
Dermatologic: Rash and erythema.
GI: Nausea and vomiting, anorexia, constipation, diarrhea, flatulence, and abdominal pain.
Hematologic: Leukopenia (mild, onset by day 7, nadir by day 14, recovery by day 21), pancytopenia, and thrombocytopenia.
Miscellaneous: Edema, arthralgia, dyspnea, pain, fever, chills, malaise, hypotension, tachycardia, and local injection site hypersensitivity.

Special Considerations

Hypersensitivity reactions, including life-threatening anaphylaxis, may occur during therapy. Therefore, appropriate precautions should be taken prior to pegaspargase administration to prevent allergic or other unwanted reactions, particularly in patients with a previous known hypersensitivity to L-asparaginase. All patients should be observed for one hour

	after pegaspargase administration. Appropriate agents for maintaining an airway and treatment of a hypersensitivity reaction (e.g., epinephrine, fluids, oxygen, antihistamines, IV corticosteroids) should be readily available.
Monitoring Parameters	Monitoring is recommended prior to initiation of therapy and at periodic intervals during therapy unless otherwise specified. • CBC with differential: Recommended prior to initiation of therapy, prior to each subsequent dose, and at periodic intervals during therapy. • Platelet count: Recommended prior to initiation of therapy, prior to each subsequent dose, and at periodic intervals during therapy. • Serum amylase: Recommended at periodic intervals during therapy. • Liver function tests: ALT, AST, alkaline phosphatase, total bilirubin, LDH. • Fibrinogen, PT, and PTT. • Blood glucose determinations. • Monitor for onset of abdominal pain and mental status changes.
Indications	Pegaspargase is indicated in patients with acute lymphoblastic leukemia who require L-asparaginase in their treatment regimen but have developed hypersensitivity to the native forms of L-asparaginase; generally used in combination. Use as a single agent should only be undertaken when multiagent chemotherapy is judged to be inappropriate for the patient.
Dosage Adjustment Recommendations	NCI Common Toxicity Criteria Grade 2–4 reactions are considered dose-limiting toxicities and require discontinuation of asparaginase.
Pharmacokinetics	L-asparaginase levels detectable for up to 15 days after IV administration; half-life ranges from approximately three to five days; systemically degraded, only trace amounts found in urine.
Manufacturer	Rhône-Poulenc Rorer Pharmaceuticals Inc., Collegeville, PA

Pentostatin

Other Names	NiPent®, 2'-deoxycoformycin, DCF, deoxycoformycin
Classification	Antimetabolite; purine analogue.
Mechanism	Inhibits adenosine deaminase; prevents adenosine deaminase from controlling intracellular adenosine levels through irreversible deamination of deoxyadenosine and adenosine. Adenosine exhibits greatest activity in lymphoid tissue.
Vesicant Information	Not classified as a vesicant or an irritant.
Preparation and Mixture	Transfer 5 ml of Sterile Water for Injection, USP, to the vial containing pentostatin, and mix thoroughly to obtain complete dissolution yielding a concentration of 2 mg/ml. May be further diluted with 25 or 50 ml of 5% Dextrose Injection, USP, or Sodium Chloride for Injection, 0.9%, USP.
Administration	IV by rapid injection over three to five minutes or diluted into larger volume and given over 20–30 minutes.

Storage and Stability	Store intact vials under refrigeration. Reconstituted and diluted solutions may be stored at room temperature exposed to ambient light and should be used within eight hours. Some data suggest solutions of pentostatin are stable at room temperature for 24 hours diluted in 5% Dextrose Injection, USP or 48 hours diluted in Sodium Chloride for Injection, 0.9%, USP.
How Supplied	Supplied as a sterile, lyophilized white to off-white powder in single-dose vials containing 10 mg of pentostatin.
Dosage	Recommended dosage is 4 mg/m^2 every other week administered as a bolus injection or IV infusion. It is recommended that patients receive hydration with 500–1,000 ml of 5% dextrose in 0.45% NS or equivalent before pentostatin administration. An additional 500 ml of 5% Dextrose Injection, USP, or equivalent should be administered after pentostatin administration.
Compatibility Information	Compatible with D$_5$W, lactated Ringer's Solution, and NS. Information also available on compatibility of pentostatin and fludarabine, ondansetron, paclitaxel, and sargramostim.
Contraindications/ Precautions	Contraindicated in patients who have demonstrated hypersensitivity. Risk versus benefit should be considered in patients with preexisting bone marrow depression, active infection, recent or existing chicken pox or herpes zoster infection, history of gout or uric acid nephropathy, renal function impairment, or cardiovascular function impairment.

Drug Interactions

Agent	Effect
Allopurinol	Concomitant use may cause increased incidence of skin rash, although causality with the combination has not been established.
Fludarabine	Concurrent use not recommended because of possible increased risk of fatal pulmonary toxicity.
Vidarabine	Biochemical studies have shown an enhancement of vidarabine's effects by pentostatin, which could result in an increase in toxicity of both agents.

Toxicity/Side Effects

Acute and/or Potentially Life-Threatening: Cardiac effects, including angina, myocardial infarction, CHF, and acute arrhythmias have been reported. These cardiac events tend to occur in patients with preexisting cardiovascular conditions; fatalities have occurred. In addition, high doses of pentostatin have been associated with CNS toxicity, including seizures, coma, and death. Infections (bacterial, viral, or fungal) may occur even in the absence of leukopenia and may be life-threatening.

Serious: Although hepatic enzyme elevations usually are transient and asymptomatic, severe hepatotoxicity has occurred requiring withdrawal of pentostatin. Maculopapular skin rashes are occasionally severe and may worsen with continued treatment, necessitating withdrawal of therapy.

Other:
Dermatologic: Dry skin, eczema, and pruritus.

GI: Nausea and vomiting, anorexia, diarrhea, flatulence, constipation, stomatitis, and weight loss.

Hematologic: Leukopenia, thrombocytopenia, and anemia.

Neurologic: Fever, headache, fatigue, amnesia, ataxia, neuralgia, confusion, dizziness, insomnia, anxiety, depression, and paresthesia.

Pulmonary: Bronchitis, dyspnea, lung edema, pneumonia, pharyngitis, rhinitis, and laryngeal edema.

Miscellaneous: Myalgia, cough, allergic reaction, chest pain, peripheral edema, dysuria, thrombophlebitis, arthralgia, weakness, vision changes, and renal toxicity.

Special Considerations	Nausea and/or vomiting may occur; antiemetic prophylaxis with a serotonin antagonist in combination with dexamethasone recommended. In addition, it is recommended that antiemetics (e.g., metoclopramide in combination with dexamethasone or prochlorperazine) be prescribed for 48–72 hours after pentostatin administration. Hydration with 500–1,000 ml of 5% dextrose in 0.45% NS or equivalent before pentostatin administration is recommended. An additional 500 ml of 5% dextrose, equivalent should be administered after pentostatin administration. High-dose pentostatin is not recommended because of risk of renal, hepatic, pulmonary, and CNS toxicity. Pentostatin appears to have immunosuppressant activity; significant reductions in T and B cells occur during treatment and up to months to years after treatment. Patients are at increased risk for infection.
Monitoring Parameters	Monitoring is recommended prior to initiation of therapy and at periodic intervals during therapy unless otherwise specified. • CBC with differential: Recommended prior to initiation of therapy, prior to each subsequent dose, and at periodic intervals during therapy. • Platelet count: Recommended prior to initiation of therapy, prior to each subsequent dose, and at periodic intervals during therapy. • Hemoglobin and/or hematocrit: Recommended prior to initiation of therapy, prior to each subsequent dose, and at periodic intervals during therapy. • Renal function tests: CrCl, actual or calculated, and/or SCr recommended prior to initiation of therapy, prior to each subsequent dose, and at periodic intervals during therapy. • Serum uric acid.
Indications	Indicated as single-agent treatment for both untreated and alpha-interferon-refractory hairy cell leukemia patients with active disease, as defined by clinically significant anemia, neutropenia, thrombocytopenia, or disease-related symptoms. Also used in the treatment of ALL and CLL and cutaneous T cell lymphoma.
Dosage Adjustment Recommendations	If CNS toxicity or severe skin rash occurs, it is recommended that pentostatin be withheld or discontinued. If elevated SCr occurs, it is recommended that pentostatin be withheld and CrCl determined. Insufficient data are available to recommend a starting dose or a subsequent dose for patients with renal function impairment (CrCl < 60 ml/minute). Patients with impaired renal function should be treated only when the potential benefit justifies the potential risk. Dosage reduction in this setting is recommended.

No dosage adjustment is necessary in patients starting therapy with anemia, thrombocytopenia, or neutropenia; however, if during therapy, the neutrophil count falls below 200 cells/mm^3 in a patient whose neutrophil count was > 500 cells/mm^3 initially, therapy should be withheld until counts have recovered to predose levels.

Pharmacokinetics	Distributes rapidly to body tissues. Low protein binding. Crosses blood-brain barrier and achieves CSF levels 10%–12.5% of serum concentrations within 24 hours. Half-life of 5–15 hours with renal impairment prolonging plasma half-life. Eliminated primarily renally with 50%–96% recovered in the urine within 24 hours.
Manufacturer	Supergen, Inc., Pleasanton, CA

Plicamycin

Other Names	Mithracin®, mithramycin
Classification	Miscellaneous; antidote, hypercalcemia.
Mechanism	Antineoplastic mechanism unknown; however, it has been shown that plicamycin forms a complex with DNA in the presence of magnesium or other divalent cations, thereby inhibiting DNA-dependent or DNA-directed RNA synthesis. In addition, plicamycin is a potent osteoclast inhibitor; inhibits bone resorption; may inhibit parathyroid hormone's effect on osteoclasts.
Vesicant Information	Classified as a vesicant. If extravasation occurs, leave needle in place, aspirate any residual drug and blood in IV tubing, needle, and suspected infiltration site. Remove the needle. May consider edetate calcium disodium (EDTA) therapy, although efficacy not established. Apply ice pack to area for 20–30 minutes every six hours for first 24–48 hours.
Preparation and Mixture	Dilute powder with 4.9 ml of sterile water for injection to yield a final concentration of 500 mcg/ml. Shake to dissolve. For IV infusion, the dose should be further diluted in 1,000 ml of 5% Dextrose Injection, USP, or Sodium Chloride for Injection, 0.9%, USP.
Administration	For IV infusion administered over four to six hours. May be administered as a direct IVP injection over 20–30 minutes but is not recommended, as it may be associated with a higher incidence and greater severity of GI toxicities.
Storage and Stability	Store intact vials under refrigeration; vials are stable at room temperature for up to three months. Reconstituted solutions are stable at room temperature for 24 hours and under refrigeration for 48 hours. Diluted solutions are stable at room temperature for 24 hours.
How Supplied	Supplied in single-use vials as a freeze-dried preparation containing 2,500 mcg of plicamycin.
Dosage	Common regimens include 15–25 mcg/kg/day for 8–10 days (testicular cancer); 15 mcg/kg once daily for 10 days (Paget's disease); 25 mcg/kg every other day for three weeks (blastic chronic granulocytic leukemia).

Additional course of therapy may be administered at monthly intervals. In the treatment of hypercalcemia, 25 mcg/kg as a single dose repeated in 48 hours if no response, daily for three days, or every other day for three to eight doses; may be repeated at intervals of one week or more until desired effect has been achieved.

Compatibility Information	Compatible with D_5W, NS, and sterile water for injection.
Contraindications/ Precautions	Contraindicated in patients with thrombocytopenia, thrombocytopathy, coagulation disorder, or an increase in susceptibility to bleeding from other causes. Mithramycin should not be administered to any patient with impairment of bone marrow function. Plicamycin is contraindicated in women who are or may become pregnant. In addition, risk versus benefit should be considered in patients with a recent or existing chicken pox or herpes zoster infection or patients with severe renal and/or hepatic function impairment.

Drug Interactions	**Agent**	**Effect**
	Anticoagulants, heparin, thrombolytics, NSAIDs, aspirin, dipyridamole, dextran, sulfinpyrazone, valproic acid	Concurrent use of any of these agents with plicamycin may increase the risk of hemorrhage.
	Calcium-containing preparations or vitamin D	Concurrent use with plicamycin may antagonize the calcium antagonist effect of plicamycin.
	Hepatotoxic agents	Concurrent use may increase risk of hepatotoxicity.
	Nephrotoxic agents	Concurrent use may increase risk of nephrotoxicity.

Toxicity/Side Effects	**Acute and/or Potentially Life-Threatening:** Hemorrhagic diathesis, or coagulopathy, because of clotting factor abnormalities and thrombocytopenia, occurs occasionally and may be fatal; incidence more frequent with doses > 30 mcg/kg/day and/or more than 10 doses. May consist of a single or several episodes of epistaxis and progress no further or may progress to more widespread hemorrhage. Facial flushing, epistaxis, and a prolonged PT are frequent signs of this syndrome. Associated drug-related mortality is approximately 1.6% with significantly higher mortality with higher doses of plicamycin. Monitor PT, PTT, AST, and ALT through course of therapy. An acute adverse drug reaction, nausea and/or vomiting, occurs within one to four hours of administration and may continue for 24 hours. Incidence and severity of GI side effects may increase with too rapid a rate of IV administration.
	Serious: Renal toxicity, manifested by proteinuria, elevated SCr levels, and azotemia.
	Other: Dermatologic: Alopecia, facial flushing, acneiform skin rash, hyperpigmentation, and toxic epidermal necrolysis.

Endocrine: Electrolyte abnormalities (e.g., hypocalcemia, hypophosphatemia, hypokalemia, hypomagnesemia).

GI: Anorexia, stomatitis, and diarrhea.

Hematologic: Leukopenia and anemia occur infrequently.

Miscellaneous: Fever, headache, weakness, lethargy, pain and soreness or swelling at injection site, depression, malaise, and drowsiness.

Special Considerations	Plicamycin is moderately to highly emetogenic, depending on dose and schedule; antiemetic prophylaxis consisting of a serotonin antagonist in combination with dexamethasone is warranted. An as-needed antiemetic (e.g., prochlorperazine) also is recommended, as nausea and/or vomiting may persist up to 24 hours. Rapid direct IV injection should be avoided because it may be associated with a greater incidence and severity of GI side effects. Consider plicamycin treatment in cases of hypercalcemia or hyperuricemia unresponsive to conventional treatment.
Monitoring Parameters	Monitoring is recommended prior to initiation of therapy and at periodic intervals during therapy unless otherwise specified. • CBC with differential: Recommended prior to initiation of therapy, prior to each subsequent dose, and at periodic intervals during therapy. • Platelet count: Recommended prior to initiation of therapy, prior to each subsequent dose, and at periodic intervals during therapy. • Hemoglobin and/or hematocrit: Recommended prior to initiation of therapy, prior to each subsequent dose, and at periodic intervals during therapy. • PT, PTT, and/or bleeding time. • Serum chemistry panel (with particular attention to calcium, potassium, and phosphorous). • Renal function tests: CrCl, actual or calculated, and/or SCr recommended prior to initiation of therapy, prior to each subsequent dose, and at periodic intervals during therapy. • Liver function tests: ALT, AST, alkaline phosphatase, total bilirubin, LDH.
Indications	Indicated in the treatment of carefully selected hospitalized patients with malignant tumors of the testis in whom successful treatment by surgery and/or radiation therapy is impossible. Also, on the basis of limited clinical experience, it may be considered in the treatment of certain symptomatic patients with hypercalcemia and hyperuricemia associated with a variety of advanced neoplasms. Plicamycin also used in the treatment of Paget's disease.
Dosage Adjustment Recommendations	Plicamycin requires dosage adjustment in patients with renal function impairment (see Appendix B). It also is recommended to reduce dose of plicamycin to 12.5 mcg/kg/day in the treatment of hypercalcemia in patients with hepatic dysfunction. The occurrence of thrombocytopenia or a significant prolongation of the PT or bleeding time is an indication for the termination of therapy.
Pharmacokinetics	Concentrated in the Kupffer cells of the liver, in renal tubular cells, and along formed bone surfaces. It may localize in areas of bone resorption. Crosses the blood-brain barrier and enters the CSF. Onset of action for decreasing calcium levels is 24 hours with peak effect seen within 48–72

	hours. Primarily eliminated renally with 90% of drug excreted in the urine within 24 hours.
Manufacturer	Bayer Corporation Pharmaceutical Division, West Haven, CT

Procarbazine

Other Names	Matulane®
Classification	Alkylating agent; miscellaneous.
Mechanism	Unclear; thought to affect preformed DNA, RNA, and protein synthesis; cause chromosomal breakage, and inhibit methylation of RNA.
Vesicant Information	Not classified as a vesicant or an irritant. Procarbazine is commercially available as an oral product.
Preparation and Mixture	No preparation or admixture necessary. Procarbazine is commercially available as an oral product.
Administration	Oral.
Storage and Stability	Store below 40°C (104°F), preferably between 15°–30°C (59°–86°F) unless otherwise specified. Drug will decompose if exposed to moisture. Store in a tight, light-resistant container. Protect from light. Capsules are generally stable at room temperature for two years.
How Supplied	Supplied as capsules containing 50 mg procarbazine hydrochloride.
Dosage	As a single-agent in the treatment of Hodgkin's lymphoma, 2–4 mg/kg/day rounded to the nearest 50 mg given in single or divided doses for seven days, then 4–6 mg/kg/day until leukopenia (< 4,000/mm^3), thrombocytopenia (< 100,000/mm^3), or maximum response occurs. When maximum response is obtained, maintenance therapy of 1–2 mg/kg/day is recommended. In MOPP (mechlorethamine, Oncovin®, procarbazine, prednisone) chemotherapy, dosed at 100 mg/m^2/day on days 1–14 of a 28-day cycle. All doses are based on actual body weight; however, the estimated lean body weight is used if patient is obese or if a weight gain has occured because of edema.
Compatibility Information	Not applicable. Procarbazine is commercially available as an oral product.
Contraindications/ Precautions	Contraindicated in patients with known hypersensitivity to the drug or inadequate marrow reserve, as demonstrated by bone marrow aspiration. Risk versus benefit should be considered in patients with cardiac arrhythmias, cerebrovascular or cardiovascular disease, coronary insufficiency, infection, existing or recent chicken pox or herpes zoster infection, hepatic or renal function impairment (dosage reduction recommended; use not recommended in severe function impairment), severe or frequent headaches, bone marrow depression, paranoid schizophrenia, and parkinsonism. In addition, caution should be used in patients with diabetes mellitus (insulin or oral hypoglycemic requirement may be altered) or epilepsy (pattern or epileptiform seizures may be changed) and in patients

who have undergone sympathectomy (may be more sensitive to the hypotensive effects of procarbazine).

Drug Interactions	The following drug interactions have been selected based on clinical relevance and importance; list is not inclusive. Refer to other sources for more detailed information.

Agent	Effect
Alcohol	Concurrent use with procarbazine may result in a disulfiram-like reaction (e.g., nausea, vomiting, sweating, headache, respiratory difficulties, hypotension, flushing) and additive CNS depression and postural hypotension; also, beer, ale, and wine may contain tyramine, which may induce a hypertensive crisis.
Barbiturates, narcotics, phenothiazines, and other CNS depressants	Concomitant use may potentiate CNS depression.
Sympathomimetic agents (e.g., epinephrine, amphetamines), tricyclic antidepressants (refer to individual drug package insert), fluoxetine, and foods containing tyramine (e.g., beer, yogurt, yeast, wine, cheese, pickled herring, chicken liver, bananas)	Concurrent use may cause hypertensive crisis, intracranial bleeding, or headache.

Toxicity/Side Effects	**Acute and/or Potentially Life-Threatening:** Hypertensive crisis manifested by severe chest pain, severe headache, fast or slow heart beat, increased sweating, increased sensitivity to light, and, possibly, with fever or cold, clammy skin. In addition, procarbazine is a moderately to highly emetogenic agent with severe acute nausea and vomiting occurring frequently; may be dose-limiting. Onset is within 24 hours with a variable duration.

Serious: CNS manifestations commonly occur and include mental depression, hallucinations, manic reactions, nightmares, insomnia, disorientation, seizures, confusion, and CNS stimulation.

Other:
Dermatologic: Alopecia, hyperpigmentation, pruritus, dermatitis, and hypersensitivity rash.
Endocrine: Amenorrhea and disulfiram-like reaction.
GI: Anorexia, abdominal pain, stomatitis, constipation, diarrhea, and dysphagia.
Hematologic: Myelosuppressive; may be dose-limiting; leukopenia, thrombocytopenia, and anemia; onset within two weeks, nadir at approximately 21 days and recovery at day 28; hemolytic anemia.
Neurologic: Headache, nervousness, irritability, paresthesia, decreased reflexes, neuropathy, foot drop, tremors, and insomnia. |

	Miscellaneous: Weakness, arthralgia, myalgia, nystagmus, pleural effusion, cough, diplopia, photophobia, flu-like syndrome, and second malignancies.
Special Considerations	Avoid tyramine-containing foods, alcoholic beverages, alcohol-containing products, over-the-counter cough and cold medicines, and other medications unless prescribed. Treatment of hypertensive crisis includes discontinuation of procarbazine, administration of phentolamine to lower blood pressure, and application of external cooling if fever present. Caution must be exercised for up to 14 days after discontinuation of procarbazine; during this period, food and drug contraindications must be observed. Procarbazine is moderately to highly emetogenic. Premedication with a serotonin antagonist with dexamethasone is warranted. Avoid the use of phenothiazines. Procarbazine may impair judgment and coordination. Avoid prolonged exposure to sun.
Monitoring Parameters	Monitoring is recommended prior to initiation of therapy and at periodic intervals during therapy unless otherwise specified. • CBC with differential: Recommended prior to initiation of therapy, prior to each subsequent dose, and at periodic intervals during therapy. • Platelet count: Recommended prior to initiation of therapy, prior to each subsequent dose, and at periodic intervals during therapy. • Hemoglobin and/or hematocrit: Recommended prior to initiation of therapy, prior to each subsequent dose, and at periodic intervals during therapy. • Liver function tests: ALT, AST, alkaline phosphatase, total bilirubin, LDH. • Renal function tests: CrCl, actual or calculated, and/or SCr recommended prior to initiation of therapy, prior to each subsequent dose, and at periodic intervals during therapy. • Bone marrow aspiration studies: Recommended at initiation of therapy and at time of maximum hematologic response to ensure adequate bone marrow reserve.
Indications	Procarbazine is indicated for use in combination with other anticancer drugs for the treatment of stage III and IV Hodgkin's disease. Other uses include non-Hodgkin's lymphoma, brain tumors, and malignant melanoma.
Dosage Adjustment Recommendations	Dosage adjustment is recommended in patients with hepatic or renal impairment; however, no guidelines are set forth by the manufacturer. Prompt cessation of procarbazine therapy is recommended if any of the following occur: • CNS signs or symptoms (e.g., paresthesias, neuropathies, confusion). • Leukopenia (WBC count < 4,000 cells/mm^3). • Thrombocytopenia (platelet count <100,000 cells/mm^3). • Hypersensitivity reaction. • Stomatitis; the first small ulceration or persistent spot soreness around the oral cavity. • Diarrhea.
Pharmacokinetics	Rapidly and completely absorbed following oral administration. Crosses the blood-brain barrier and distributes into CSF. Metabolized in the liver

and kidneys and eliminated in the urine and through respiratory tract as unchanged drug (< 5%) and metabolites.

Manufacturer	Sigma-Tau Pharmaceuticals, Inc., Gaithersburg, MD

Streptozocin

Other Names	Zanosar®
Classification	Alkylating agent; nitrosourea.
Mechanism	Selective inhibition of DNA synthesis via formation of DNA intrastrand cross-links. Cell-cycle non specific. Unique feature of a chemical sugar D-glucopyranose, which enhances uptake in the islet cells.
Vesicant Information	Irritant.
Preparation and Mixture	Reconstitute with 9.5 ml NaCl or sterile water to a concentration of 100 mg/ml. Can further dilute in 100–250 ml of solution.
Administration	Administer IVP, IVPB (over 15–30 minutes), or continuous IV over six hours. Infuse in D_5W or NS.
Storage and Stability	Store intact vials under refrigeration. Reconstituted and diluted solutions stable for 48 hours at room temperature (22°–25°C; 72°–77°F) and 96 hours under refrigeration (2°–8°C; 36°–46°F). Protect from light.
How Supplied	Supplied as 1-g vials of powder for injection.
Dosage	Usual dose in combination therapy is 500 mg/m² daily for five days every four to six weeks until maximum benefit or toxicity is achieved. Each cycle in four- to six-week intervals. As a single agent, dosed at 1,000 mg/m² weekly for two weeks. May escalate dose in subsequent courses. Also, dosed weekly for six weeks followed by a four-week observation period.
Compatibility Information	The reader is referred to other resources on admixture for detailed information.
Contraindications/ Precautions	No known contraindications. Use caution in patients with impaired kidney and liver function.

Drug Interactions	Agent	Effect
	Other nephrotoxic drugs	Potentiate renal toxicity and failure.
	Doxorubicin	When used concomitantly with doxorubicin, result is prolonged half-life; may see prolonged leukopenia and thrombocytopenia.
	Phenytoin	May decrease the effectiveness of streptozocin.
	Corticosteroids	Avoid concomitant use of corticosteroids with streptozocin.

Toxicity/Side Effects	**Acute and/or Potentially Life-Threatening:** Renal dysfunction occurs in 65% of patients; dose-related and cumulative. May be severe or fatal. Manifested by proteinuria, decreased CrCl, increased BUN, hypophosphatemia, and renal tubular acidosis. Highly emetogenic. Onset of nausea and vomiting within one to three hours and lasting up to 12 hours.
	Serious: Hypoglycemia because of an acute release of insulin. Keep $D_{50}W$ at bedside.
	Other: GI: Diarrhea (10%) and increased liver function tests and jaundice. Hematologic: Mildly myelosuppressive; neutropenia, thrombocytopenia (nadir at two weeks with recovery at three weeks). Neurologic: Depression, confusion, and lethargy. Miscellaneous: Hypoalbuminemia, secondary malignancy, and pain at injection site.
Special Considerations	Too-rapid IVP infusion can cause venous irritation and burning sensation. Recommend infusing over at least 30–60 minutes.
Monitoring Parameters	Monitoring is recommended prior to initiation of therapy and at periodic intervals during therapy unless otherwise specified. • CBC with differential: Recommended prior to initiation of therapy, prior to each subsequent dose, and at periodic intervals during therapy. • Platelet count: Recommended prior to initiation of therapy, prior to each subsequent dose, and at periodic intervals during therapy. • Hemoglobin and/or hematocrit: Recommended prior to initiation of therapy, prior to each subsequent dose, and at periodic intervals during therapy. • Liver function tests: ALT, AST, alkaline phosphatase, total bilirubin, LDH. • Renal function tests: CrCl, actual or calculated, and/or SCr recommended prior to initiation of therapy, prior to each subsequent dose, and at periodic intervals during therapy. • Blood glucose: Monitor at regular intervals during therapy. • Inspect site for stinging and burning during peripheral line or implanted port infusion.
Indications	FDA-approved in the treatment of islet cell carcinoma of the pancreas. Off-label uses include carcinoid tumors, lung and colorectal cancer, Hodgkin's disease, and Zollinger-Ellison tumors.
Dosage Adjustment Recommendations	May increase dose to 1,500 mg/m² if no toxicity and/or positive treatment response. Dose reduction necessary in renal impairment (see Appendix B).
Pharmacokinetics	Metabolized in the liver. Biphasic plasma elimination initial half-life of five minutes with the terminal half-life of up to 40 minutes. Multiorgan distribution (e.g., pancreas, kidneys, liver, intestines). Majority renally excreted as metabolites.
Manufacturer	Pharmacia & UpJohn, Peapack, NJ

Temozolomide

Other Names	Temodar®
Classification	Imidazotetrazine derivative.
Mechanism	Temozolomide is a pro-drug that is rapidly converted at physiologic pH to its active form, monomethyl 5-triazino imidazole carboxamide (MTIC). MTIC has cytotoxic and antiproliferative activity against tumor cells through DNA methylation.
Vesicant Information	Not classified as a vesicant or an irritant. Temozolomide is available commercially as an oral product.
Preparation and Mixture	No preparation or admixture necessary. Temozolomide is available commercially as an oral product.
Administration	Oral.
Storage and Stability	Store in tightly sealed bottles away from children at controlled room temperature 15°–30°C (59°–86°F).
How Supplied	Commercially available as 5-mg (green imprint), 20-mg (brown imprint), 100-mg (blue imprint), and 250-mg (black imprint) gelatin capsules in bottles of 5 or 20 capsules.
Dosage	The initial dose is 150 mg/m²/day on days 1–5 of 28-day treatment cycle. Subsequent dosing is based on nadir neutrophil and platelet counts of previous cycle and neutrophil and platelet counts at the time of the next treatment (see dosage adjustment recommendations).
Compatibility Information	Not applicable. Temozolomide is available commercially as an oral product.
Contraindications/ Precautions	Contraindicated if known hypersensitivity to temozolomide or dacarbazine because both drugs are metabolized to MTIC. Caution should be exercised in patients with severe renal or hepatic impairment.
Drug Interactions	Valproic acid decreases temozolomide clearance by 5%.
Toxicity/Side Effects	**Acute and/or Potentially Life-Threatening:** None noted. **Serious:** Hematologic: the dose-limiting toxicity is leukopenia and thrombocytopenia, which are noncumulative and occur within the first few treatment cycles. Nadir counts occur late in the treatment cycle (day 22–29) and recover in 14 days. In clinical trials, women experienced a higher rate of grade 4 neutropenia (ANC < 500 cells/mm³) and thrombocytopenia (< 20,000 cells/mcl) in first cycle of therapy than did men. **Other:** Dermatologic: Rash and pruritus. GI: Nausea and vomiting is the most frequent side effect (up to 70% of treated patients). The nausea and vomiting generally is self-limiting or easily treated with standard antiemetics. Constipation, diarrhea, anorexia, and mucositis also are seen. Genitourinary: Urinary incontinence and urinary tract infection.

Neurologic: Convulsions, hemiparesis, headache, dizziness, abnormal coordination, amnesia, insomnia, ataxia, anxiety, dysphasia, depression, abnormal gait, and confusion have been seen.

Miscellaneous: Fatigue, asthenia, edema (peripheral), back pain, and adrenal hypercorticism.

Special Considerations	Temozolomide can be given with or without food. Consistency of administration with respect to food is recommended because food does affect absorption. Taking on an empty stomach may reduce nausea and vomiting. Antiemetic therapy may be given prior to or following administration of temozolomide. It also is recommended to administer at bedtime. Patients should be advised not to open capsules. If capsules are accidentally opened, avoid inhaling or exposing skin to contents.
Monitoring Parameters	Monitoring is recommended prior to initiation of therapy and at periodic intervals during therapy unless otherwise specified. • CBC with differential: Recommended prior to initiation of therapy; obtain on day 22 (21 days after first dose) during treatment and weekly until ANC is > 1,500/mcl, prior to each subsequent dose, and at periodic intervals during therapy. • Platelet count: Recommended prior to initiation of therapy, prior to each subsequent dose, and at periodic intervals during therapy. • Hemoglobin and/or hematocrit: Recommended prior to initiation of therapy, prior to each subsequent dose, and at periodic intervals during therapy. • Liver function tests: ALT, AST, alkaline phosphatase, total bilirubin, LDH; skin color (hyperbilirubinemia) should be monitored periodically during therapy. • Serum chemistry profile: Recommended prior to initiation of therapy, prior to each subsequent dose, and at periodic intervals during therapy.
Indications	Temozolomide is indicated for the treatment of adult patients with refractory anaplastic astrocytoma (i.e., patients with first relapse who have experienced disease progression on a drug regimen containing a nitrosourea and procarbazine). Off-label uses include malignant glioma and metastatic melanoma.

Dosage Adjustment Recommendations

Day 1	Administer 150 mg/m^2/day for five days (starting dose) or 200 mg/m^2/day for five days.
Day 22 and day 29 (day 1 of next cycle)	Measure ANC and platelets. If ANC < 1,000 or platelets < 50,000, postpone therapy until ANC > 1,500 and platelets ≥ 100,000; reduce dose by 50 mg/m^2 for subsequent cycle. If ANC 1,000–1,500 or platelets 50,000–100,000, postpone therapy until ANC > 1,500 and platelets > 100,000; maintain initial dose. If ANC ≥ 1,500 and platelets ≥ 100,000, increase dose to or maintain dose at 200 mg/m^2/day for five days for subsequent cycle.

Temozolomide therapy can be continued until disease progression.

Pharmacokinetics	Well absorbed orally. Peak concentrations occur in one hour. Administration with high-fat meals prolongs time to peak concentration and decreases peak plasma concentration. Volume of distribution is 0.4 l/kg. Total protein binding is 15%. Crosses blood-brain barrier to an unknown extent. Temozolomide is spontaneously hydrolyzed at physiologic pH to its active form, MTIC. MTIC is further hydrolyzed to the active alkylating form. Cytochrome P-450 enzymes play a minor role in metabolism. Approximately 37.7% of the dose is excreted in the urine. Overall clearance is 5.5 l/hr/minute. Women clear temozolomide 5% slower than men.
Manufacturer	Schering Corporation, Kenilworth, NJ

Teniposide

Other Names	VM-26, Vumon®
Classification	Antimicrotubule; semisynthetic podophyllotoxin-derivative antineoplastic agent.
Mechanism	Teniposide causes single- and double-stranded breaks in DNA leading to inhibition of DNA synthesis. This effect is through the inhibition of type II topoisomerases. It kills cells in the G_2 and late S phases of replication.
Vesicant Information	Classified as a vesicant.
Preparation and Mixture	Teniposide doses should be diluted in NS or D_5W to a final concentration of 0.1, 0.2, 0.4, or 1 mg/ml. Because teniposide solution contains Cremophor®, which can leach DEHP from PVC containers and tubing, solutions should be administered using containers and tubing made of polyolefin, polypropylene, or glass.
Administration	Teniposide is administered by IV infusion over a minimum of 30–60 minutes and must not be given by rapid IV injection.
Storage and Stability	Vials should be stored under refrigeration and protected from light. Solutions diluted to 0.1, 0.2, or 0.4 mg/ml are stable for 24 hours at room temperature, and 1-mg/ml solutions should be used within four hours of preparation. Solutions should be prepared in non-PVC containers.
How Supplied	Vials of teniposide 10 mg/ml are available in a solution of dehydrated alcohol, benzyl alcohol, and polyoxyl 35 castor oil.
Dosage	Vary according to protocol; doses of 165 mg/m² to 250 mg/m² have been studied.
Compatibility Information	No data available.
Contraindications/ Precautions	Teniposide is contraindicated in patients with a history of hypersensitivity to the drug or polyoxyl 35 castor oil. Patients should be monitored closely for at least 60 minutes after the start of the infusion for signs of hypotension or hypersensitivity reactions. Medications for the treatment of anaphylaxis (e.g., epinephrine, corticosteroids, IV fluids) should be readily

	available during administration of teniposide infusions. Down syndrome people with may be sensitive to the myelosuppressive effects of teniposide.
Drug Interactions	**Agent** **Effect** Phenobarbital, phenytoins May significantly increase the metabo- and fosphenytoin lism of etoposide. Teniposide is > 99% protein-bound, and taking sodium salicylate, sulfamethizole, or tolbutamide has been shown to displace teniposide from plasma proteins, which can lead to increased toxicities.
Toxicity/Side Effects	**Acute and/or Potentially Life-Threatening:** Hypersensitivity reaction may occur (e.g., chills, fever, flushing of face, hives, hyper- or hypotension, tachycardia, trouble breathing, SOB, wheezing). **Serious:** None noted. **Other:** Anemia, neutropenia, and thrombocytopenia may be significant and are characterized by early onset and delayed recovery. In addition, mucositis, skin rash, neurotoxicity, mild to moderate nausea and vomiting, diarrhea, alopecia, and hepatic and/or renal function impairment may occur.
Special Considerations	Polyoxyl 35 castor oil used in the formulation of teniposide is known to cause hypotension and hypersensitivity reactions, including anaphylaxis, and patients must be monitored for symptoms of these reactions. Considered a moderate emetogen; administer a prophylactic antiemetic (e.g., serotonin antagonist, dexamethasone, or the combination) as well as an as-needed antiemetic (e.g., prochlorperazine).
Monitoring Parameters	Monitoring is recommended prior to initiation of therapy and at periodic intervals during therapy unless otherwise specified. • CBC with differential: Recommended prior to initiation of therapy, prior to each subsequent dose, and at periodic intervals during therapy. • Hemoglobin and/or hematocrit: Recommended prior to initiation of therapy, prior to each subsequent dose, and at periodic intervals during therapy. • Platelet count: Recommended prior to initiation of therapy, prior to each subsequent dose, and at periodic intervals during therapy. • Renal function tests: CrCl, actual or calculated, and/or SCr recommended prior to initiation of therapy, prior to each subsequent dose, and at periodic intervals during therapy. • Liver function tests: ALT, AST, alkaline phosphatase, total bilirubin, LDH.
Indications	ALL; also certain types of lymphomas and a wide variety of solid tumors.
Dosage Adjustment Recommendations	For significant renal impairment, dose reductions may be warranted. Dosage adjustments are required for hepatic dysfunction. For patients with Down syndrome, a 50% dosage reduction is recommended.
Pharmacokinetics	Plasma elimination is triphasic, with half-lives of 45 minutes, 4 hours, and 20 hours. Teniposide is extensively metabolized by the liver.
Manufacturer	Bristol-Myers Squibb Oncology/Immunology Division, Princeton, NJ

Thalidomide

Other Names	Thalomid®
Classification	Miscellaneous; immunomodulatory.
Mechanism	Immunomodulatory agent with a spectrum of activity that is not fully characterized. Thought to modulate tumor necrosis factor-alpha production.
Vesicant Information	Not classified as a vesicant or an irritant. Thalidomide is commercially available as an oral product.
Preparation and Mixture	No preparation or admixture necessary. Thalidomide is commercially available as an oral product.
Administration	Oral.
Storage and Stability	Store at 15°–30°C (59°–86°F). Protect from light. This drug must not be repackaged.
How Supplied	Supplied as hard, white, opaque gelatin capsules containing 50 mg of thalidomide and imprinted with the following: "Celgene" and "do not get pregnant." Packaged in boxes containing six prescription packs of 14 capsules each.
Dosage	Investigationally in the oncology setting, doses range from 100 mg/day up to 1,200 mg/day. Lower doses used in combination with other cancer therapies (e.g., chemotherapy, biologics such as interferons).
Compatibility Information	Not applicable. Thalidomide is commercially available as an oral product.
Contraindications/ Precautions	Pregnancy category X. Contraindicated in pregnant women and women capable of becoming pregnant as well as in patients who have demonstrated hypersensitivity to the drug or any of its components. Risk versus benefit should be considered prior to initiating thalidomide therapy in women of childbearing potential. Thalidomide has been associated with the development of neuropathy. Caution should be used when combining thalidomide with other drugs known to cause peripheral neuropathy.

Drug Interactions	**Agent**	**Effect**
	Barbiturates, alcohol, chlorpromazine, reserpine	Thalidomide enhances sedative potential.
	Drugs causing peripheral neuropathy	Potential to enhance development of neuropathy.
	Drugs that interfere with hormonal contraceptives	May reduce efficacy of contraception.

Toxicity/Side Effects	**Acute and/or Potentially Life-Threatening:** Human teratogenicity. Severe, life-threatening human birth defects are associated with thalidomide use. Because of this, thalidomide is only approved for marketing under a special restricted drug distribution program. In addition, pregnancy testing should occur within 24 hours prior to initiating thalidomide therapy, weekly during the first month of treatment, and then monthly thereafter in

women with regular menstrual cycles. If menstrual cycles are irregular, testing should occur at every-two-week intervals.

Other: Thalidomide use is associated with drowsiness/somnolence, peripheral neuropathy, dizziness/orthostatic hypotension, neutropenia, anemia, constipation, hypersensitivity, and increase in HIV viral load. Other adverse reactions that have occurred have not been causally related to thalidomide; however, asthenia and nausea seem to increase in incidence with higher doses.

Special Considerations	Hypersensitivity has been reported (erythematous macular rash, fever, tachycardia, and hypotension). If severe, may necessitate interruption of therapy. If reaction recurs when thalidomide is resumed, therapy should be discontinued. The potential for teratogenicity if fetal exposure occurs should be discussed at length with all patients. Thalidomide should be taken only as prescribed, and adherence to the provisions of the restricted drug distribution program is essential. Effective contraception must be used at least one month prior to beginning thalidomide therapy, during thalidomide therapy, and for one month after the discontinuation of thalidomide therapy. Two reliable forms of contraception must be used simultaneously unless continuous abstinence from heterosexual sexual intercourse is chosen method of birth control. Men taking thalidomide should use barrier form of contraception when engaging in sexual intercourse with women of childbearing potential. Pregnancy testing should occur within 24 hours prior to initiating thalidomide therapy, weekly during the first month of treatment, and then monthly thereafter in women with regular menstrual cycles. If menstrual cycles are irregular, testing should occur at every-two-week intervals. If pregnancy does occur during treatment, thalidomide must be discontinued immediately. Suspected fetal exposure must be reported immediately to the FDA via the MedWATCH system and to the manufacturer. Patients should be warned that the drug might make them drowsy and dizzy. Caution should be exercised when going from a lying to standing position too quickly. Patients should report any signs/symptoms of peripheral neuropathy to their physician. Patients should not donate blood or sperm while on thalidomide therapy.
Monitoring Parameters	Monitoring is recommended prior to initiation of therapy and at periodic intervals during therapy unless otherwise specified. • CBC with differential: Withhold initiation of therapy if ANC < 750/mm³; if ANC drops below 750/mm³ during therapy, re-evaluation of regimen and possible withholding continued therapy are indicated. • HIV viral load: If applicable. • Pregnancy testing: As outlined above. • Peripheral neurosensory assessment: At periodic intervals.
Indications	FDA-approved for the acute treatment of the cutaneous manifestations of moderate to severe erythema nodosum leprosum. Investigationally, thalidomide is being studied in numerous oncology settings, including renal cell carcinoma, multiple myeloma, melanoma, glioblastoma, and pediatric malignancies.
Dosage Adjustment Recommendations	It is recommended to withhold initiation of thalidomide therapy if ANC < 750/mm³. In addition, if the ANC drops and persists below 750/mm³ at

	any time during treatment, regimen should be re-evaluated and continued treatment possibly withheald.
Pharmacokinetics	The absolute bioavailability of thalidomide is not well characterized. Poor solubility in aqueous media may account for the lack of C_{max} dose proportionality and increased T_{max} values, suggesting a hindering in the rate of absorption. Coadministration with a high fat content meal causes minor changes in C_{max} and AUC concentrations, although an increase in T_{max} does occur. The exact metabolic route and fate of thalidomide are not known in humans. Half-life is approximately five to seven hours.
Manufacturer	Celgene Corporation, Warren, NJ

Thioguanine

Other Names	6-thioguanine, 2-amino-6-mercaptopurine, Thioguanine®
Classification	Antimetabolite; purine antagonist.
Mechanism	Thioguanine ribonucleotides are incorporated into DNA and RNA, resulting in blockade of syntheses and utilization of purine nucleotides.
Vesicant Information	Not classified as a vesicant or an irritant. Thioguanine is available commercially as an oral product.
Preparation and Mixture	No preparation or admixture necessary. Thioguanine is available commercially as an oral product.
Administration	Oral in single or divided daily doses.
Storage and Stability	Store at room temperature.
How Supplied	Available as 40-mg scored tablets.
Dosage	As a single agent, dose is 2 mg/kg/day with increases to 3 mg/kg/day after four weeks if inadequate response. In other combination therapies for ALL, doses vary from 80 mg/m^2/day to 200 mg/m^2/day in either daily or weekly schedules. Refer to specific treatment regimens for correct dosage.
Compatibility Information	Not applicable. Thioguanine is available commercially as an oral product.
Contraindications/ Precautions	Risk versus benefit should be considered in patients with existing bone marrow suppression, liver or kidney dysfunction, or infection.
Drug Interactions	None noted.
Toxicity/Side Effects	**Acute and/or Potentially Life-Threatening:** None noted. **Serious:** Uric acid nephropathy, hepatotoxicity, hepatic fibrosis, and toxic hepatitis have been reported rarely. **Other:** Leukopenia, thrombocytopenia, anemia, alopecia, photosensitivity, liver enzyme elevations, nausea, vomiting, stomatitis, diarrhea, hyperuricemia, and rash.

Special Considerations	Actions of thioguanine may be delayed; prompt discontinuation of therapy is recommended at the first sign of myelosuppression. Because of the potential for the development of uric acid nephropathy in patients with leukemia and/or lymphoma, adequate oral hydration, allopurinol, and, possibly, alkalinization of the urine all may be necessary as preventative measures. Produces a low percentage of nausea and vomiting; consider an as-needed antiemetic (e.g., prochlorperazine).
Monitoring Parameters	Monitoring is recommended prior to initiation of therapy and at periodic intervals during therapy unless otherwise specified. • CBC with differential: Recommended prior to initiation of therapy, prior to each subsequent dose, and at periodic intervals during therapy. • Hemoglobin and/or hematocrit: Recommended prior to initiation of therapy, prior to each subsequent dose, and at periodic intervals during therapy. • Platelet count: Recommended prior to initiation of therapy, prior to each subsequent dose, and at periodic intervals during therapy. • Renal function tests: CrCl, actual or calculated, and/or SCr recommended prior to initiation of therapy, prior to each subsequent dose, and at periodic intervals during therapy. • Liver function tests: ALT, AST, alkaline phosphatase, total bilirubin, LDH. • Serum uric acid.
Indications	Indicated in the remission induction, remission consolidation, and maintenance therapy for ANLL.
Dosage Adjustment Recommendations	Dosage must be adjusted based on clinical response and toxicity for each individual patient. In addition, prompt discontinuation of therapy is recommended at the first sign of myelosuppression because of the delayed effects of the drug.
Pharmacokinetics	Oral thioguanine is slowly and poorly absorbed (30%), and peak levels are reached approximately eight hours after dosing. Thioguanine is metabolized by the liver with an elimination half-life of up to 11 hours.
Manufacturer	Glaxo Wellcome Inc., Research Triangle Park, NC

Thiotepa

Other Names	TESPA, Thioplex®
Classification	Alkylating agent; miscellaneous (aziridine).
Mechanism	Thiotepa interferes with DNA replication and transcription of RNA.
Vesicant Information	Not classified as a vesicant or an irritant.
Preparation and Mixture	Thiotepa should be reconstituted by adding 1.5 ml sterile water for injection to each 15 mg vial. Solutions should be further diluted in NS prior to IV administration.
Administration	IVP, short IV infusion, IM injection, continuous IV infusion, intravesical instillation for superficial bladder cancer, intratumoral injection.

Storage and Stability	Intact vials should be stored under refrigeration and protected from light. Solutions of 1–3 mg/ml thiotepa are stable for 24 hours at room temperature or 48 hours under refrigeration, and solutions at 5 mg/ml are stable for 24 hours at room temperature or under refrigeration.
How Supplied	Supplied as a lyophilized powder in 15-mg vials.
Dosage	Usual doses of 0.3–0.4 mg/kg repeated every one to four weeks. Higher doses of up to 125 mg/m^2/day for four days are used in some HCT regimens. In papillary carcinoma of the bladder, 60 mg of thiotepa in 30–60 ml of sodium chloride injection is instilled into the bladder by catheter and retained for two hours.
Compatibility Information	Thiotepa may be mixed with 2% procaine hydrochloride and/or 0.1% epinephrine hydrochloride injection for use in local administration. For further dilution, NS, D$_5$W, or lactated Ringer's solution may be used.
Contraindications/ Precautions	Myelosuppression can occur, even from absorption during intravesical irrigation. Risk versus benefit should be considered for patients with bone marrow depression, hepatic impairment, renal impairment, or infection.
Drug Interactions	None noted.
Toxicity/Side Effects	**Acute and/or Potentially Life-Threatening:** Hypersensitivity reactions, including rash, urticaria, laryngeal edema, asthma, anaphylactic shock, and wheezing. **Serious:** None noted. **Other:** GI: Nausea, vomiting, abdominal pain, and anorexia. Hematologic: Myelosuppression (e.g., leukopenia, thrombocytopenia, anemia). Miscellaneous: Fatigue, weakness, dysuria, and chemical or hemorrhagic cystitis with intravesical therapy; dizziness, headache, and alopecia.
Special Considerations	Prompt discontinuation of therapy or dosage reduction is recommended at the first sign of a sudden, large decrease in leukocyte or platelet count. Because of the potential for the development of uric acid nephropathy in patients with leukemia or lymphoma, adequate oral hydration, allopurinol, and, possibly, alkalinization of the urine may be necessary as preventative measures. Considered a moderately low emetogen; consider an as-needed antiemetic (e.g., prochlorperazine).
Monitoring Parameters	Monitoring is recommended prior to initiation of therapy and at periodic intervals during therapy unless otherwise specified. • CBC with differential: Recommended prior to initiation of therapy, prior to each subsequent dose, and at periodic intervals during therapy. • Hemoglobin and/or hematocrit: Recommended prior to initiation of therapy, prior to each subsequent dose, and at periodic intervals during therapy. • Platelet count: Recommended prior to initiation of therapy, prior to each subsequent dose, and at periodic intervals during therapy. • Renal function tests: CrCl, actual or calculated, and/or SCr recommended prior to initiation of therapy, prior to each subsequent dose, and at periodic intervals during therapy.

	• Liver function tests: ALT, AST, alkaline phosphatase, total bilirubin, LDH. • Serum uric acid.
Indications	Thiotepa is approved for adenocarcinoma of the breast, adenocarcinoma of the ovary, superficial papillary carcinoma of the urinary bladder, lymphomas (e.g., lymphosarcoma, Hodgkin's disease), and controlling intracavitary effusions secondary to diffuse or localized neoplastic diseases of various serosal cavities. It also is being studied in the treatment of numerous other malignancies.
Dosage Adjustment Recommendations	Thiotepa is 85% renally eliminated, and dose reductions may be required (see Appendix B).
Pharmacokinetics	Thiotepa is metabolized to the active metabolite, triethylenephosphoramide (TEPA), by the cytochrome P450 microsomal enzyme system of the liver. The elimination of thiotepa is biphasic; initial half-life of 12 minutes and a terminal half-life of 1.2–2.9 hours. The elimination half-life of TEPA is 3-21 hours.
Manufacturer	Immunex Corporation, Seattle, WA

Topotecan hydrochloride

Other Names	Hycamtin®
Classification	Miscellaneous; topoisomerase 1 inhibitor.
Mechanism	Topotecan binds to and stabilizes the DNA topoisomerase cleavable complex, thereby preventing the topoisomerase from religating single-strand breaks, which then leads to apoptosis.
Vesicant Information	Not classified as a vesicant or an irritant, although mild local reactions such as erythema and bruising have been reported.
Preparation and Mixture	Reconstitute the vial with 4 ml of sterile water for injection. The dose should then be further diluted in 50–250 ml of NS or D_5W.
Administration	IV infusion over 30 minutes.
Storage and Stability	Reconstituted vials are stable for 24 hours at room temperature. Solutions diluted to 10 or 500 mcg/ml in NS or D_5W in Viaflex® (Baxter International Inc., Deerfield, IL) IV bags are reported stable up to four days at room temperature.
How Supplied	Lyophilized light yellow to greenish powder in single-dose vials containing 4 mg each.
Dosage	Usual dose 1.5 mg/m² daily for five days with cycles repeated every three weeks.
Compatibility Information	No data available for admixture with other medications.
Contraindications/ Precautions	Doses should be held or reduced for bone marrow depression or significant renal impairment. Risk versus benefit should be considered for patients with infection or renal insufficiency.

Drug Interactions	**Agent**	**Effect**
	Filgrastim (G-CSF)	Concomitant use can prolong the duration of neutropenia; therefore, it should be delayed until 24 hours after the therapy is completed.

Toxicity/Side Effects	**Acute and/or Potentially Life-Threatening:** None noted.
	Serious: Severe myelosuppression, including neutropenia, thrombocytopenia, and anemia, occurs in a significant number of patients. Topotecan should only be administered in patients with adequate bone marrow reserve (i.e., baseline ANC $\geq$ 1,500/ mm^3, platelet count $\geq$ 100,000 /mm^3; subsequent courses ANC $\geq$ 1,000/mm^3, platelet count $\geq$ 100,000/mm^3).
	Other: GI: Nausea, vomiting, and diarrhea. Neurologic: Headache and paresthesia. Miscellaneous: Liver enzyme elevations, alopecia, and mild local erythema and bruising.

Special Considerations	Care should be taken to avoid extravasation; drug has been associated with mild local reactions, such as erythema and bruising. Topotecan is considered a moderately low emetogen; consider an as-needed antiemetic (e.g., prochlorperazine).

Monitoring Parameters	Monitoring is recommended prior to initiation of therapy and at periodic intervals during therapy unless otherwise specified. • CBC with differential: Recommended prior to initiation of therapy, prior to each subsequent dose, and at periodic intervals during therapy. • Hemoglobin and/or hematocrit: Recommended prior to initiation of therapy, prior to each subsequent dose, and at periodic intervals during therapy. • Platelet count: Recommended prior to initiation of therapy, prior to each subsequent dose, and at periodic intervals during therapy. • Renal function tests: CrCl, actual or calculated, and/or SCr recommended prior to initiation of therapy, prior to each subsequent dose, and at periodic intervals during therapy.

Indications	Indicated in the treatment of metastatic ovarian cancer after failure of initial or subsequent chemotherapy. Also indicated in the second-line treatment of small cell lung cancer. Investigationally studied in the treatment of several other cancers, including acute leukemia.

Dosage Adjustment Recommendations	Dosage adjustments are needed in renal insufficiency (see Appendix B).

Pharmacokinetics	Topotecan has a multiexponential elimination, primarily renal, with a terminal half-life of two to three hours.

Manufacturer	SmithKline Beecham Pharmaceuticals, Philadelphia, PA

Tretinoin

Other Names	Vesanoid®, all-trans retinoic acid, ATRA
Classification	Retinoid.

Mechanism	The exact mechanism of action is unknown; however, tretinoin induces cytodifferentiation and decreased proliferation of acute promyelocytic cells in culture and in vivo. Complete responses are characterized by an initial maturation of primitive promyelocytes derived from the leukemic clone, followed by a repopulation of the peripheral blood and bone marrow by normal, polyclonal hematopoietic cells.
Vesicant Information	Not classified as a vesicant or an irritant. Tretinoin is commercially available as an oral product.
Preparation and Mixture	No preparation or admixture necessary. Tretinoin is commercially available as an oral product.
Administration	Oral.
Storage and Stability	Store capsules at 15°–30°C (59°–86°F). Protect from light.
How Supplied	Vesanoid is supplied as 10 mg capsules in bottles of 100. The capsules are two-tone (lengthwise), orange-yellow and reddish-brown and imprinted with the following: VESANOID 10 ROCHE.
Dosage	The recommended dose for APL is 45 mg/m^2/day administered as two evenly divided daily doses until complete remission (CR) is achieved. Treatment should be discontinued 30 days after CR has been achieved or after 90 days of treatment, whichever occurs first.
Compatibility Information	Not applicable. Tretinoin is commercially available as an oral product.
Contraindications/ Precautions	Contraindicated in patients with a known hypersensitivity to retinoids or sensitivity to parabens, which are used as preservatives in the gelatin capsules. Risk versus benefit should be considered in patients with preexisting leukocytosis. Tretinoin may cause a rapid increase in the leukocyte count during therapy, which increases the risk of life-threatening complications in a patient with preexisting leukocytosis. Tretinoin is teratogenic; there is a high-risk of a severely deformed infant being born to a woman receiving tretinoin therapy during pregnancy.
Drug Interactions	Limited clinical data are available on potential drug interactions, however, the potential for interactions exist as tretinoin is metabolized by the hepatic P450 system. Caution should be used when coadministering tretinoin with hepatic P450 system inducers (rifampicin, glucocorticoids, phenobarbital) or inhibitors (erythromycin, ketoconazole, cimetidine, and others), although to date there are no data to suggest that co-use increases or decreases the efficacy or safety of tretinoin.
Toxicity/Side Effects	**Acute and/or Potentially Life-Threatening:** Retinoic acid-APL syndrome, which is characterized by fever, dyspnea, weight gain, radiographic pulmonary infiltrates, and pleural or pericardial effusions and occasionally accompanied by impaired myocardial contractility and episodic hypotension, may occur in up to 25% of patients. This syndrome may be severe, requiring endotracheal intubation and mechanical ventilation. Multiorgan failure and death have occurred. High-dose steroids (e.g.,

dexamethasone 10 mg intravenously every 12 hours for three days or to the resolution of symptoms) should be initiated immediately upon suspicion of syndrome. The syndrome generally occurs during the first month of therapy. In addition, rapidly evolving leukocytosis, in the presence or absence of the retinoic acid-APL syndrome, may lead to an increase in life-threatening complications.

Serious: A number of cardiovascular events have been reported and may be severe in nature and include arrhythmias, cardiac failure, cardiac arrest, myocardial infarction, ischemia, stroke, myocarditis, pericarditis, and pulmonary hypertension.

Other: Most patients will experience retinoid drug-related toxicity, especially headache, fever, weakness, and fatigue. These are seldom permanent or irreversible and rarely require interruption of tretinoin therapy. Other retinoid-related toxicities included skin/mucous membrane dryness, pruritus, rash, bone pain, increased sweating, mucositis, nausea and vomiting, visual disturbances, and alopecia.

Cardiovascular: As noted above, and flushing, hypotension, enlarged heart, heart murmur, and hypertension.
Dermatologic: As noted above, and cellulitis.
GI: Abdominal pain, GI hemorrhage and/or ulceration, diarrhea, constipation, ascites, pancreatitis, anorexia, and dyspepsia.
Hematologic: Leukocytosis, disseminated intravascular coagulation, and hemorrhage.
Neurologic: Dizziness, paresthesia, depression, confusion, agitation, cerebral hemorrhage, intracranial hypertension (pseudotumor cerebri), hallucination, and rarely cerebellar disorders, convulsions, coma, hemiplegia, hyporeflexia, encephalopathy, dementia, somnolence, and slowed speech.
Miscellaneous: Earache, feeling of fullness in ear, hearing loss, hypercholesteremia, hypertriglyceridemia, elevated liver function tests, dysuria, renal insufficiency and failure, infections, myalgia, facial edema, pallor, peripheral edema, and respiratory difficulties (outlined above) including pneumonia, wheezing, rales, upper/lower respiratory disorders, effusions, and infiltrates.

Special Considerations	Doses should be evenly divided in two daily doses. May take with or without regard to meals. Take missed dose as soon as possible; contact physician if not remembered until prior to next dose. Women of childbearing age need to have a negative pregnancy test within one week prior to the initiation of tretinoin therapy, use two reliable forms of contraception during and for one month after discontinuation of tretinoin therapy, and be fully informed of the risk to the fetus if they become pregnant. Notify physician immediately if symptoms of retinoic acid-APL syndrome develop. Consideration should be given to the addition of full-dose chemotherapy on days 1 and 2 of tretinoin therapy if the patient presents with a WBC count greater than $5 \times 10^9/l$ or per package insert when WBC count rises quickly during therapy.

Monitoring Parameters	Monitoring is recommended prior to initiation of therapy and at periodic intervals during therapy unless otherwise specified. • CBC with differential: Obtain at baseline; and should be monitored frequently during therapy. • Liver function tests: Obtain at baseline, should be monitored frequently during therapy; tretinoin therapy should be discontinued if liver function test values are elevated more than five times the upper limit of normal. • Lipid studies: Obtain at baseline, and should be monitored frequently during therapy. • Coagulation tests: PT and INR; should be monitored frequently during therapy. • Pregnancy testing: Prior to initiation of therapy and periodically thereafter if clinically indicated.
Indications	Indicated for the induction of remission in patients with French-American-British classification M3 (including the M3 variant), characterized by the presence of the t(15,17) translocation and/or presence of the PML-RAR$_a$ gene who are refractory to, or who have relapsed from, anthracycline chemotherapy, or for whom anthracycline-based chemotherapy is contraindicated. Tretinoin therapy is for the induction of remission only.
Dosage Adjustment Recommendations	Temporary withdrawal of tretinoin therapy should be considered if liver function test values exceed five times the upper limit of normal.
Pharmacokinetics	Well absorbed after oral administration; greater than 95% bound to plasma proteins. Undergoes hepatic metabolism by the cytochrome P450 enzyme system with an elimination half-life of one to two hours. Eliminated by renal and fecal routes.
Manufacturer	Roche Laboratories Inc., Nutley, NJ

Valrubicin

Other Names	Valstar®
Classification	Antineoplastic antibiotic, doxorubicin analogue.
Mechanism	Valrubicin and its metabolites arrest cells in the G_2 phase of cell division by causing chromosomal damage though the inhibition of topoisomerase II.
Vesicant Information	Valrubicin has not demonstrated vesicant properties.
Preparation and Mixture	After allowing vials to warm to room temperature, withdraw contents of four vials (200 mg per 5-ml vial) and dilute with 55 ml of NS to provide 75 ml of solution for instillation. Because valrubicin solution contains Creomophor®, which can leach DEHP from PVC containers and tubing, solutions should be administered using containers and tubing made of polyolefin, polypropylene, or glass.
Administration	Solution should be instilled into urethral catheter by gravity flow into the bladder and allowed to remain for two hours. After two hours, the patient should void the bladder contents.

Storage and Stability	Unopened vials should be stored under refrigeration. Diluted solutions are stable for 12 hours at room temperature.
How Supplied	Commercially available as a preservative-free nonaqueous solution containing valrubicin 40 mg/ml (200 mg/5 ml) in 50% Cremophor and 50% dehydrated alcohol.
Dosage	Instill 800 mg intravesically once weekly for six weeks.
Compatibility Information	No data available; therefore, valrubicin should not be mixed with any other medications or IV fluids.
Contraindications/ Precautions	Therapy is contraindicated in patients with known hypersensitivity to anthracyclines or Cremophor. To avoid the chance of toxic systemic exposure, valrubicin should not be instilled into a perforated bladder or under other conditions that compromise the integrity of the bladder mucosa. Patients who have undergone transurethral resection of the bladder should have therapy delayed until the integrity of the bladder mucosa has recovered. Therapy should be avoided in patients with concurrent urinary tract infections.
Drug Interactions	No drug interaction studies were conducted, as very little valrubicin is expected to be absorbed following bladder instillation.
Toxicity/Side Effects	**Acute and/or Potentially Life-Threatening:** If bladder mucosa is not intact, drug absorption may lead to myelosuppression. **Serious:** Irritable bladder may present during and following instillation. **Other:** Red-tinged urine may persist for up to 24 hours following instillation. Patient may be prone to urinary tract infections.
Special Considerations	As with other cytotoxic agents, procedures for the safe handling and disposal of valrubicin should be followed. Spills should be cleaned up with undiluted chlorine bleach.
Monitoring Parameters	• Monitor urine for prolonged passage of red-tinged urine. • If perforation of the bladder wall is suspected or occurs during retention of valrubicin, monitor blood counts weekly for three weeks for possible myelosuppression.
Indications	Valrubicin is indicated for the intravesical treatment of patients with bacillus Calmette-Guérin-resistant cancer of the urinary bladder for which surgical removal of the bladder is not an option.
Dosage Adjustment Recommendations	None noted.
Pharmacokinetics	Following instillation, concentrations in bladder tissue exceeded levels that cause 90% cytotoxicity to bladder cells in culture. During the two-hour retention time, only nanogram quantities of valrubicin are absorbed into the blood, although some valrubicin metabolites were detected in the blood. More than 98% of valrubicin is recovered as the parent compound after voiding of an administered dose.
Manufacturer	Medeva Pharmaceuticals, Inc., Rochester, NY

Vinblastine sulfate

Other Names	Vincaleukoblastine sulfate, Velban®
Classification	Antimicrotubule; vinca alkaloid antineoplastic agent.
Mechanism	By binding to tubulin, vinblastine inhibits microtubule assembly and causes cellular metaphase arrest.
Vesicant Information	Classified as a vesicant; if infiltrated application of hot compresses may be warranted.
Preparation and Mixture	Vials of powder should be reconstituted with bacteriostatic or non-bacteriostatic water for injection.
Administration	IVP or infusion only; DO NOT administer intrathecally.
Storage and Stability	Vials of solution and powder should be stored in a refrigerator and protected from light. Vials of reconstituted powder are stable for 28 days under refrigeration.
How Supplied	Vials containing 10 mg as a lyophilized powder and 1 mg/ml injectable solution.
Dosage	Doses vary depending on the specific treatment regimen. The manufacturer suggests the adult dosage is 3.7 mg/m^2, and the pediatric dosage is 2.5 mg/m^2 as a single dose. Doses are increased weekly by about 1.8 mg/m^2 in adults and 1.25 mg/m^2 in pediatric patients, according to their hematologic response up to a maximum dose of 18.5 mg/m^2 (adults) or 12.5 mg/m^2 (pediatric patients). Dosages generally are reduced in patients who have had recent radiation therapy or chemotherapy.
Compatibility Information	Incompatible with IV phenytoin. Velban can reduce absorption or increase metabolism and elimination of anticonvulsants.
Contraindications/ Precautions	Contraindicated in patients who are severely leukopenic. Use with caution in patients with hepatic impairment; dose adjustments are needed for elevations in bilirubin.
Drug Interactions	Drugs that inhibit cytochrome P-450 isoenzyme CYP3A may impair metabolism of vinblastine; therefore, caution should be taken when using these agents together.
Toxicity/Side Effects	**Acute and/or Potentially Life-Threatening:** May cause severe and life-threatening myelosuppression. Nadir usually occurs on day 7–10 with recovery by day 17. IT use may result in death; DO NOT administer intrathecally. **Serious:** Severe local tissue inflammation and necrosis if extravasated. Hot compresses may be warranted. **Other:** Cardiovascular: Hypertension, Raynaud's phenomena. Dermatologic: Alopecia, rash, photosensitivity, and dermatitis. GI: Moderately emetogenic; nausea and vomiting occur in 30%–60% of patients and are easily controlled with conventional antiemetics (e.g.,

	serotonin antagonists, dexamethasone, phenothiazines); diarrhea, constipation, stomatitis, abdominal cramps, paralytic ileus, metallic taste, and hemorrhagic colitis. Hematologic: Myelosuppression is dose-limiting (see page 220); anemia and thrombocytopenia. Neurologic: Headache, malaise, depression, seizures, paresthesia, and neurotoxicity (e.g., peripheral neuropathy, loss of deep tendon reflexes, weakness, urinary retention, tachycardia, orthostatic hypotension, convulsions) with high doses. Miscellaneous: Myalgia, hyperuricemia, vestibular manifestations (e.g., dizziness, nystagmas and vertigo), hearing impairment, acute bronchospasm, and SOB.
Special Considerations	Must only be given IV. Vinblastine can cause tissue damage if given by IM or SC injection and has been fatal when given intrathecally.
Monitoring Parameters	Monitoring is recommended prior to initiation of therapy and at periodic intervals during therapy unless otherwise specified. • CBC with differential. Recommended prior to initiation of therapy, prior to each subsequent dose, and at periodic intervals during therapy. • Hemoglobin and/or hematocrit: Recommended prior to initiation of therapy, prior to each subsequent dose, and at periodic intervals during therapy. • Platelet count: Recommended prior to initiation of therapy, prior to each subsequent dose, and at periodic intervals during therapy. • Liver function tests: ALT, AST, alkaline phosphatase, total bilirubin, LDH. • Bowel sounds: Assess frequently. • Serum uric acid levels: Recommended prior to initiation of therapy and at periodic intervals during initial therapy. • Peripheral neurosensory assessment: Prior to each dose.
Indications	Hodgkin's disease, non-Hodgkin's lymphoma, carcinoma of the testis, KS, bladder carcinoma, choriocarcinoma, and breast cancer.
Dosage Adjustment Recommendations	Vinblastine is metabolized and excreted in the bile and feces, and a dose reduction is recommended for elevations in direct bilirubin (see Appendix A).
Pharmacokinetics	Vinblastine has rapid clearance from the blood. Metabolized by the liver to an active metabolite. Undergoes biliary excretion with < 1% eliminated unchanged in the urine.
Manufacturer	Eli Lilly and Company, Indianapolis, IN

Vincristine sulfate

Other Names	Oncovin®, Vincasar PFS®, Vincristine Sulfate Injection, Vincrex®
Classification	Antimicrotubule agent; plant alkaloid from the periwinkle plant.
Mechanism	Cell-cycle specific at S and M phase. Protein binding stopping mitosis during metaphase.

Vesicant Information	Classified as a vesicant; if infiltrated, application of hot compresses may be warranted.
Preparation and Mixture	Dilute 1-mg sterile vial with 10 ml sterile water or NS to a final concentration of 0.1 mg/ml.
Administration	IV. Peripheral slow IVP over one to two minutes, central line IVP over one minute. May be infused in 50 ml D_5W or NS over 15 minutes. Caution to avoid extravasation. Do not give intrathecally.
Storage and Stability	Store intact vials under refrigeration. Diluted solutions in NS or D_5W stable for 21 days at room temperature and under refrigeration. Protect from light.
How Supplied	Supplied as 1-mg, 2-mg, and 5-mg sterile vials.
Dosage	Single dose: $0.4–1.4$ mg/m² every week. Total not to exceed 2 mg/wk. Infusion dose is 0.5/mg/m²/day for five days. Some regimens use vincristine infused with doxorubicin over 96 hours.
Compatibility Information	Compatible with bleomycin, cisplatin, fluorouracil, leucovorin, MTX, mitomycin-C, cyclophosphamide, doxorubicin.
Contraindications/ Precautions	DO NOT administer intrathecally. Contraindicated in patients with hypersensitivity to vincristine or any component and in patients with demyelinating form of Charcot-Marie-Tooth syndrome. Risk versus benefit should be considered in patients who are pregnant, are lactating, and/ or have underlying neuropathy.

Drug Interactions	Agent	Effect
	MTX	Increased cellular uptake of MTX.
	Phenytoin	Decreased serum levels of phenytoin with concomitant use.
	Digoxin	Decreased bioavailability of digoxin with concomitant use.
	Calcium channel blockers	Increased cellular uptake of vincristine.
	Mitomycin	Increased frequency of bronchospasms and SOB with previous or simultaneous use.
	Asparaginase	Decreased liver clearance of vincristine.

Toxicity/Side Effects	**Acute and/or Potentially Life-Threatening:** FATAL if given intrathecally.
	Serious: Tissue irritation and necrosis may develop if extravasated. Hot compresses indicated. Peripheral neuropathy may be severe and may include loss of deep tendon reflexes in the lower extremities, numbness, tingling, pain, paresthesias of the fingers and toes (i.e., stocking and glove distribution), foot drop, and wrist drop. In addition, paralytic ileus and seizures also may develop.
	Other: Cardiovascular: Hypo- or hypertension. Dermatologic: Alopecia, phlebitis, and rash.

	GI: Constipation, stomatitis, abdominal cramps, anorexia, metallic taste, bloating, diarrhea, and mild nausea and vomiting. Genitourinary: Urinary retention, dysuria, and uric acid neuropathy. Hematologic: Occasional mild leukopenia and thrombocytopenia (onset 7 days, nadir 10 days, and recovery 21 days). Neurologic: Motor difficulties, headache, cranial nerve paralysis, fever, depression, vocal cord paralysis. Pulmonary: SOB and bronchospasms. Reproductive: Azoospermia and amenorrhea. Miscellaneous: Hyperuricemia, SIADH, extraocular muscle paresis, photophobia, and diplopia.
Special Considerations	Administer intravenously only. Patient may develop paralytic ileus. Use prophylactic stool softener.
Monitoring Parameters	Monitoring is recommended prior to initiation of therapy and at periodic intervals during therapy unless otherwise specified. • CBC with differential: Recommended prior to initiation of therapy, prior to each subsequent dose, and at periodic intervals during therapy. • Hemoglobin and/or hematocrit: Recommended prior to initiation of therapy, prior to each subsequent dose, and at periodic intervals during therapy. • Platelet count: Recommended prior to initiation of therapy, prior to each subsequent dose, and at periodic intervals during therapy. • Liver function tests: ALT, AST, alkaline phosphatase, total bilirubin, LDH. • Assess bowel sounds frequently. • Serum uric acid levels: Recommended prior to initiation of therapy and at periodic intervals during initial therapy. • Peripheral neurosensory assessment: Prior to each dose.
Indications	FDA-approved for Hodgkin's disease and non-Hodgkin's lymphoma; cervical, testicular, bladder, and head and neck carcinoma; and non-small cell lung cancer. Other uses include neuroblastoma, Wilms' tumor, rhabdomyosarcoma, multiple myeloma, and breast cancer.
Dosage Adjustment Recommendations	Dose reduction necessary in hepatic impairment (see Appendix A). Hold if WBC < 4,000/mm^3.
Pharmacokinetics	Primarily excreted via the liver with 80% excreted via bile and feces, and 20% excreted in the urine. Minimal penetration into the blood-brain barrier. Initial half-life is five minutes with terminal half-life of 85 hours. Binds RBCs and platelets.
Manufacturer	Oncovin®, Eli Lilly and Company, Indianapolis, IN; Vincasar PFS®, Adria Laboratories, Kalamazoo, MI; Vincristine Sulfate Injection, Lymphomed, Inc., Rosemont, IL; Vincrex®, Bristol-Myers Squibb Oncology/Immunology Division, Princeton, NJ

Vinorelbine tartrate

Other Names	3′, 4′-didehydro-4′-deoxy-c′-norvincaleukoblastine, Navelbine®
Classification	Antimicrotubule; semisynthetic vinca alkaloid antineoplastic agent.

Mechanism	By binding to tubulin, vinorelbine inhibits microtubule assembly and causes cellular metaphase arrest.
Vesicant Information	Classified as a vesicant.
Preparation and Mixture	Injections should be further diluted in a syringe to 1.5–3 mg/ml with NS or D$_5$W or diluted in an IV bag between 0.5–2 mg/ml with D$_5$W, NS, 50/50 mixture of D$_5$W and NS, Ringer's solution, or lactated Ringers solution.
Administration	Infuse over 6–10 minutes and follow by flushing the line with at least 75–125 ml of compatible IV fluid.
Storage and Stability	Unopened vials should be stored under refrigeration and protected from light. The product should not be frozen. Diluted vinorelbine may be used for up to 24 hours under normal room light when stored in polypropylene syringes or PVC bags under refrigeration or at room temperature.
How Supplied	Available as a 10-mg/ml clear, colorless to pale-yellow solution in 10-mg/1 ml and 50-mg/5 ml vials.
Dosage	Recommended dose is 30 mg/m² repeated weekly.
Compatibility Information	No compatibility data available.
Contraindications/Precautions	Contraindicated in patients with ANC < 1,000 cells/ml prior to therapy.
Drug Interactions	**Agent** **Effect** Mitomycin Acute pulmonary reactions have been reported when vinorelbine is used with mitomycin. Cisplatin Increased incidence of granulocytopenia when vinorelbine used in combination with cisplatin.
Toxicity/Side Effects	**Acute and/or Potentially Life-Threatening:** None noted. **Serious:** Acute SOB and severe bronchospasm have been reported, although rare. May require treatment with supplemental oxygen, bronchodilators, and/or corticosteroids. **Other:** Dermatologic: Alopecia. GI: Nausea, vomiting, constipation, diarrhea, stomatitis, abdominal cramps, anorexia, and metallic taste. Hematologic: Myelosuppression (e.g., neutropenia, thrombocytopenia, anemia) can be moderate to severe with onset within four days, nadir at day 7–10, and recovery within 14–21 days. Miscellaneous: Peripheral neuropathy, paresthesia, injection site reactions, transient elevations of liver enzymes, chest pain, dyspnea, fatigue, myalgia, and rash.
Special Considerations	Considered a mild emetogen; consider an as-needed antiemetic (e.g., prochlorperazine). Fatal if given intrathecally. Because of possibility of extravasation, a central line should be placed for ease of administration.

Monitoring Parameters	Monitoring is recommended prior to initiation of therapy and at periodic intervals during therapy unless otherwise specified. • CBC with differential: Recommended prior to initiation of therapy, prior to each subsequent dose, and at periodic intervals during therapy. • Hemoglobin and/or hematocrit: Recommended prior to initiation of therapy, prior to each subsequent dose, and at periodic intervals during therapy. • Platelet count: Recommended prior to initiation of therapy, prior to each subsequent dose, and at periodic intervals during therapy. • Liver function tests: ALT, AST, alkaline phosphatase, total bilirubin, LDH.
Indications	FDA-approved for use in the treatment of non-small cell lung cancer and breast cancer. Vinorelbine is being investigated in several other malignancies.
Dosage Adjustment Recommendations	Dose reductions are made for hematologic toxicity or hepatic insufficiency. For total bilirubin 2.1–3 mg/dl, use 15 mg/m² (50% dose); for total bilirubin > 3 mg/dl, use 7.5 mg/m² (25% dose) (see Appendix A). For ANC 1,000–1,499 cells/ml, use 15 mg/m² (50% dose); if ANC < 1,000 cells/ml, hold dose and recheck ANC in one week. Discontinue treatment if three consecutive doses are held because of ANC < 1,000 cells/ml. If moderate to severe neurotoxicity develops, discontinue treatment.
Pharmacokinetics	Not readily absorbed from GI tract; must be given intravenously. Extensive hepatic metabolism with a triphasic elimination (feces 46%; urine 18%) and a half-life of 27.7–43.6 hours.
Manufacturer	Glaxo Wellcome Inc., Research Triangle Park, NC

Hormonal Therapies

Aminoglutethimide

Other Name	Cytadren®
Classification	Hormonal agent.
Mechanism	Blocks the enzymatic conversion of cholesterol to delta-5-pregnenolone, thereby reducing the synthesis of adrenal glucocorticoids, mineralocorticoids, estrogens, aldosterone, and androgens.
Vesicant Information	Not classified as a vesicant or an irritant. Aminoglutethimide is commercially available as an oral product.
Preparation and Mixture	No preparation or admixture necessary. Aminoglutethimide is commercially available as an oral product.
Administration	Oral.
Storage and Stability	Do not store above 30°C (86°F). Protect from light.
How Supplied	Commercially available in 250-mg white, round, scored tablets in bottles of 100. The tablets are imprinted with the following: CIBA 24.
Dosage	Common regimen of 250 mg every six hours; may be increased in increments of 250 mg daily at one- to two-week intervals to a total daily dose of 2 g/day. Hydrocortisone 20–30 mg/day is usually sufficient for endogenous steroid replacement. Occasionally, mineralocorticoid (e.g., fludrocortisone) replacement therapy may be necessary.
Compatibility Information	Not applicable. Aminoglutethimide is commercially available as an oral product.
Contraindications/ Precautions	Contraindicated in patients with a known hypersensitivity to aminoglutethimide or any component and glutethimide. Risk versus benefit should be considered in patients with hepatic or renal function impairment, hypothyroidism, infection, or recent or existing chicken pox or herpes zoster infection.

Drug Interactions	**Agent**	**Effect**
	Dexamethasone	Concomitant use increases metabolism of dexamethasone.
	Digitoxin	Increases clearance of digitoxin after three to eight weeks of concomitant therapy.
	Propanolol	Case report of enhanced aminoglutethimide toxicity (e.g., rash, lethargy).
	Theophylline	Increases metabolism of theophylline.
	Warfarin	Diminishes anticoagulant effect of warfarin; monitor PT and adjust warfarin as necessary.

Toxicity/Side Effects	**Acute and/or Potentially Life-Threatening:** None noted.
	Serious: Adrenocortical hypofunction: patients should be monitored closely, particularly under conditions of stress (e.g., surgery, trauma, acute illness); hydrocortisone and mineralocorticoid therapy as indicated. Orthostatic or persistent hypotension also may occur and is related to aminoglutethimide's ability to suppress aldosterone production.
	Other: Most adverse effects diminish in incidence and severity after few weeks of therapy.
	Cardiovascular: Hypotension, occasionally orthostatic, and tachycardia. Dermatologic: Measles-like rash may appear on face and/or palms of hands; withdraw aminoglutethimide therapy if severe or persistent. GI: Nausea, vomiting, and anorexia. Neurologic: Headache, dizziness, drowsiness, and lethargy. Miscellaneous: Myalgia, masculinization and hirsutism in females, hypothyroidism, and nephrotoxicity.
Special Considerations	Administration of aminoglutethimide in divided doses reduces incidence of nausea and vomiting. Drowsiness, dizziness, and lethargy may be more pronounced in the elderly. Take missed dose as soon as possible if remembered within two to four hours, otherwise skip dose and take scheduled six-hour dose. Do not double-dose. Masculinization is reversible upon drug discontinuation.
Monitoring Parameters	No monitoring parameters recommended.
Indications	Indicated in the treatment of breast cancer and suppression of adrenal function in selected patients with Cushing's syndrome. May also be used in the treatment of prostate and adrenal cortical carcinoma.
Dosage Adjustment Recommendations	Dosage reduction may be necessary for significant CNS side effects and renal insufficiency. It is recommended that aminoglutethimide be withdrawn for severe skin rash or for mild to moderate skin rash that persists longer than five to eight days.
Pharmacokinetics	Well absorbed orally; the onset of action and of adrenal suppression is approximately three to five days; half-life is 7–15 hours, although aminoglutethimide induces its own metabolism with chronic administration; up to 50% of drug excreted unchanged in the urine; drug does cross the placenta (pregnancy category D).
Manufacturer	Novartis Pharmaceutical Corporation, East Hanover, NJ

Anastrozole

Other Names	Arimidex®
Classification	Antiestrogen, nonsteroidal selective aromatase inhibitor.
Mechanism	Anastrozole is a potent and selective aromatase inhibitor. Aromatase is required for the conversion of androstenedione to estrone, which is

	ultimately converted to estradiol. Anastrozole inhibits the enzyme aromatase, resulting in a significant reduction in estradiol. Many breast cancer tumors have estrogen receptors that are stimulated by estrogens.
Vesicant Information	Not classified as a vesicant or an irritant. Anastrozole is commercially available as an oral product.
Preparation and Mixture	No preparation or admixture necessary. Anastrozole is commercially available as an oral product.
Administration	Oral.
Storage and Stability	Store at controlled room temperature 20°–25°C (68°–77°F).
How Supplied	White, biconvex 1-mg tablets.
Dosage	One tablet (1 mg) taken orally once daily, without regard to food.
Compatibility Information	Not applicable. Anastrozole is commercially available as an oral product.
ContraIndications/ Precautions	Contraindicated in patients with known hypersensitivity to the drug or in women who are pregnant or breast-feeding. Risk versus benefit should be considered in patients with cardiac function impairment, renal or hepatic function impairment, prostatic hyperplasia, coronary artery disease, or a history of myocardial infarction.
Drug Interactions	No clinically significant drug interactions reported.
Toxicity/Side Effects	**Acute and/or Potentially Life-Threatening:** Thromboembolism.
	Serious: Chest pain, dyspnea, hypertension, and thrombophlebitis.
	Other:
	GI: GI disturbances, nausea, and increased cholesterol levels.
	Endocrine: Peripheral edema, hot flashes, and vaginal bleeding.
	Miscellaneous: Anemia, weakness, bone pain, tumor pain, myalgia, cough, dizziness, dry mouth, flushing, headache, skin reactions, and alopecia.
Special Considerations	It is unlikely that women will respond to anastrozole if they are estrogen-receptor negative or did not respond to tamoxifen.
Monitoring Parameters	No monitoring parameters recommended.
Indications	Anastrozole is recommended for the treatment of postmenopausal women with advanced breast cancer who have progressed on tamoxifen therapy or as first-line therapy for advanced hormone-receptor positive breast cancer in postmenopausal women.
Dosage Adjustment Recommendations	No dosage adjustment recommended for patients with renal or hepatic dysfunction.
Pharmacokinetics	Well absorbed orally; moderately bound to plasma proteins (40%); extensively metabolized in the liver; reaches steady-state levels in seven days; eliminated primarily through the biliary route with limited renal excretion.
Manufacturer	Zeneca Pharmaceuticals, Wilmington, DE

Bicalutamide

Other Name	Casodex®
Classification	Nonsteroidal antiandrogen.
Mechanism	Bicalutamide binds to androgen receptors, competitively inhibiting binding of dihydrotestosterone and testosterone. In prostate cancer, bicalutamide inhibits tumor growth and causes tumor regression.
Vesicant Information	Not classified as a vesicant or an irritant. Bicalutamide is commercially available as an oral product.
Preparation and Mixture	No preparation or admixture necessary. Bicalutamide is commercially available as an oral product.
Administration	Oral.
Storage and Stability	Store at controlled room temperature 20°–25°C (68°–77°F).
How Supplied	50-mg white, film-coated tablet.
Dosage	One tablet daily, given orally at the same time each day. May be given with or without food. Bicalutamide therapy should be initiated at the same time luteinizing hormone-releasing hormone (LHRH) treatment is started.
Compatibility Information	Not applicable. Bicalutamide is commercially available as an oral product.
Contraindications/ Precautions	Contraindicated in patients who are hypersensitive to bicalutamide, pregnant, or nursing. Risk versus benefit should be considered in patients with moderate to severe hepatic function impairment.
Drug Interactions	**Agent** **Effect** Warfarin Bicalutamide has been shown to displace warfarin from its protein-binding sites. It is recommended to monitor the PT closely if bicalutamide is started in a patient stabilized on warfarin; adjust warfarin dose as necessary.
Toxicity/Side Effects	**Acute and/or Potentially Life-Threatening:** None noted. **Serious:** CHF, angina, hypertension, and increased liver enzyme tests. **Other:** GI: Diarrhea. Endocrine: Hot flashes, breast pain, gynecomastia, edema, hypochromic and iron deficiency anemia, and hyperglycemia. Neurologic: Anxiety, depression, and confusion. Miscellaneous: Myalgia, leg cramps, urinary symptoms, fever, and infection.
Special Considerations	None.

Monitoring Parameters	Monitor liver function tests at beginning of therapy and periodically during therapy.
Indications	Bicalutamide is indicated for use in combination with a LHRH analogue (e.g., goserelin, leuprolide) for the treatment of advanced prostate cancer.
Dosage Adjustment Recommendations	Bicalutamide requires no dosing adjustment in patients with renal dysfunction. Caution should be used in patients with severe hepatic dysfunction because the drug may accumulate.
Pharmacokinetics	Bicalutamide is well absorbed orally; highly protein-bound (96%); extensively metabolized in the liver; eliminated in the urine and feces.
Manufacturer	Zeneca Pharmaceuticals, Wilmington, DE

Estradiol

Other Names	Oral: Estrace®; IM (estradiol valerate): Delestrogen®, Dioval®, Duragen®, Valergen®
Classification	Estrogen.
Mechanism	Estradiol reduces the release of gonadotropin-releasing hormone, resulting in a decrease in follicle-stimulating hormone (FSH) and luteinizing hormone (LH) release from the pituitary. Ultimately, the gonadal production of testosterone is decreased.
Vesicant Information	Not classified as a vesicant or an irritant.
Preparation and Mixture	No preparation or mixture required.
Administration	IM injection, oral.
Storage and Stability	Store between 15°–30°C (59°–86°F).
How Supplied	Oral: 0.5-mg, 1-mg, and 2-mg round, scored tablets; IM (estradiol valerate): 10 mg per ml, 20 mg per ml, and 40 mg per ml.
Dosage	Inoperable breast cancer: orally 10 mg three times per day with food for a minimum of three months; inoperable prostate cancer: orally 1–2 mg three times per day, IM 30 mg once every one to two weeks.
Compatibility Information	Estradiol valerate should not be mixed with any other drugs or solutions.
Contraindications/ Precautions	Contraindicated in patients who are pregnant, breast-feeding, or with undiagnosed abnormal genital bleeding. Estradiol should be used with caution in patients with a history of thromboembolic disorders. Risk versus benefit should be considered in patients with endometriosis, gallbladder disease, pancreatitis, hepatic function impairment, or hyperlipoproteinemia.

Drug Interactions	Agent	Effect
	Anticoagulants	Estrogens may reduce the effectiveness of anticoagulants. Monitor PT closely in patients receiving warfarin; adjust dose accordingly.
	Corticosteroids	Estrogens may increase the pharmacologic and toxic effects of corticosteroids. Corticosteroid dosage reduction may be necessary.

Toxicity/Side Effects	**Acute and/or Potentially Life-Threatening:** Thromboembolic events, myocardial infarction.
	Serious: Hypercalcemia, hypertension, peripheral edema, and pancreatitis.
	Other: GI: Nausea, anorexia, and bloating. Endocrine: Gynecomastia, breast pain, breast tenderness, amenorrhea, and breakthrough bleeding. Miscellaneous: Headache, increased libido (females), decreased libido (males), and intolerance to contact lenses.
Special Considerations	Estrogens have been reported to increase the risk of endometrial carcinoma in postmenopausal women. Estrogens may worsen cancer-related hypercalcemia.
Monitoring Parameters	No monitoring parameters recommended.
Indications	Used in the treatment of inoperable breast and prostate cancers.
Dosage Adjustment Recommendations	Estradiol should not be used in patients with severe liver disease. Dosage reduction is recommended in patients with mild liver disease. No specific dosage reduction recommendations are published.
Pharmacokinetics	Estradiol is readily absorbed from the GI tract; primarily metabolized in the liver; 80% protein bound; extensive enterohepatic recirculation occurs; primarily eliminated in urine with some drug eliminated in feces.
Manufacturer	Estrace®, Bristol-Myers Squibb Company, Princeton, NJ; Delestrogen®, E.R. Squibb & Sons, Inc., Princeton, NJ; Dioval®, Keene Pharmaceuticals, Keene, TX; Duragen®, Integra Lifesciences, Ltd., Plainsboro, NJ; Valergen®, Hyrex Pharmaceuticals, Memphis, TN.

Estrogens, conjugated

Other Names	Premarin®
Classification	Estrogen.
Mechanism	Conjugated estrogens reduce the release of gonadotropin-releasing hormone resulting in a decrease in FSH and LH release from the pituitary. Ultimately, the gonadal production of testosterone is decreased.

Vesicant Information	Not classified as a vesicant or an irritant. Conjugated estrogens are commercially available as an oral product.
Preparation and Mixture	No preparation or admixture necessary. Conjugated estrogens are commercially available as an oral product.
Administration	Oral.
Storage and Stability	Store between 15°–30°C (59°–86°F) in a well-closed container.
How Supplied	0.3-mg, 0.625-mg, 0.9-mg, 1.25-mg, and 2.5-mg oval tablets.
Dosage	Breast cancer: 10 mg by mouth three times per day for at least three months; prostate cancer: 1.25 mg–2.5 mg, by mouth three times per day.
Compatibility Information	Not applicable. Conjugated estrogens are commercially available as an oral product.
Contraindications/ Precautions	Contraindicated in patients who are pregnant or breast-feeding or have undiagnosed abnormal genital bleeding or a history of hypersensitivity reactions to estrogens. Conjugated estrogens should be used with caution in patients with a history of thromboembolic disorders. Risk versus benefit should be considered in patients with endometriosis, gallbladder disease, pancreatitis, hepatic function impairment, or hyperlipoproteinemia.

Drug Interactions	**Agent**	**Effect**
	Anticoagulants	Estrogens may reduce the effectiveness of anticoagulants. Monitor PT closely in patients receiving warfarin; adjust warfarin dose as necessary.
	Corticosteroids	Estrogens may increase the pharmacologic and toxic effects of corticosteroids. Corticosteroid dosage reduction may be necessary.

Toxicity/Side Effects	**Acute and/or Potentially Life-Threatening:** Thromboembolic events, myocardial infarction. **Serious:** Hypercalcemia, hypertension, peripheral edema, and pancreatitis. **Other:** GI: Nausea, anorexia, and bloating. Endocrine: Gynecomastia, breast pain, breast tenderness, amenorrhea, and breakthrough bleeding. Miscellaneous: Headache, increased libido (females), decreased libido (males), and intolerance to contact lenses.
Special Considerations	Estrogens have been reported to increase the risk of endometrial carcinoma in postmenopausal women. Estrogens may worsen cancer-related hypercalcemia.
Monitoring Parameters	No monitoring parameters recommended.

Indications	Conjugated estrogens are indicated in the treatment of inoperable and progressing breast cancer in selected males and postmenopausal females and in inoperable and progressing prostate cancer.
Dosage Adjustment Recommendations	Use with caution in patients with hepatic dysfunction. Conjugated estrogens should not be used in patients with severe or acute hepatic dysfunction. Mild hepatic dysfunction may require dose reductions. No specific dosage reduction recommendations are published.
Pharmacokinetics	Well absorbed from the GI tract; metabolized in the liver; excreted in the urine and bile.
Manufacturer	Wyeth-Ayerst Pharmaceuticals, Philadelphia, PA

Exemestane

Other Names	Aromasin®
Classification	Steroidal aromatase inactivator.
Mechanism	Suppresses plasma estrogen through irreversible inhibition of aromatase.
Vesicant Information	Not classified as a vesicant or an irritant. Exemestane is available commercially as an oral product.
Preparation and Mixture	No preparation or admixture necessary. Exemestane is available commercially as an oral product.
Administration	Oral.
Storage and Stability	Store in tightly sealed bottles at controlled room temperature 15°–30°C (59°–86°F).
How Supplied	Commercially available as 25-mg tablets in bottles of 30. The tablets are round, biconvex, off-white to gray in color, and imprinted with the number 7663 in black on one side.
Dosage	25 mg orally once daily after a meal.
Compatibility Information	Not applicable. Exemestane is available commercially as an oral product.
Contraindications/ Precautions	Contraindicated if known hypersensitivity to the product. Precaution should be exercised in patients with cardiovascular disease or hyperlipidemia, coadministration of estrogens, GI disorders, moderate to severe hepatic insufficiency, premenopausal status, or pregnancy.
Drug Interactions	No significant drug interactions reported.
Toxicity/Side Effects	**Acute and/or Potentially Life-Threatening:** None noted. **Serious:** Hypertension. **Other:** Most commonly seen side effects include nausea, fatigue, hot flashes, pain, depression, insomnia, anxiety, and dyspnea. Other effects reported include vomiting, edema, flu-like symptoms, dizziness, headache, abdominal pain, anorexia, and coughing.

Special Considerations	Should be taken after meals.
Monitoring Parameters	No monitoring parameters recommended.
Indications	Exemestane is indicated to treat advanced metastatic breast cancer in postmenopausal women who have not responded to tamoxifen therapy.
Dosage Adjustment Recommendations	No dosing adjustment is recommended for renal or hepatic dysfunction.
Pharmacokinetics	Exemestane is rapidly absorbed orally, with a 42% bioavailability. Giving dose following a high-fat meal significantly increases plasma levels. Exemestane is 90% protein bound. Metabolized by the liver and excreted in the urine and feces. The elimination half-life is 24 hours.
Manufacturer	Pharmacia & Upjohn, Peapack, NJ

Fluoxymesterone

Other Names	Halotestin®
Classification	Androgen.
Mechanism	Large doses of androgens appear to inhibit gonadotropin-releasing hormone release and subsequent estrogen production.
Vesicant Information	Not classified as a vesicant or an irritant. Fluoxymesterone is commercially available as an oral product.
Preparation and Mixture	No preparation or admixture necessary. Fluoxymesterone is commercially available as an oral product.
Administration	Oral.
Storage and Stability	Store at controlled room temperature 15°–30°C (59°–86°F).
How Supplied	2-mg, 5-mg, and 10-mg tablets.
Dosage	The dose for female breast cancer is 10–40 mg per day in divided doses, taken with food.
Compatibility Information	Not applicable. Fluoxymesterone is available commercially as an oral product.
Contraindications/ Precautions	Contraindicated in pregnancy; known hypersensitivity to the drug; severe cardiac, renal, or hepatic dysfunction; or in males with prostate or breast cancer. Risk versus benefit should be considered in patients with cardiac function impairment, coronary artery disease, history of myocardial infarction, diabetes mellitus, or prostatic hyperplasia.

Drug Interactions	**Agent** Anticoagulants	**Effect** Fluoxymesterone may increase the toxicity of oral anticoagulants. The doses of warfarin may need to be reduced with concomitant fluoxymesterone administration.
	Antidiabetic agents	Fluoxymesterone may increase toxicity of antidiabetic agents, including insulin and sulfonylureas. Doses of these agents may need to be reduced with concomitant fluoxymesterone administration.
Toxicity/Side Effects	**Acute and/or Potentially Life-Threatening:** None noted. **Serious:** Electrolyte abnormalities, hypercalcemia, jaundice, and hepatic dysfunction. **Other:** GI: Nausea and vomiting. Endocrine: Edema, acne, hypoglycemia, menstrual irregularities, amenorrhea, breast soreness, virilism, changes in libido, and hirsutism. Miscellaneous: Headache and anxiety.	
Special Considerations	Fluoxymesterone is a controlled substance. Monitor liver function tests periodically.	
Monitoring Parameters	No monitoring parameters recommended.	
Indications	Fluoxymesterone is indicated for palliative treatment of advanced breast cancer in females. It also is used for the treatment of anemia, hypogonadism, and delayed puberty in males.	
Dosage Adjustment Recommendations	Avoid using in patients with severe renal or hepatic dysfunction.	
Pharmacokinetics	Rapidly absorbed; time to peak concentration is one to two hours; undergoes hepatic metabolism; half-life of 9–13 hours; excreted in the urine.	
Manufacturer	Pharmacia & Upjohn, Peapack, NJ	

Flutamide

Other Names	Eulexin®
Classification	Nonsteroidal antiandrogen.
Mechanism	Flutamide binds to androgen receptors, competitively inhibiting binding of dihydrotestosterone and testosterone. In prostate cancer, flutamide inhibits tumor growth and causes tumor regression.
Vesicant Information	Not classified as a vesicant or an irritant. Flutamide is commercially available as an oral product.
Preparation and Mixture	No preparation or admixture necessary. Flutamide is commercially available as an oral product.

Administration	Oral.
Storage and Stability	Store between 2°–30°C (36°–86°F). Protect the unit-dose packages from excessive moisture.
How Supplied	Available as 125-mg, two-toned capsules.
Dosage	Two capsules (250 mg) by mouth three times per day for a total daily dose of 750 mg with or without food.
Compatibility Information	Not applicable. Flutamide is commercially available as an oral product.
Contraindications/ Precautions	Contraindicated in patients with a known hypersensitivity. Risk versus benefit should be considered in patients with hepatic function impairment.

Drug Interactions

Agent	Effect
Warfarin	Flutamide has been shown to displace warfarin from its protein-binding sites. If flutamide is initiated in a patient stabilized on warfarin, the PT should be monitored closely; adjust warfarin dose as necessary.

Toxicity/Side Effects	**Acute and/or Potentially Life-Threatening:** None noted. **Serious:** Hypertension, hepatitis, jaundice, hemolytic and macrocytic anemia. **Other:** GI: Diarrhea. Endocrine: Hot flashes, gynecomastia, and edema. Miscellaneous: Urine discoloration, decreased libido, impotence, photosensitivity, and skin reactions.
Special Considerations	Liver function tests should be monitored routinely.
Monitoring Parameters	See above.
Indications	Flutamide is indicated for use in combination with an LHRH analogue (e.g., goserelin, leuprolide) for the management of locally confined stage B_2-C and stage D_2 metastatic carcinoma of the prostate.
Dosage Adjustment Recommendations	The half-life of the active metabolite is slightly prolonged in patients with CrCl < 29 ml/minute. Flutamide requires no dosing adjustment in patients with chronic renal failure. Caution should be used in patients with severe hepatic dysfunction.
Pharmacokinetics	Flutamide is rapidly and completely absorbed following oral administration; rapidly and extensively metabolized to active alpha-hydroxylated metabolite; highly protein-bound (94%–96%); half-life of five to six hours; excreted primarily in urine with limited fecal excretion.
Manufacturer	Schering Corporation, Kenilworth, NJ

Goserelin acetate implant

Other Names	Zoladex®
Classification	Gonadotropin-releasing hormone analogue.
Mechanism	Goserelin suppresses secretion of LH and FSH, resulting in a decrease in testosterone levels and pharmacologic castration.
Vesicant Information	Not a vesicant or an irritant.
Preparation and Mixture	No preparation necessary.
Administration	Administer the appropriate dosage as an SC injection into the upper abdominal wall using aseptic technique under the supervision of a physician.
Storage and Stability	Store at controlled room temperature (do not exceed 25°C [77°F]).
How Supplied	Zoladex 3.6-mg implant and Zoladex 10.8-mg implant. Both dosages are prepared in a disposable syringe device fitted with a 14-gauge needle.
Dosage	Advanced prostate cancer: 3.6-mg implant every 28 days or 10.8-mg implant every 12 weeks. Although a delay of a few days is permissible, an effort should be made to adhere to the 28-day or 12-week dosing schedule.
Compatibility Information	Not applicable. Goserelin is given as an SC injection.
Contraindications/ Precautions	Contraindicated in women who are or may become pregnant while taking this drug or patients with spinal cord compression. Risk versus benefit should be considered in patients with abnormal, undiagnosed uterine bleeding or urinary tract obstruction or a history of urinary tract obstruction.
Drug Interactions	No drug interactions reported.
Toxicity/Side Effects	During the first few weeks of therapy, patients may experience a transient increase in testosterone levels and worsening of signs and symptoms of disease. Bone and tumor pain, temporary weakness and paresthesia of the lower limbs, and urinary obstructive symptoms have been reported.
	Acute and/or potentially life threatening: Cardiac arrhythmias and palpitations, pulmonary embolism, and anaphylaxis (e.g., SOB, rash, itching, hypotension).
	Other:
	GI: Nausea, vomiting, constipation, and diarrhea.
	Endocrine: Prostate carcinoma disease flare, endometrial disease flare, hot flashes, edema, swelling and tenderness of breasts, amenorrhea, and irregular vaginal bleeding.
	Neurologic: Blurred vision, dizziness, headache, trouble sleeping, and personality and behavioral changes.

	Miscellaneous: Decreased libido, decrease in size of testicles, impotence, injection site reaction, and weight gain.
Special Considerations	During the first few weeks of therapy, patients may experience a transient increase in testosterone levels and worsening of signs and symptoms of disease.
Monitoring Parameters	No monitoring parameters recommended.
Indications	Goserelin is indicated for the treatment of advanced prostate cancer, advanced breast cancer, and endometriosis. Goserelin also has been used in the treatment of ovarian cancer.
Dosage Adjustment Recommendations	No recommended dosing adjustments are necessary for patients with renal or hepatic dysfunction.
Pharmacokinetics	Peak mean concentrations (3 ng/ml) are reached approximately 15 days after administration; low-protein binding (< 30 %); hepatic metabolism and urinary excretion.
Manufacturer	Zeneca Pharmaceuticals, Wilmington, DE

Letrozole

Other Names	Femara®
Classification	Antiestrogen, nonsteroidal selective aromatase inhibitor.
Mechanism	Letrozole is a potent and selective aromatase inhibitor. Aromatase is required for the conversion of androstenedione to estrone. Letrozole inhibits the enzyme aromatase, resulting in a significant reduction in estradiol. Many breast cancer tumors have estrogen receptors that are stimulated by estrogens.
Vesicant Information	Not classified as a vesicant or an irritant. Letrozole is commercially available as an oral product.
Preparation and Mixture	No preparation or admixture necessary. Letrozole is commercially available as an oral product.
Administration	Oral.
Storage and Stability	Store at 25°C (77°F). Excursions permitted to 15°–30°C (59°–86°F).
How Supplied	Dark yellow, film-coated, round, 2.5-mg tablets.
Dosage	One 2.5-mg tablet daily, without regard to meals.
Compatibility Information	Not applicable. Letrozole is commercially available as an oral product.
Contraindications/ Precautions	Contraindicated in patients with known hypersensitivity to the drug or in women who are pregnant or breast-feeding. Risk versus benefit should be considered in patients with hepatic or renal function impairment.

Drug Interactions	No clinically significant drug interactions reported.
Toxicity/Side Effects	**Acute and/or Potentially Life-Threatening:** Thromboembolism. **Serious:** Chest pain and hypertension. **Other:** GI: Nausea, vomiting, constipation, diarrhea, abdominal pain, anorexia, and dyspepsia. Endocrine: Peripheral edema, vaginal bleeding, and hot flashes. Miscellaneous: Dyspnea, coughing, arthralgia, skin reactions, headache, dizziness, and depression.
Special Considerations	It is unlikely that women will respond to letrozole if they are estrogen-receptor negative or have not responded to tamoxifen.
Monitoring Parameters	No monitoring parameters recommended.
Indications	Letrozole is recommended for the treatment of postmenopausal women with advanced breast cancer who have progressed on tamoxifen therapy.
Dosage Adjustment Recommendations	No dosage adjustment is necessary for patients with CrCl $\geq$ 10 ml/minute or with mild to moderate hepatic dysfunction. Letrozole should be used with caution in patients with severe hepatic dysfunction.
Pharmacokinetics	Letrozole is rapidly and completely absorbed orally; weakly bound to plasma proteins; metabolized in the liver; steady-state levels attained in two to six weeks; renal elimination.
Manufacturer	Novartis Pharmaceuticals Corporation, East Hanover, NJ

Leuprolide

Other Names	Lupron®, Lupron Depot®, Lupron Depot®-3 Month 22.5 mg, Lupron Depot®-4 Month 30 mg, Viadur® (leuprolide acetate implant)
Classification	Gonadotropin-releasing hormone analogue.
Mechanism	Continuous administration of leuprolide suppresses secretion of gonadotropin-releasing hormone, resulting in a decrease in testosterone levels and pharmacologic castration.
Vesicant Information	Not classified as a vesicant or an irritant.
Preparation and Mixture	Vial and ampule: Withdraw the appropriate volume of the supplied diluent (1 ml for 7.5-mg depot, 1.5 ml for 22.5-mg depot) and inject it into the vial of lyophilized microspheres. Shake well. The resulting suspension will appear milky. Withdraw the contents of the vial and inject immediately. Do not dilute with any fluid other than the diluent provided. Prefilled dual chamber syringe: Attach the white plunger to the end stopper. Remove and discard the tab around the base of the needle. Release the diluent by slowly pushing the plunger until the first stopper is at the blue line in the middle of the barrel. Shake gently.

Administration	Administer dose in one IM injection using a 23-gauge or larger needle. Leuprolide implant is a titanium device that is implanted in the upper arm.
Storage and Stability	Prior to reconstitution, store at controlled room temperature 20°–25°C (68°–77°F). Upon reconstitution, the suspension is stable for 24 hours. Product does not contain a preservative.
How Supplied	Vial and ampule: Depot 7.5 mg, Depot-3 Month 22.5 mg, Depot-4 Month 30 mg. Prefilled dual-chamber syringe: Depot 7.5 mg, Depot-3 Month 22.5 mg, Depot-4 Month 30 mg.
Dosage	Advanced prostate cancer (depot formulations): 7.5 mg IM monthly (28–33 days), 22.5 mg IM every three months (84 days), or 30 mg IM every four months (16 weeks). The titanium implant delivers a controlled rate of leuprolide over 12 months.
Compatibility Information	Leuprolide should not be mixed with any other medication or solution.
Contraindications/ Precautions	Contraindicated in women who are or may become pregnant while taking this drug or patients with spinal cord compression. Risk versus benefit should be considered in patients with abnormal, undiagnosed uterine bleeding or urinary tract obstruction or a history of urinary tract obstruction.
Drug Interactions	No significant drug interactions reported.
Toxicity/Side Effects	During the first two weeks of therapy, patients may experience a transient increase in testosterone levels and worsening of signs and symptoms of disease. Temporary weakness and paresthesia of the lower limbs, bone pain, and urinary obstruction have been reported. **Acute and/or Potentially Life-Threatening:** Cardiac arrhythmias or palpitations (up to 19% in males) and anaphylaxis. **Serious:** See above. **Other:** GI: Nausea, vomiting, constipation, and diarrhea. Endocrine: Prostate carcinoma disease flare, endometrial disease flare, hot flashes, edema, swelling and tenderness of breasts, amenorrhea, irregular vaginal bleeding. Neurologic: Blurred vision, dizziness, headache, trouble sleeping, and personality and behavioral changes. Miscellaneous: Decreased libido, decrease in size of testicles, impotence, injection site reaction, and weight gain.
Special Considerations	During the first two weeks of therapy, patients may experience a transient increase in testosterone levels and worsening of signs and symptoms of disease.
Monitoring Parameters	No monitoring parameters recommended.

Indications	Leuprolide is indicated for the treatment of advanced prostate cancer, endometriosis, and precocious puberty. It also has been used in the treatment of breast, ovarian, and endometrial cancers.
Dosage Adjustment Recommendations	No dose adjustment recommendations for patients with renal or hepatic dysfunction.
Pharmacokinetics	Depot formulation provides peak plasma levels within four hours of administration with steady plasma concentrations through the dosing interval (one to three weeks) because of constant rate of release; 90% bioavailability; volume of distribution 27 l; moderate protein binding 46%; terminal half-life of three hours; metabolized to inactive peptides.
Manufacturer	Lupron®, Lupron Depot®, Lupron Depot®-3 Month 22.5 mg, Lupron Depot®-4 Month 30 mg, TAP Pharmaceuticals Inc., Deerfield, IL; Viadur® (leuprolide acetate implant), Alza Corporation, Palo Alto, CA

Medroxyprogesterone acetate

Other Names	Provera®, Depo-Provera®
Classification	Progestational agent.
Mechanism	The mechanism of action in patients with cancer has not been clearly defined. Medroxyprogesterone, like all progestins, appears to affect the serum concentration of other hormones, particularly estrogen. Progestins are thought to have antiestrogenic activity by decreasing the quantity of estrogen receptors or reducing the availability or stability of the hormone receptor complex. In addition, they may directly inhibit tumor growth, suppress the release of gonadotropins from the pituitary, and inhibit the growth of hormone-sensitive tumors.
Vesicant Information	Medroxyprogesterone is not considered a vesicant or an irritant.
Preparation and Mixture	No preparation or mixture is required. Medroxyprogesterone acetate is available as an aqueous suspension.
Administration	Shake well prior to administration. Medroxyprogesterone is administered IM for the treatment of patients with cancer.
Storage and Stability	Store at controlled room temperature. Protect from freezing.
How Supplied	Depo-Provera is available as 400-mg/ml aqueous suspension in 2.5 ml and 10-ml multidose vials.
Dosage	400–1,000 mg given IM weekly.
Compatibility Information	Medroxyprogesterone acetate aqueous suspension should not be mixed with any other drugs.
Contraindications/ Precautions	Contraindicated in the following situations: known or suspected pregnancy; undiagnosed vaginal bleeding; known or suspected malignancy of the breast; active thrombophlebitis, current or past history of thromboembolic

	disorders, or cerebral vascular disease; liver dysfunction or disease; known sensitivity to medroxyprogesterone.
Drug Interactions	**Agent** **Effect** Aminoglutethimide May decrease the effectiveness of medroxyprogesterone by increasing hepatic metabolism.
Toxicity/Side Effects	**Acute and/or Potentially Life-Threatening:** Pulmonary embolism. **Serious:** Jaundice. **Other:** Endocrine: Edema, changes in menstrual flow, and amenorrhea. Miscellaneous: Weakness, depression, fever, insomnia, changes in weight, acne, hirsutism, alopecia, thrombophlebitis, and skin reactions.
Special Considerations	Patients should be instructed to notify their physician if sudden loss of vision or migraine headache occurs.
Monitoring Parameters	No monitoring parameters recommended.
Indications	Medroxyprogesterone acetate is indicated as adjunctive therapy and palliative treatment of inoperable, recurrent, and metastatic endometrial or renal carcinoma. It also has been used in the treatment of advanced breast cancer.
Dosage Adjustment Recommendations	Because of the possibility of medroxyprogesterone causing fluid retention, patients with renal dysfunction should be observed carefully. Patients with hepatic dysfunction should not receive this drug.
Pharmacokinetics	Following IM administration, peak plasma concentrations were reached within two to seven hours; 90% bound to plasma proteins; metabolized in the liver; excreted in urine and feces.
Manufacturer	Pharmacia & Upjohn, Inc., Peapack, NJ

Megestrol acetate

Other Names	Megace®
Classification	Progestational agent.
Mechanism	The mechanism of action in patients with cancer has not been clearly defined. Megestrol acetate, like all progestins, appears to affect the serum concentration of other hormones, particularly estrogen. Progestins are thought to have antiestrogenic activity by decreasing the quantity of estrogen receptors or reducing the availability or stability of the hormone receptor complex. In addition, they may directly inhibit tumor growth, suppress the release of gonadotropins from the pituitary, and inhibit the growth of hormone-sensitive tumors.
Vesicant Information	Not classified as a vesicant or an irritant. Megestrol is commercially available as an oral product.

Preparation and Mixture	No preparation or admixture necessary. Megestrol is commercially available as an oral product.
Administration	Oral.
Storage and Stability	Store between 15°–25°C (59°–77°F) in a well-closed container.
How Supplied	Megestrol acetate is available as 20-mg and 40-mg white, scored tablets. Megestrol is also available as a 40-mg/ml suspension.
Dosage	For the treatment of cachexia: 800 mg (20-ml suspension) per day as a single daily dose. For the treatment of advanced breast cancer: 160 mg per day in divided doses. For the treatment of endometrial cancer: 40–320 mg per day in divided doses.
Compatibility Information	Not applicable. Megestrol is commercially available as an oral product.
Contraindications/ Precautions	Contraindicated during pregnancy or breast-feeding or in patients with a history of hypersensitivity to the drug. Megestrol should be used with caution in patients with a history of thrombophlebitis.
Drug Interactions	No significant drug interactions have been reported.
Toxicity/Side Effects	**Acute and/or Potentially Life-Threatening:** Pulmonary embolism. **Serious:** Hepatotoxicity. **Other:** GI: Nausea and vomiting. Endocrine: Edema, abnormal menstrual bleeding, amenorrhea, and hyperglycemia. Neurologic: Depression, headache, and insomnia. Miscellaneous: Weight gain, weakness, fever, dyspnea, alopecia, rash, thrombophlebitis, and carpal tunnel syndrome.
Special Considerations	Megestrol should be taken orally with or without food. Shake suspension well before use. A minimum of two months of continuous therapy is required for assessing efficacy in patients with cancer.
Monitoring Parameters	No monitoring parameters recommended.
Indications	Megestrol is indicated for the palliative treatment of advanced carcinoma of the breast or endometrium (i.e., recurrent, inoperable, or metastatic disease). The oral suspension is indicated for the treatment of HIV-related cachexia. Megestrol also has been used in the treatment of cancer-related cachexia as well as in the treatment of ovarian, prostate, and renal cell cancer.
Dosage Adjustment Recommendations	No dosage adjustments are recommended for patients with renal or hepatic dysfunction.
Pharmacokinetics	Megestrol is well absorbed orally and metabolized in the liver. Primarily eliminated in the urine. Some drug is eliminated in the feces and bile.
Manufacturer	Bristol-Myers Squibb Oncology/Immunology Division, Princeton, NJ

Mitotane

Other Names	Lysodren®
Classification	Antiadrenal agent.
Mechanism	The exact mechanism of action is unknown. Mitotane causes adrenal cortical atrophy, with cytotoxic effects on mitochondria in adrenal cortical cells. The production of cortisol is reduced. Peripheral cortisol and androgen metabolism also are altered.
Vesicant Information	Not classified as a vesicant or an irritant. Mitotane is commercially available as an oral product.
Preparation and Mixture	No preparation or admixture necessary. Mitotane is commercially available as an oral product.
Administration	Oral.
Storage and Stability	Store at controlled room temperature.
How Supplied	500-mg scored tablets.
Dosage	Initially, 2–6 g per day in 3–4 divided doses should be given. The dose should be titrated up to 9–10 g per day based on clinical response and adverse effects. Mitotane should not be taken with high-fat foods.
Compatibility Information	Not applicable. Mitotane is available commercially as an oral product.
Contraindications/ Precautions	Contraindicated in patients who are breast-feeding or who are hypersensitive to the drug. Safety during pregnancy has not been established. Only use during pregnancy when the potential benefits outweigh the risks. Risk versus benefit should be considered in patients with hepatic function impairment or infection.

Drug Interactions	**Agent**	**Effect**
	Corticosteroids	The metabolism of corticosteroids may be increased during concomitant therapy with mitotane. The dosage of corticosteroids may need to be increased.
	Warfarin	The metabolism of warfarin may be increased during concomitant therapy with mitotane. The dosage of warfarin may need to be increased.

Toxicity/Side Effects	**Acute and/or Potentially Life-Threatening:** None noted.
	Serious: Visual disturbances, hematuria, hemorrhagic cystitis, albuminuria, and hypertension.
	Other: GI: Anorexia, nausea, vomiting, and diarrhea. Miscellaneous: Depression, dizziness, skin reactions, flushing, orthostatic hypotension, generalized aching, and fever.

Special Considerations	Mitotane should be temporarily discontinued immediately following trauma or shock. Behavioral and neurological testing should be performed routinely in patients receiving long-term, high-dose therapy. These patients are at risk of developing brain damage. Patients may require adrenal steroid replacement if adrenal insufficiency develops.
Monitoring Parameters	No monitoring parameters recommended.
Indications	Mitotane is indicated in the treatment of inoperable adrenal cortical carcinoma of both functional and nonfunctional types.
Dosage Adjustment Recommendations	No dosage adjustment necessary in patients with renal compromise. Patients with hepatic dysfunction may require dosage reduction.
Pharmacokinetics	Approximately 40% absorbed orally; hepatic metabolism; 60% of dose excreted unchanged in stool, also excreted in urine; remainder stored in body fat.
Manufacturer	Bristol-Myers Squibb Oncology/Immunology Division, Princeton, NJ

Nilutamide

Other Names	Nilandron®
Classification	Nonsteroidal antiandrogen.
Mechanism	Nilutamide is a nonsteroidal antiandrogen that inhibits androgen uptake and binds to androgen receptors competitively inhibiting binding of androgen in target tissues. In prostate cancer, nilutamide inhibits tumor growth and causes tumor regression.
Vesicant Information	Not classified as a vesicant or an irritant. Nilutamide is commercially available as an oral product.
Preparation and Mixture	No preparation or admixture necessary. Nilutamide is commercially available as an oral product.
Administration	Oral.
Storage and Stability	Store between 15°–30°C (59°–86°F). Protect from light.
How Supplied	50-mg white, biconvex tablets.
Dosage	300 mg once a day for 30 days, then 150 mg once a day thereafter with or without food.
Compatibility Information	Not applicable. Nilutamide is commercially available as an oral product.
Contraindications/ Precautions	Contraindicated in patients with severe hepatic impairment, severe respiratory insufficiency, or hypersensitivity to the drug. Risk versus benefit should be considered in patients with severe respiratory function impairment or hepatic function impairment.
Drug Interactions	Nilutamide can delay the elimination and increase the serum concentration of the following drugs: fosphenytoin, phenytoin, theophylline, and

	warfarin. If nilutamide must be given with one of these agents, frequent monitoring is recommended.
Toxicity/Side Effects	**Acute and/or Potentially Life-Threatening:** Hepatotoxicity. **Serious:** Pneumonia, upper respiratory tract infections, interstitial pneumonitis, and hypertension. **Other:** GI: Nausea, constipation, and anorexia. Endocrine: Gynecomastia and hot flashes. Neurologic: Headache, insomnia, and depression. Miscellaneous: Decreased libido, impotence, diaphoresis, weakness, fever, rash, and ocular photosensitivity.
Special Considerations	Advise patients to report to their physician any of the following effects: dyspnea, jaundice, dark urine, fatigue, and abdominal pain. Patients should not consume alcoholic beverages while taking nilutamide.
Monitoring Parameters	Monitoring is recommended prior to initiation of therapy or at periodic intervals during therapy. • Liver function tests: ALT, AST, alkaline phosphatase. • Renal function tests: BUN, SCr.
Indications	Nilutamide is indicated with surgical or medical castration in the treatment of metastatic prostate cancer in patients with normal liver and respiratory function.
Dosage Adjustment Recommendations	No dosage adjustment necessary for patients with renal dysfunction. Patients with severe hepatic dysfunction should not receive this drug.
Pharmacokinetics	Nilutamide is well absorbed orally; undergoes extensive hepatic metabolism; moderate plasma protein binding (84%); primarily eliminated in urine, with limited fecal elimination.
Manufacturer	Hoechst Marion Roussel, Kansas City, MO

Raloxifene

Other Names	Evista®
Classification	Selective estrogen receptor modulator.
Mechanism	Raloxifene binds to estrogen receptors, resulting in different effects depending on the receptor location. It has estrogenic effects in the bone (increasing bone mineral density) and on lipid metabolism (decreasing in total and low-density lipoprotein [LDL] cholesterol levels). Raloxifene is an estrogen receptor antagonist in uterine and breast tissues.
Vesicant Information	Not classified as a vesicant or an irritant. Raloxifene is commercially available as an oral product.
Preparation and Mixture	No preparation or mixture necessary. Raloxifene is commercially available as an oral product.
Administration	Oral.

Storage and Stability	Store at controlled room temperature 20°–25°C (68°–77°F).
How Supplied	60-mg white, elliptical, film-coated tablets.
Dosage	One 60-mg tablet by mouth once daily. It may be given at any time of the day without regard to meals.
Compatibility Information	Not applicable. Raloxifene is commercially available as an oral product.
Contraindications/ Precautions	Contraindicated in women who are pregnant or nursing or who have a history of venous thrombotic events or hypersensitivity reactions to raloxifene.

Drug Interactions	**Agent**	**Effect**
	Cholestyramine	Significantly reduces the absorption of raloxifene and should not be used concurrently.
	Warfarin	Raloxifene may decrease the PT in patients taking warfarin. Monitor PT closely.
	Protein-bound drugs	Raloxifene is highly protein-bound. Caution should be used when raloxifene is administered with other highly protein-bound drugs, such as clofibrate, indomethacin, ibuprofen, naproxen, and diazepam.

Toxicity/Side Effects	**Acute and/or Potentially Life-Threatening:** Deep vein thrombosis and pulmonary embolism. **Serious:** Retinal thrombosis and chest pain. **Other:** Hot flashes, leg cramps, migraine, fever, depression, insomnia, weight gain, edema, and infection.
Special Considerations	The greatest risk for thromboembolic events occurs during the first four months of treatment. Raloxifene should be discontinued at least 72 hours prior to prolonged immobilization.
Monitoring Parameters	No monitoring parameters recommended.
Indications	Raloxifene is indicated for the prevention of osteoporosis in postmenopausal women. Raloxifene also is under investigation for the treatment of estrogen-receptor positive patients with breast cancer, as well as in the prevention of breast cancer in high-risk postmenopausal women.
Dosage Adjustment Recommendations	Raloxifene dose may need to be reduced in patients with severe hepatic dysfunction. No dosage reducation necessary in patients with renal dysfunction.
Pharmacokinetics	Raloxifene is rapidly absorbed orally; only 2% bioavailability because of extensive presystemic glucuronide conjugation; volume of distribution of 2,348 l/kg; 95% protein-bound; half-life of approximately 32 hours; extensive first-pass metabolism; primarily excreted in the feces; limited urinary elimination.
Manufacturer	Eli Lilly and Company, Indianapolis, IN

Tamoxifen

Other Names	Nolvadex®
Classification	Nonsteroidal antiestrogen.
Mechanism	Tamoxifen competitively binds to estrogen receptors in tumors and other tissues. Antiestrogenic effects are seen on the breast, whereas estrogenic effects are seen on the bones, lipids, and endometrium.
Vesicant Information	Not classified as a vesicant or an irritant. Tamoxifen is commercially available as an oral product.
Preparation and Mixture	No preparation or admixture necessary. Tamoxifen is commercially available as an oral product.
Administration	Oral.
Storage and Stability	Store at controlled room temperature.
How Supplied	10-mg and 20-mg tablets.
Dosage	20–40 mg per day. Doses above 20 mg should be given in divided doses. In the adjuvant setting, five years of tamoxifen is the recommended duration of treatment. The tamoxifen regimen used in the chemoprevention studies was 20 mg a day for five years.
Compatibility Information	Not applicable. Tamoxifen is available commercially as an oral product.
Contraindications/ Precautions	Contraindicated in patients with a known hypersensitivity to the drug; patients who are pregnant or breast-feeding; patients with a history of deep vein thrombosis or pulmonary embolism; and in patients that require concomitant anticoagulant therapy. Risk versus benefit should be considered in patients with visual disturbances, cataracts, and hyperlipidemia.
Drug Interactions	**Agent** / **Effect** Warfarin — Tamoxifen may increase the risk of bleeding in patients stabilized on warfarin therapy. Monitor PT; dose of warfarin may need to be reduced. Estrogens — May interfere with tamoxifen's therapeutic effect.
Toxicity/Side Effects	**Acute and/or Potentially Life-Threatening:** Endometrial cancer, deep vein thrombosis, and pulmonary embolism. **Serious:** Visual disturbances (e.g., ocular toxicity including retinopathy, keratopathy, cataracts, optic neuritis) and hypercalcemia. **Other:** GI: Nausea, vomiting, and weight gain. Endocrine: Hot flashes, menstrual irregularities, vaginal bleeding, and vaginal discharge.

	Miscellaneous: Increased bone and tumor pain (associated with good tumor response), transient leukopenia and thrombocytopenia, rash, and depression.
Special Considerations	An initial disease flare can occur. Patients should be advised of the potential for a transient increase in bone pain, tumor pain, and hot flashes. Because of tamoxifen's estrogenic activity in the uterus, endometrial changes, including hyperplasia, polyps, and cancer, can occur. Gynecologic and ophthalmologic examinations recommended at regular intervals.
Monitoring Parameters	No monitoring parameters recommended.
Indications	Tamoxifen is indicated for the treatment of metastatic breast cancer in females and males. In the adjuvant setting, tamoxifen is indicated for the treatment of node-negative premenopausal and postmenopausal women and node-positive postmenopausal women. It also is indicated to reduce the incidence of breast cancer in high-risk patients.
Dosage Adjustment Recommendations	No dosing adjustment recommendations.
Pharmacokinetics	Rapidly absorbed orally; steady-state levels attained in four to six weeks; 99% protein-bound; hepatic metabolism; elimination half-life seven days; eliminated primarily through biliary/fecal route; limited renal elimination.
Manufacturer	Zeneca Pharmaceuticals, Wilmington, DE

Testosterone

Other Names	Testosterone injectable (aqueous) suspension: Andro®, Histerone®; testosterone propionate; testosterone cypionate: Andro-Cyp®, Andronate®, Depotest®, Duratest®; testosterone enenthate: Andro L.A.®, Durathate®; oral (methyltestosterone): Android®, Testred®, Virilon®; various generic testosterone formulations also are available.
Classification	Androgen.
Mechanism	Large doses of androgens appear to inhibit gonadotropin-releasing hormone release and subsequent estrogen production.
Vesicant Information	Testosterone is not considered a vesicant or an irritant. Inflammation and pain at the site of injection have been reported.
Preparation and Mixture	Shake the IM formulations well prior to administration.
Administration	IM injection, oral.
Storage and Stability	Store between 15°–30°C (59°–86°F).
How Supplied	Testosterone injectable suspension: 25 mg per ml, 50 mg per ml, or 100 mg per ml; testosterone propionate: 100 mg per ml; testosterone cypionate and

	testosterone enanthate: 100 mg per ml and 200 mg per ml; methyltestoster-one: 10-mg and 25-mg tablets, 10-mg buccal tablets, and 25-mg capsules.
Dosage	Testosterone injectable suspension and testosterone propionate: 50–100 mg IM two or three times per week; testosterone cypionate and testoster-one enanthate: 200–400 mg IM every two to four weeks; methyltestoster-one: 50 mg orally one to two times daily.
Compatibility Information	Testosterone should not be mixed with any other drug or fluid.
Contraindications/ Precautions	Contraindicated in patients with severe renal or cardiac disease, male patients with breast or prostate cancer, pregnant or breast-feeding women, and patients with a history of hypersensitivity to the drug. Risk versus benefit should be considered in patients with cardiac function impair-ment, coronary artery disease, history of myocardial infarction, diabetes mellitus, or prostatic hyperplasia.
Drug Interactions	**Agent** **Effect** Warfarin — The toxicity and anticoagulant effects of war-farin may be enhanced. Monitor PT; dosage reduction of warfarin may be warranted. Antidiabetic agents — The dosage of antidiabetic agents may need to be adjusted because of the increases or decreases in blood sugar that may occur with testosterone.
Toxicity/Side Effects	**Acute and/or Potentially Life-Threatening:** None noted. **Serious:** Hepatic dysfunction, jaundice, hypercalcemia, and leukopenia. **Other:** GI: Nausea, vomiting, and diarrhea. Endocrine: Amenorrhea, virilism, acne, flushing, and edema. Miscellaneous: Changes in libido, dizziness, abnormal hair growth, head-ache, infection, stomach pain, and trouble sleeping.
Special Considerations	Take oral product with food. Hepatic neoplasms have been associated with long-term, high-dose androgen use. Monitor liver function tests pe-riodically. Testosterone is a controlled substance.
Monitoring Parameters	Monitoring recommended prior to initiating therapy and at periodic intervals. See above.
Indications	Testosterone is indicated in the treatment of inoperable female breast cancer. It also is used in the treatment of hypogonadism in males.
Dosage Adjustment Recommendations	The dosage may need to be reduced in patients with renal or hepatic dysfunction.
Pharmacokinetics	The pharmacokinetic profile of testosterone varies depending on the ester, dosage form, and route of administration; high first-pass metabolism with oral administration; very highly protein-bound (99%) (80% to sex hormone-binding globulin and 19% to albumin); metabolized in the liver; enanthate and cypionate esters are longer-acting than propionate ester and base; metabolites are excreted in the urine with some fecal elimination.

Manufacturer	Andro®, Novavax, Inc., Columbia, MD; Histerone®, Roberts Pharmaceuticals, Eatontown, NJ; Andro-Cyp®, Keene Pharmaceuticals, Keene, TX; Andronate®, Pasadena Research Labs, San Clemente, CA; Depotest®, Hyrex Pharmaceuticals, Memphis, TN; Duratest®, Roberts Pharmaceuticals, Eatontown, NJ; Andro L.A.®, Forest Pharmaceuticals, St. Louis, MO; Durathate®, Roberts Pharmaceuticals, Eatontown, NY; Android®, Testred®, ICN Pharmaceuticals, Inc., Costa Mesa, CA; Virilon®, Star Pharmaceuticals, Inc., Pompano Beach, FL

Toremifene

Other Names	Fareston®
Classification	Nonsteroidal antiestrogen.
Mechanism	Toremifene competitively binds to estrogen receptors in tumors and other tissues. In breast cancer, toremifene works by blocking the tumor growth-stimulating effects of estrogen.
Vesicant Information	Not classified as a vesicant or an irritant. Toremifene is commercially available as an oral product.
Preparation and Mixture	No preparation or admixture necessary. Toremifene is commercially available as an oral product.
Administration	Oral.
Storage and Stability	Store at 25°C (77°F). Protect from heat and light.
How Supplied	60-mg round white tablet.
Dosage	One tablet by mouth once daily. May be taken with or without food.
Compatibility Information	Not applicable. Toremifene is commercially available as an oral product.
Contraindications/ Precautions	Contraindicated in patients with a known hypersensitivity to the drug, patients who are pregnant or breast-feeding, and patients with a history of thromboembolic disease. Caution should be used in patients with pre-existing endometrial hyperplasia.

Drug Interactions	Agent	Effect
	Warfarin	Toremifene may increase the risk of bleeding in patients stabilized on warfarin therapy.
	Erythromycin, ketoconazole	May inhibit the metabolism of toremifene, resulting in increased levels of toremifene.
	Carbamazepine, phenobarbital, phenytoin	May induce the metabolism of toremifene, decreasing its effectiveness.
	Thiazide diuretics	Decrease the renal excretion of calcium; may increase the risk of developing hypercalcemia.

Toxicity/Side Effects	**Acute and/or Potentially Life-Threatening:** Thromboembolic events, cardiac failure, and myocardial infarction. **Serious:** Visual disturbances, hypercalcemia, endometrial hyperplasia, and hepatotoxicity. **Other:** GI: Nausea and vomiting. Endocrine: Hot flashes, menstrual irregularities, vaginal discharge, and vaginal bleeding. Miscellaneous: Sweating, dizziness, and headache.
Special Considerations	An initial disease flare can occur. Patients should be advised of the potential for a transient increase in bone pain, tumor pain (associated with a good response), hypercalcemia, and hot flashes.
Monitoring Parameters	No monitoring parameters recommended.
Indications	Toremifene is indicated for the treatment of metastatic breast cancer in patients with estrogen-receptor positive or estrogen-receptor unknown tumors.
Dosage Adjustment Recommendations	No dosage adjustment necessary for renal dysfunction. Patients with hepatic dysfunction may require dose reductions. No specific recommendations have been published.
Pharmacokinetics	Well absorbed; 99.5 % protein-bound; steady-state levels attained in four to six weeks; hepatically metabolized; elimination half-life of five days; eliminated primarily through the fecal route, limited renal elimination.
Manufacturer	Schering Corporation, Kenilworth, NJ

Biotherapeutics

Aldesleukin

Other Names	Proleukin®, interleukin-2, IL-2
Classification	Biological response modifier.
Mechanism	Promotes proliferation, differentiation, and recruitment of T and B cells, natural killer cells, and thymocytes; cytolytic activity in a subset of lymphocytes; stimulation of lymphokine-activated killer cells and tumor-infiltrating lymphocytes.
Vesicant Information	Not classified as a vesicant or an irritant.
Preparation and Mixture	Reconstitution and dilution other than those recommended by the manufacturer may alter the delivery and/or pharmacology of IL-2. SC or IM injection: 1. Reconstitute with 1.2 ml Sterile Water for Injection, USP, directed at the side of the vial. Gently swirl; DO NOT SHAKE. No further dilution necessary for SC or IM administrations. Final concentration is 18 million IU per 1 ml. IV infusion: 1. The reconstituted dose should be diluted with D_5W in a glass or PVC bag. DO NOT dilute with NS. 2. Bolus doses may be diluted in 50–100 ml of D_5W and administered over 15–30 minutes; continuous infusions usually diluted in 250–500 ml D_5W. Concentrations of IL-2 should not fall below 30 mcg/ml (500,000 IU/ml) or exceed 70 mcg/ml (1.2 million IU/ml). Dilution of IL-2 outside this recommended concentration range should be avoided. 3. DO NOT filter. 4. Concentrations below 60 mcg/ml (1 million IU/ml) require the addition of 5% human albumin (1 ml for every 50 ml of D_5W) to PVC bag prior to the addition of IL-2.
Administration	IL-2 may be given SC, IM, and as an IV infusion (15-minute bolus infusion most common). IL-2 also has been administered by continuous IV infusion, which in high doses requires cardiac monitoring. Investigationally, IL-2 also has been administered intraperitoneally, via hepatic artery infusion, and by isolated limb perfusion. DO NOT dilute or piggyback with NS or bacteriostatic solutions.
Storage and Stability	Store lyophilized vials in refrigerator at 2°–8°C (36°–46°F). Reconstituted or diluted IL-2 is stable for up to 48 hours at refrigerated and room temperatures. However, because this product does not contain a preservative, the reconstituted or diluted solution should be stored in the refrigerator. Do not freeze. Refrigerated solutions should be brought to room temperature prior to administration.
How Supplied	IL-2 is a sterile, white to off-white, preservative-free, lyophilized powder packaged in vials containing 22 million IU. Proleukin for injection is supplied

	in individually boxed single-use vials. Each vial contains 22 x 10⁶ IU of IL-2. Discard unused portion.
Dosage	IL-2 is indicated in the treatment of metastatic renal cell carcinoma and metastatic melanoma. A variety of dosages and dosing regimens have been investigated. The approved dosage regimen is 600,000 IU/kg per dose as a 15-minute infusion every eight hours for a total of 14 doses; following nine days of rest, the schedule is repeated for another 14 doses, for a maximum of 28 doses per course. Prior to retreatment, patients should be evaluated for response at least four weeks after completion of a treatment course. Other dosage regimens used include 9 million–18 million units/m²/day IV continuous infusion for three to five days and repeated at intervals of one to four weeks; 5 million–9 million units/m²/day SC administered three to five times per week.
Compatibility Information	Compatible only with D_5W. Do not reconstitute or dilute with NS or bacteriostatic water for injection, as aggregation and precipitation of IL-2 may occur.
Contraindications/ Precautions	Contraindicated in patients with a known hypersensitivity to IL-2 or any component of formulation, patients with abnormal thallium stress test or pulmonary function tests, and patients with organ allografts. Retreatment is contraindicated in patients experiencing cardiac abnormalities, intubation, renal failure, seizures, and other significant toxicities while on the drug. Refer to package insert for more detailed information.

Drug Interactions

Agent	Effect
Psychotropic drugs (e.g., opioid analgesics, sedatives)	Increased CNS toxicity (sedation, confusion).
Antihypertensives	May potentiate hypotension seen with IL-2.
Glucocorticosteroids	May reduce effectiveness of IL-2.
Nephrotoxins (e.g., aminoglycosides, indomethacin), cardiotoxins (e.g., doxorubicin), hepatotoxins (e.g., MTX), myelotoxins (e.g., cytotoxic chemotherapy)	May increase toxicity in kidney, heart, liver, bone marrow systems.
Iodinated contrast media	Acute reactions, including fever, chills, nausea and vomiting, hypotension, and oliguria may occur within hours of contrast infusion; this reaction may occur within weeks to months following IL-2 administration.

Toxicity/Side Effects	Intensity of adverse effects related to dose and duration of therapy. **Acute and/or Potentially Life-Threatening:** High-dose therapy may cause hemodynamic instability (e.g., severe hypotension, tachycardia, pulmonary edema) requiring fluid and vasopressor support. A capillary leak syndrome manifested by an increase in vascular permeability (e.g., peripheral edema, ascites, pulmonary infiltrates, pleural effusion); begins

with first dose and increases in magnitude with repetitive doses; resolves after therapy ends.

Serious: Hypotension, fluid retention, and renal dysfunction (e.g., oliguria, anuria, increased SCr) are dose-limiting.

Other:

Dermatologic: Skin erythema, burning and itching; may involve entire body, although head and neck most prominent; usually begins two to three days after onset of IL-2 treatment and slowly begins to resolve within 72 hours after treatment discontinuation; desquamation follows; alopecia also may occur.

GI: Nausea, vomiting, and diarrhea.

Hematologic: Thrombocytopenia, anemia, leukopenia, and eosinophilia.

Neurologic: Transient somnolence, impaired memory, headache, dizziness, confusion, and seizures; resolves rapidly with cessation of IL-2.

Miscellaneous: Flu-like syndrome (e.g., generalized weakness, fever, chills, rigors); may respond to acetaminophen; electrolyte abnormalities, hypothyroidism, transient increases in liver enzymes, and substantial weight gain (> 10% of body weight).

Special Considerations	High-dose therapy requires cardiac monitoring and possible vasopressor support. Daily monitoring of vital signs, weight, and pulmonary function is recommended during high-dose therapy. Standard prophylactic supportive care during high-dose IL-2 therapy includes acetaminophen for constitutional symptoms (e.g., fever, chills), serotonin antagonists to reduce incidence of nausea and vomiting and H_2 antagonists (e.g., ranitidine) to reduce the risk of GI ulceration and bleeding. Avoid the use of corticosteroids (topical or systemic).
Monitoring Parameters	See above.
Indications	FDA-approved for metastatic renal cell cancer and metastatic malignant melanoma. Also studied in colorectal cancer, bladder cancer (as a continuous bladder perfusion), and ovarian cancer (intraperitoneally).
Dosage Adjustment Recommendations	There are a number of clinical situations (e.g., hypotension, decreased oxygen saturation, elevated SCr, mental status changes, grade III or IV toxicities) when IL-2 therapy should be held, discontinued, or restarted. Refer to package insert or specific protocol for detailed information on dosage adjustments.
Pharmacokinetics	IL-2 is not absorbed orally; half-life of 30–60 minutes; eliminated from the body through metabolism in the kidneys.
Manufacturer	Chiron Corporation, Emeryville, CA

Bacillus Calmette-Guérin (BCG) Vaccine

Other Names	BCG Vaccine, TICE® BCG (for vaccination), TheraCys® (for bladder instillation)
Classification	Biological response modifier; vaccine prepared from lyophilized preparation of the live, attenuated strain of *Mycobacterium bovis* (Calmette-Guérin strain).

Mechanism	BCG works by causing a local inflammatory reaction with histiocytic and leukocytic infiltration in the urinary bladder.
Vesicant Information	Not classified as a vesicant or an irritant.
Preparation and Mixture	Reconstitute BCG with 3 ml sterile water for injection without preservatives. Further dilute the product in 50 ml saline to make a total of 53 ml for intravesical instillation.
Administration	Prepared solution is instilled into an empty bladder for one to two hours as tolerated. The patient may lie in the prone and supine positions and on each side for 15 minutes each, then arise for the second hour while the suspension is retained. At the end of the retention time, the patient should void in a seated position.
Storage and Stability	Store intact ampules under refrigeration and protected from light. After reconstitution, the solution should be protected from light, refrigerated, and used within two hours. At no time should the freeze-dried or reconstituted product be exposed to direct or indirect sunlight.
How Supplied	TheraCys is available as a creamy white, dried mass in a single-use vial. Also supplied is a 3-ml diluent for reconstitution of the product and a 50-ml vial of phosphate buffered saline solution for use as the final diluent. BCG also is formulated for use as a vaccine, and the doses and vial sizes differ from this product.
Dosage	Common immunotherapy dosages of BCG by intravesical instillation in the treatment of superficial bladder cancer is $10.5 +/-8.7 \times 10^8$ colony-forming units (one vial). BCG is instilled into the bladder and allowed to remain around the site of the tumor. Induction therapy consists of repeated weekly treatments for six cycles and is followed by one treatment given 3, 6, 12, 18, and 24 months after the first induction treatment.
Compatibility Information	BCG vaccine should not be admixed with other medications or solutions.
Contraindications/ Precautions	Contraindicated in individuals with a known hypersensitivity to BCG. Also contraindicated in patients with any state of altered immune response, including prolonged treatment with immunosuppressive therapies or patients who have had a transurethral resection or traumatic bladder catheterization associated with hematuria, in the previous week. Patients with urinary tract infections or active tuberculosis should not receive BCG therapy.
Drug Interactions	Immunosuppressive therapy with corticosteroids, chemotherapeutic agents, and radiation therapy should be avoided in patients receiving live vaccines. In addition, concomitant antibiotic therapy may have potential negative effects on the activity of BCG.
Toxicity/Side Effects	**Acute and/or Potentially Life-Threatening:** Disseminated BCG infection or osteomyelitis can occur rarely and should be treated immediately with appropriate antituberculosis therapy. Symptoms of disseminated BCG infection may be hard to distinguish from bacterial sepsis or acute

	hypersensitivity reaction. Disseminated infection may occur as late as six months or more after BCG therapy.
	Serious: The most common side effect from receiving intravesical BCG is cystitis with or without hematuria. Bladder irritation, which occurs in most patients, may be severe in some patients. Symptoms begin within two to four hours after dose and may last up to 72 hours.
	Other: Fever, chills, and malaise (i.e., flu-like symptoms) are common systemic side effects. In addition, bladder contracture, hepatic function impairment, hypotension, skin rash or erythema nodosum, and leukopenia also may occur.
Special Considerations	Care should be taken by those handling BCG to avoid contact with product during admixture and administration. All equipment, materials, and containers that may have come in contact with TheraCys should be placed in plastic bags labeled "infectious waste" and then sterilized or disposed of properly. BCG should not be injected IV, IM, or SC. It is recommended that BCG therapy not be started until 7–10 days after bladder resection or biopsy because of increased risk of BCG infection. If BCG infection suspected, therapy should be withheld and antituberculosis therapy initiated immediately. Severe adverse effects may be prevented or reduced in severity by administering prophylactic isoniazid therapy (also antihistamines and NSAIDs) prior to initiation of BCG.
Monitoring Parameters	Monitoring is recommended prior to initiation of therapy and at periodic intervals during therapy unless otherwise specified. • CBC with differential: Recommended prior to initiation of therapy and at regular intervals during and after treatment. • Liver function tests: ALT, AST, alkaline phosphatase, total bilirubin, LDH recommended prior to initiation of therapy, prior to each subsequent dose, and at periodic intervals during therapy. • Urinalysis: Recommended throughout therapy for signs of cystitis.
Indications	Adjuvant therapy for treatment of superficial bladder cancer.
Dosage Adjustment Recommendations	Hold doses for immunosuppression or suspected BCG infection.
Pharmacokinetics	TheraCys contains live-attenuated mycobacteria.
Manufacturer	TheraCys®, Pasteur Merieux Connaught, Swiftwater, PA; TICE® BCG, Organon Inc., West Orange, NJ

Epoetin alfa

Other Names	Procrit®, Epogen®, epoetin alfa, erythropoietin, EPO, rHuEPO-alfa
Classification	Hematopoietic cytokine.
Mechanism	Erythropoietin increases the production of erythrocytes by stimulating the proliferation and differentiation of committed erythroid precursors.
Vesicant Information	Not classified as a vesicant or an irritant.

Preparation and Mixture	Epoetin alfa should not be further diluted or mixed with other IV solutions because albumin, a carrier protein in the epoetin alfa formulation, can adsorb to PVC containers or tubing and possibly lead to instability of epoetin alfa.
Administration	Epoetin may be given by direct IV or SC injection.
Storage and Stability	Vials should be stored under refrigeration. Exposure to light for duration of less than 24 hours does not adversely affect stability. Shaking of vials may cause denaturation of the protein with loss of biologic activity.
How Supplied	Epoetin alfa is available as an isotonic, buffered liquid for injection both as a benzyl alcohol preserved and preservative-free product. Preservative-free vials each contain 1 ml of liquid with epoetin alfa concentrations of 2,000, 3,000, 4,000, or 10,000 units/ml. Multidose, preserved vials contain 20,000 units of epoetin alfa as either 2 ml of 10,000 units/ml or 1 ml of 20,000 units/ml and as 40,000 units as 40,000 units/ml.
Dosage	Epoetin alfa 50–100 units/kg three times a week is a typical dose for anemia of chronic renal failure. For anemia caused by chemotherapy in patients with cancer, epoetin 150–300 units/kg three times a week has been used to decrease blood transfusion requirements. Alternatively, 40,000 units once a week also has been used and proven efficacious in phase IV studies; this schedule allows a more convenient dosage schedule for patients.
Compatibility Information	Epoetin alfa may be further diluted in the original vial with bacteriostatic NS preserved with benzyl alcohol prior to administration.
Contraindications/ Precautions	It has been suggested to begin therapy in patients with documented unstable angina or recent myocardial infarction at dosages lower than the normal starting dose. Blood pressure should be monitored closely during initiation of therapy, as responses to therapy may be associated with increases in blood pressure. Epoetin alfa is contraindicated in patients with uncontrolled hypertension. Epoetin alfa treatment is not appropriate for patients requiring immediate correction of severe anemia.

Drug Interactions	**Agent**	**Effect**
	Androgens	May increase the response to epoetin alfa, and lower doses may be required to give the desired increases in hematocrit.
	Probenecid	May inhibit tubular secretion of epoetin alfa in animals and may alter responses to epoetin in patients with whom both drugs are used concomitantly.

Toxicity/Side Effects	**Acute and/or Potentially Life-Threatening:** Although rare, seizures and thromboembolic events have been reported.
	Serious: See above.
	Other: Headache, arthralgia, fever, abdominal pain/cramps, rash, and paresthesia.

Special Considerations	None.
Monitoring Parameters	Monitoring is recommended prior to initiation of therapy and at periodic intervals during therapy unless otherwise specified. • Hematocrit: Should be closely monitored (i.e., one to two times a week) until it has stabilized within the desired range; then monitoring may be decreased to less frequent intervals. • CBC, differential, reticulocyte count, platelet, and other erythrocyte indices: Should be monitored regularly. • Evaluation of iron stores: Should be performed prior to and at periodic intervals during therapy.
Indications	Epoetin alfa has been used in the treatment of anemia in patients with chemotherapy-induced anemia; AZT-treated HIV infection; chronic renal failure; and other hematologic disorders causing anemia. Other uses include treatment of radiation-induced anemia and prevention of anemia in the radiation oncology setting to improve local regional control and survival.
Dosage Adjustment Recommendations	Dosage should be titrated based on patient responses. A period of time is required for erythroid progenitors to mature and be released into the circulation. As a result, the time required to elicit a clinically significant change in hematocrit/hemoglobin is essentially two to four weeks, thus, if a response (at least a 1 g/dl increase in hemoglobin) has not been seen in this time period, an increase in dose (150 units/kg to 300 units/kg for thrice weekly dosing or 40,000 units to 60,000 units for once weekly dosing) is recommended.
Pharmacokinetics	Epoetin alfa is destroyed in the GI tract and must be administered by IV or SC injection. Serum levels are higher but less sustained when administered by the IV route compared to the SC route. The half-life may range from approximately 3–13 hours.
Manufacturer	Procrit®, Ortho Biotech Products, L.P., Raritan, NJ; Epogen®, Amgen Inc., Thousand Oaks, CA

Filgrastim

Other Names	Neupogen®, granulocyte-colony-stimulating factor (G-CSF)
Classification	Hematopoietic cytokine.
Mechanism	Filgrastim increases the proliferation and differentiation of neutrophils within the bone marrow.
Vesicant Information	Not classified as a vesicant or an irritant.
Preparation and Mixture	Filgrastim may be diluted to a concentration of 5–15 mcg/ml in D_5W in which albumin has first been added to a concentration of 2 mg/ml. Albumin, which is used as a carrier protein, is not needed if filgrastim is diluted to a concentration > 15 mcg/ml. Diluted solutions are compatible with glass or plastics commonly used in syringes, IV bags, and IV pump cassettes. Dilution with NS may cause precipitation and should not be done.

Administration	Doses should be administered as a single daily SC injection, short IV infusion (15–30 minutes), or continuous IV infusion.
Storage and Stability	Intact vials should be stored in a refrigerator and should not be allowed to freeze. Undiluted filgrastim is stable in Becton-Dickinson tuberculin syringes for up to 24 hours at room temperature or for up to seven days when stored in a refrigerator. If properly diluted in D_5W, filgrastim is stable for seven days when stored in a refrigerator. Because of concerns over possible bacterial contamination, the manufacturer recommends using solutions within 24 hours of preparation.
How Supplied	Filgrastim is available as a clear, colorless, preservative-free liquid for injection. Vials contain filgrastim 300 mcg/ml in either 1 ml (300 mcg) or 1.6 ml (480 mcg) sizes. Also available in prefilled syringes with 300 mcg/0.5 ml and 480 mcg/0.8 ml sizes.
Dosage	Common dosage: 5 mcg/kg/day; for stem cell mobilization: 10 mcg/kg/day. To decrease waste, it is common practice to round the doses to fit the combinations of available vial sizes.
Compatibility Information	Filgrastim should not be admixed with any other medications.
Contraindications/Precautions	Avoid using in any patient with known hypersensitivity to *E. coli*-derived proteins, filgrastim, or any component of the product.
Drug Interactions	It is not recommended to administered filgrastim within 24 hours prior to or after doses of myelosuppressive antineoplastic medications. Medications that also may increase neutrophil counts (e.g., lithium) may potentiate the myeloproliferative effects of filgrastim.
Toxicity/Side Effects	**Acute and/or Potentially Life-Threatening:** Allergic or anaphylactic reactions, although rare, have been reported. **Serious:** See above. **Other:** Fever, rash, edema, dyspnea, bone pain (mild to moderate; dose-related; occurs in 25%–50% of patients), mild to moderate headache; injection site erythema, swelling, and pruritus.
Special Considerations	It is not recommended to administer filgrastim within 24 hours prior to or after doses of myelosuppressive antineoplastic medications. Risk versus benefit should be considered in patients with excessive leukemic myeloid blasts in the marrow or peripheral blood.
Monitoring Parameters	Monitoring is recommended prior to initiation of therapy and at periodic intervals during therapy unless otherwise specified. • CBC with differential: Monitored regularly (twice weekly after chemotherapy or thrice weekly after HCT, during therapy to monitor response). • Platelet count: Monitor at regular intervals throughout therapy. • Hemoglobin and/or hematocrit: Monitor at regular intervals throughout therapy.
Indications	Indicated to decrease the incidence of infection in patients with nonmyeloid malignancies receiving myelosuppressive anticancer therapy; to reduce

the time to neutrophil recovery and the duration of fever following induction or consolidation therapy for adults with AML; to reduce the duration of neutropenia and neutropenia-related events in patients with nonmyeloid malignancies undergoing myeloablative chemotherapy followed by marrow transplantation; for the mobilization of peripheral blood stem cells for collection; and for the chronic administration to reduce the incidence and duration of sequelae of neutropenia in patients with congenital neutropenia, cyclic neutropenia, or idiopathic neutropenia.

Dosage Adjustment Recommendations	Filgrastim dose based on neutrophil recovery.

ANC	Filgrastim Dose Adjustment
ANC > 1,000/mm^3 for three consecutive days	Reduce to 5 mcg/kg/day.
If ANC remains > 1,000/mm^3 for three more consecutive days	Discontinue filgrastim.
If ANC decreases to < 1,000/mm^3	Resume at 5 mcg/kg/day.

Pharmacokinetics	Absorption after SC dosing is 100% with peak plasma concentrations maintained up to 12 hours; elimination half-life is approximately 1.8–3.5 hours.
Manufacturer	Amgen Inc., Thousand Oaks, CA

Gemtuzumab ozogamicin

Other Names	Mylotarg®, CMA 676
Classification	Antitumor antibiotic (e.g., calicheamicin) linked to recombinant humanized IgG antibody specific for the CD33 antigen on leukemic blasts and immature normal cells of the myelomonocytic lineage but not on normal hematopoietic stem cells.
Mechanism	After binding to CD33, a complex is formed and internalized into the cell. The calicheamicin is released inside the lysosomes of the cell. Free calicheamicin then binds to DNA, resulting in DNA double-strand breaks and cell death.
Vesicant Information	Not classified as a vesicant or an irritant.
Preparation and Mixture	Drug is light-sensitive and must be protected from direct sunlight and fluorescent light during preparation and administration. The biologic safety hood fluorescent light must be turned off during dose preparation. Reconstitute each 5-mg vial with 5 ml sterile water for injection. Gently swirl the vials to speed dissolution of the drug. Withdraw the desired volume from the vials and transfer into a 100-ml IV bag of NS. The IV bag should placed into inside-UV protective wrap or bag and used immediately.
Administration	The prepared solution should be infused into a peripheral or central line over two hours. The solutions should be infused through an IV tubing

	equipped with a low protein-binding, 1.2-micron filter. Premedication with acetaminophen 650–1,000 mg and diphenhydramine 50 mg is necessary to decrease the incidence of postinfusion reactions. Acetaminophen should be repeated every four hours for two additional doses.
Storage and Stability	Store intact ampules under refrigeration and protected from light.
How Supplied	Mylotarg is supplied in 20-ml vials containing 5 mg of gemtuzumab ozogamicin lyophylized powder.
Dosage	Mylotarg 9 mg/m^2 IV should be administered as a two-hour infusion followed by one repeat dose after a 14-day period.
Compatibility Information	No compatibility information is available, and Mylotarg should only be mixed with or infused through NS.
Contraindications/ Precautions	Elevated WBC count with high blast count (> 30,000) may predispose patient to increased risk of tumor lysis syndrome. It may be desirable to lower blast count with hydroxyurea or by other means prior to starting therapy.
Drug Interactions	No studies have been performed.
Toxicity/Side Effects	**Acute and/or Potentially Life-Threatening:** Tumor lysis syndrome. **Serious:** Severe myelosuppression, including neutropenia, thrombocytopenia and anemia, oral mucositis or stomatitis (majority grade I–II), and hepatotoxicity with elevations in ALT, AST, and/or bilirubin have been seen. **Other:** Infusion-related reactions might include chills, fever, nausea, vomiting, headache, hypotension or hypertension, hypoxia, dyspnea, and hyperglycemia. Reactions generally occurred after the end of the infusion and resolved after two to four hours. Fewer reactions were seen following the second dose. Also, skin rashes, arthralgia, diarrhea, constipation, and anorexia have been reported.
Special Considerations	Mylotarg should not be given as an IVP or bolus. The use of UV light protection and filtration with a low protein-binding filter during administration is required. During clinical trials, a 1.2-micron in-line filter made of Supor® (Gelman Sciences, Inc., Ann Arbor, MI) filter material was used. Treatment with IV fluids and allopurinol are needed to prevent hyperuricemia caused by tumor lysis syndrome.
Monitoring Parameters	Monitoring is recommended prior to initiation of therapy and at periodic intervals during therapy unless otherwise specified. • CBC with differential: Recommended prior to initiation of therapy and at regular intervals after treatment. • Liver function tests: ALT, AST, alkaline phosphatase, total bilirubin, LDH recommended prior to initiation of therapy and at periodic intervals after therapy. • Electrolyte monitoring: Perform frequently immediately following treatment to detect tumor lysis syndrome.
Indications	Treatment of patients with CD33-positive AML in first relapse who are > 60 years of age.

Dosage Adjustment Recommendations	No studies have been performed in patients with bilirubin > 2 mg/dl, and, therefore, caution should be exercised in patients with hepatic dysfunction.
Pharmacokinetics	The elimination half-life of total and unbound calicheamicin are approximately 45 and 100 hours, respectively, after dose number one. After the second dose, the half-life of bound calicheamicin was increased to approximately 60 hours.
Manufacturer	Wyeth Laboratories, Philadelphia, PA

Interferon alfa

Other Name	Alfa interferon, leukocyte interferon; interferon alfa-2a, Roferon-A®; interferon alfa-2b, Intron A®
Classification	Biological response modifier, antineoplastic and antiviral activities.
Mechanism	The mechanism of activity has not been fully elucidated. Endogenous interferons are secreted by peripheral blood leukocytes in response to viral infection or biological inducers. Interferon alfa is known to exhibit antiviral and antitumor activity. Interferon alfa has been shown to induce antiproliferative and immunomodulatory responses in human cells in culture.
Vesicant Information	Not classified as a vesicant or an irritant.
Preparation and Mixture	Interferon alfa-2a and 2b are available as solution for injection and sterile powder for injection, which should be reconstituted with the provided diluent.
Administration	Therapy may be given as SC injection, IM injection, IV infusion, or intralesional injection for *Condylomata acuminata*. Refer to specific treatment regimens for methods of administration.
Storage and Stability	Interferon alfa vials should be stored under refrigeration. Reconstituted vials of interferon alfa-2a and 2b are stable 30 days under refrigeration. After reconstitution, interferon alfa-2a is stable for 24 hours, and interferon alfa-2b is stable for one to two days at room temperature.
How Supplied	Interferon alfa-2b is available as a white- to cream-colored powder for injection and as solution for injection. Each vial of powder for injection is supplied with diluent in 3-, 5-, 10-, 18-, 25-, and 50-million IU strengths. Single-use vials of solution are available in 3-, 5-, and 10-million IU strengths. Multidose vials are supplied in strengths of 18 million IU, containing 22.8 million IU/3.8 ml to dispense 6 x 3 million IU doses, and 25 million IU, containing 32 million IU/3.2 ml to dispense 5 x 5 million IU doses. Multidose pens for injection also are available in 18-, 20-, and 60-million IU strengths containing 22.5 million IU/1.5 ml, 37.5 million IU/1.5 ml, and 75 million IU/1.5 ml of interferon alfa-2b. Interferon alfa-2a is available in 3-, 6-, 9-, 18-, and 26-million IU vials.
Dosage	Doses will vary depending on the disease to be treated and each specific interferon subtype selected. Check with each individual treatment protocol

	for specific recommendations. Doses range from 3 million units/day up to 36 million units/week. Recommended dosing for melanoma (interferon alfa-2b) includes an induction phase of 20 million units/m^2 as an IV infusion for five consecutive days per week for four weeks, followed by a maintenance phase of 10 million units/m^2 three times per week subcutaneously for 48 weeks.
Compatibility Information	Interferons should not be mixed with any other medications.
Contraindications/ Precautions	Interferon alfa may increase the activity of the immune system and worsen autoimmune diseases.
Drug Interactions	Interferon alfa may depress microsomal enzymes involved in the hepatic cytochrome P-450 system, and metabolism inhibition of some medications may occur.
Toxicity/Side Effects	Most side effects are dose-related and are mild to moderate in nature. **Acute and/or Potentially Life-Threatening:** Depression and suicidal behavior, including suicidal ideation and suicide attempts, have been reported in association with interferon alfa therapy. Patients with a history of a preexisting psychiatric condition should not be treated with interferon alfa therapy. Hepatotoxicity, pulmonary infiltrates, and rare autoimmune disorders have occurred and have resulted in fatalities. **Serious:** Acute serious hypersensitivity reactions (e.g., urticaria, angioedema, bronchoconstriction, anaphylaxis) have been reported, although rarely, with interferon alfa therapy. **Other:** Cardiovascular: Tachycardia, arrhythmias, chest pain, hypotension, and supraventricular tachycardia. Dermatologic: Alopecia, dry skin, and rash. Endocrine: Hypothyroidism and increased uric acid levels. GI: Xerostomia, nausea, vomiting, diarrhea, abdominal cramps, weight loss, metallic taste, anorexia, and stomatitis. Hematologic: Mildly myelosuppressive (e.g., neutropenia, thrombocytopenia, anemia). Neurologic: Headache, delirium, dizziness, somnolence, visual disturbances, confusion, depression, sensory neuropathy, and electroencephalogram (EEG) changes. Miscellaneous: Liver abnormalities (may occur at higher doses), myalgia, arthralgia, proteinuria, flu-like symptoms (e.g., fever, chills, malaise), rigors, diaphoresis, cough, and neutralizing antibodies.
Special Considerations	Multidose vials and pens of solution are overfilled with volumes and interferon amounts greater than labeled on the vial to allow for wastage during transfer into syringes. Interferon alfa is considered a mild to moderate emetogen, depending on dose; consider prophylactic and as-needed antiemetics (e.g., serotonin antagonists, prochlorperazine).
Monitoring Parameters	Monitoring is recommended prior to initiation of therapy and at periodic intervals during therapy unless otherwise specified.

- CBC with differential: Recommended prior to initiation of therapy, prior to each subsequent dose, and at periodic intervals during therapy.
- Hemoglobin and/or hematocrit: Recommended prior to initiation of therapy, prior to each subsequent dose, and at periodic intervals during therapy.
- Platelet count: Recommended prior to initiation of therapy, prior to each subsequent dose, and at periodic intervals during therapy.
- Cardiac function: ECG recommended prior to the initiation of therapy and at periodic intervals during therapy in patients with cardiac disease.
- Neuropsychiatric monitoring: Recommended in patients receiving high-dose therapy.

Indications	Interferon alfa-2b is indicated for hairy cell leukemia, malignant melanoma, and follicular lymphoma. Interferon alfa-2a is indicated for hairy cell leukemia and for therapy of minimally treated patients with chronic phase, Philadelphia chromosome positive CML. Interferons are being studied in many other cancers, including renal cell carcinoma and bladder cancer.
Dosage Adjustment Recommendations	Refer to individual package inserts; dosage adjustments recommended for interferon alfa based on toxicity and tolerability.
Pharmacokinetics	The elimination half-life for interferon alfa-2a and interferon alfa-2b are 3.7–8.5 hours and 2–3 hours, respectively. The renal tubules are responsible for the degradation of interferons.
Manufacturer	Roferon-A®, Roche Pharmaceuticals, Humaco, PR ; Intron-A®, Schering Corporation, Kenilworth, NJ

Oprelvekin

Other Name	Interleukin 11, Neumega®
Classification	Hematopoietic cytokine.
Mechanism	Oprelvekin is a thrombopoietic growth factor that directly stimulates the proliferation of hematopoietic stem cells and megakaryocyte progenitor cells and induces megakaryocyte maturation, resulting in increased platelet production.
Vesicant Information	Not classified as a vesicant or an irritant.
Preparation and Mixture	Reconstitute vial with 1 ml of sterile water for injection. During reconstitution, the diluent should be directed at the side of the vial and the contents gently swirled. Excessive or vigorous agitation should be avoided.
Administration	Give SC as a single injection in the abdomen, thigh, or hip (upper arm if not self-injecting). Dosing should be initiated 6–24 hours after the completion of chemotherapy.
Storage and Stability	The lyophilized powder and diluent should be stored under refrigeration. The reconstituted solution contains no preservatives, and the manufacturer recommends using the solution within three hours of mixing.

How Supplied	Single-use vials containing 5 mg of oprelvekin as a sterile, lyophilized powder.
Dosage	The recommended dose of oprelvekin in adults is 50 µg/kg given once daily beginning 6–24 hours after the completion of chemotherapy.
Compatibility Information	No data are available for mixing oprelvekin with other medications.
Contraindications/ Precautions	Oprelvekin should be used with caution in patients with a history of atrial arrhythmia. Transient atrial arrhythmias have occurred in approximately 10% of patients. Mild to moderate peripheral edema and SOB on exertion can occur within the first week of treatment and may continue for the duration of administration.
Drug Interactions	Drug interactions between oprelvekin and other drugs have not been fully evaluated.
Toxicity/Side Effects	In general, adverse events in clinical trials were similar between treated and placebo patients. **Acute and/or Potentially Life-Threatening:** None noted. **Serious:** Mild to moderate fluid retention and transient atrial arrhythmias have occurred and reversed spontaneously after discontinuation of therapy. **Other:** Cardiovascular: Tachycardia, syncope, palpitations, edema, and vasodilation. GI: Nausea, vomiting, mucositis, and diarrhea. Miscellaneous: Headache, fever, dizziness, dyspnea, pleural effusion, and rash.
Special Considerations	Dosing should be continued until the post-nadir platelet count is 50,000 cells/mm^3. In controlled clinical studies, doses were administered in courses of 10–21 days. Dosing beyond 21 days per treatment course is not recommended.
Monitoring Parameters	Monitoring is recommended prior to initiation of therapy and at periodic intervals during therapy unless otherwise specified. • CBC with differential: Recommended prior to initiation of therapy, prior to each subsequent dose, and at periodic intervals during therapy. • Hemoglobin and/or hematocrit: Recommended prior to initiation of therapy, prior to each subsequent dose, and at periodic intervals during therapy. • Platelet count: Recommended during time of expected nadir and until recovery has occurred; post-nadir platelet counts ≥ 50,000.
Indications	Oprelvekin has been studied for the prevention of severe thrombocytopenia following single or repeated sequential cycles of various myelosuppressive chemotherapy regimens.
Dosage Adjustment Recommendations	Titrate dose to individual patient response.
Pharmacokinetics	The bioavailability of oprelvekin > 80% with a terminal half-life of 6.9±1.7 hours.
Manufacturer	Genetics Institute, Cambridge, MA

Rituximab

Other Name	Rituxan®
Classification	Monoclonal antibody, chimeric murine/human origin.
Mechanism	A genetically engineered chimeric murine/human monoclonal antibody directed against the CD20 antigen found on the surface of normal and malignant B lymphocytes. The Fc domain of rituximab recruits immune effector functions to mediate B cell lysis in vitro.
Vesicant Information	Not classified as a vesicant or an irritant.
Preparation and Mixture	Withdraw the dose of rituximab, and dilute to a final concentration of 1–4 mg/ml into an infusion bag containing either D_5W or NS.
Administration	The first infusion should be administered IV at an initial rate of 50 mg/hour. If adverse reactions do not occur, increase the infusion rate in 50 mg/hour increments every 30 minutes to a maximum of 400 mg/hour. Subsequent infusions may be started at 100 mg/hour and increased in 100 mg/hour increments every 30 minutes to a maximum of 400 mg/hour. DO NOT give as an IVP or bolus.
Storage and Stability	Vials should be stored under refrigeration and protected from direct sunlight. Diluted solutions for infusion are stable under refrigeration for 24 hours and at room temperature for an additional 12 hours.
How Supplied	Rituximab is a sterile, clear, colorless, preservative-free, 10 mg/ml liquid supplied in either 100-mg (10-ml) or 500-mg (50-ml) single-use vials.
Dosage	Most commonly, 375 mg/m^2 is given as a weekly IV infusion for four doses.
Compatibility Information	Rituximab should not be admixed with other medications.
Contraindications/ Precautions	Rituximab is contraindicated for patients with known hypersensitivity or anaphylactic reactions to murine proteins or to any component of this product.
Drug Interactions	There are no known drug interactions.
Toxicity/Side Effects	**Acute and/or Potentially Life-Threatening:** Infusion-related reactions of fever and chills/rigors occurred in the majority of patients during the first dose. Other frequent infusion-related symptoms included nausea, urticaria, fatigue, headache, pruritus, bronchospasm, dyspnea, angioedema, rhinitis, vomiting, hypotension, flushing, and pain at disease sites. These reactions usually occur within one-half to two hours of the start of the infusion and have been noted to be significant in a number of patients. Symptoms often resolve with slowing or interruption of the infusion and with initiation of routine supportive care (e.g., IV saline, diphenhydramine, acetaminophen). **Serious:** None noted.

	Other: Anemia, thrombocytopenia, neutropenia, conjunctivitis, hypertension, peripheral edema, pain at injection site, headache, abdominal pain, nausea, pruritus, rash, and, rarely, cardiovascular events (e.g., angina, arrhythmias, bradycardia).
Special Considerations	Premedication, consisting of acetaminophen and diphenhydramine, should be considered before each infusion of rituximab. Premedication may attenuate infusion-related events. As transient hypotension may occur during infusions, consideration should be given to withholding antihypertensive medications 12 hours prior to treatments. Severe reactions may require treatment with epinephrine. Consider an as-needed antiemetic (e.g., prochlorperazine).
Monitoring Parameters	Monitoring is recommended prior to initiation of therapy and at periodic intervals during therapy unless otherwise specified. • CBC with differential: Recommended prior to initiation of therapy, prior to each subsequent dose, and at periodic intervals during therapy. • Hemoglobin and/or hematocrit: Recommended prior to initiation of therapy, prior to each subsequent dose, and at periodic intervals during therapy. • Platelet count: Recommended prior to initiation of therapy, prior to each subsequent dose, and at periodic intervals during therapy. • Cardiac function tests: Recommended at periodic intervals.
Indications	Treatment of patients with relapsed or refractory low-grade or follicular, CD20 positive, B cell non-Hodgkin's lymphoma.
Dosage Adjustment Recommendations	None noted.
Pharmacokinetics	Studies of doses of 375 mg/m² as an IV infusion for four doses demonstrated a mean serum half-life of 59.8 hours (range 11.1–104.6 hours) after the first infusion and 174 hours (range 26–442 hours) after the fourth infusion.
Manufacturer	Genentech, Inc., South San Francisco, CA

Sargramostim

Other Name	Granulocyte-macrophage-colony-stimulating factor (GM-CSF), Leukine®
Classification	Hematopoietic cytokine.
Mechanism	Sargramostim stimulates the proliferation and differentiation of hematopoietic progenitor cells. It induces partially committed progenitor cells to divide and differentiate in the granulocyte-macrophage pathways.
Vesicant Information	Not classified as a vesicant or an irritant.
Preparation and Mixture	Vials of lyophilized powder should be reconstituted with 1 ml of sterile water for injection or bacteriostatic water for injection. For IV infusions, sargramostim may be further diluted in NS. If the final concentration of sargramostim is < 10 mcg/ml, then albumin must be added to the NS at a

	concentration of 0.1% (e.g., 1 ml of 5% albumin added to 50 ml NS) prior to the addition of sargramostim.
Administration	SC injection, continuous IV infusion, or short IV infusion (usually two to four hours).
Storage and Stability	Vials of powder and solution should be stored under refrigeration. Once entered, vials of Leukine liquid and Leukine powder reconstituted with preserved water for injection can be stored up to 20 days in the refrigerator. Vials reconstituted with sterile water for injection should be used shortly after reconstitution.
How Supplied	Sargramostim 500 mcg/ml is supplied in vials as a clear, colorless, benzyl alcohol-preserved injectable solution. It also is available as a lyophilized powder in vials containing either 250 or 500 mcg.
Dosage	250 mcg/m²/day; dosages may be increased up to 500 mcg/m²/day in situations of graft failure following HCT. To decrease waste, it is common practice to round the doses to fit the combinations of available vial sizes.
Compatibility Information	It is not recommended to mix sargramostim with any other medication.
Contraindications/ Precautions	Sargramostim is contraindicated in patients with excessive leukemic myeloid blasts in the bone marrow or peripheral blood and patients with known hypersensitivity to sargramostim, yeast-derived products, or other components of the product. It also is contraindicated for concomitant use with chemotherapy and radiotherapy. Monitor the patient for signs of respiratory distress after the first dose.
Drug Interactions	Medications that may potentiate the myeloproliferative effects of sargramostim, such as lithium and corticosteroids, should be used with caution.
Toxicity/Side Effects	**Acute and/or Potentially Life-Threatening:** First-dose reaction, although rare, may occur and includes flushing, hypotension, and syncope. Capillary leak syndrome (e.g., fluid retention, peripheral edema, pericardial and/or pleural effusions) also has been reported and associated with higher doses of sargramostim. In addition, allergic or anaphylactic reactions have been reported. **Serious:** See above. **Other:** Fever, rash, edema, dyspnea, bone pain (mild to moderate; dose-related; occurs in 20%–50% of patients), mild to moderate headache, injection site erythema, swelling, and pruritus.
Special Considerations	Systemic side effects (e.g., fever, bone pain, asthenia) usually are prevented or reversed by analgesics or antipyretics.
Monitoring Parameters	Monitoring is recommended prior to initiation of therapy and at periodic intervals during therapy unless otherwise specified. • CBC with differential: Monitored regularly (twice weekly after chemotherapy or thrice weekly after HCT during therapy to monitor response). • Platelet count: Monitor at regular intervals throughout therapy.

	• Hemoglobin and/or hematocrit: Monitor at regular intervals throughout therapy.
Indications	Indicated to reduce the time to neutrophil recovery and the duration of fever following induction or consolidation therapy for adults with AML; to reduce the duration of neutropenia and neutropenia-related events in patients with nonmyeloid malignancies undergoing myeloablative chemotherapy followed by HCT; for the mobilization of peripheral blood stem cells for collection; and for use in HCT failure or engraftment delay.
Dosage Adjustment Recommendations	None noted.
Pharmacokinetics	Peak levels after IV administration occur during or immediately after the infusion and one to three hours after SC administration; elimination half-life is two hours following IV administration and three hours following SC injection.
Manufacturer	Immunex Corporation, Seattle, WA

Trastuzumab

Other Name	Herceptin®
Classification	Monoclonal antibody; humanized.
Mechanism	Trastuzumab selectively binds to the extracellular domain of the human epidermal growth factor receptor 2 protein (HER2), leading to the inhibition of proliferation of tumor cells that overexpress HER2.
Vesicant Information	Not classified as a vesicant or an irritant.
Preparation and Mixture	Reconstitute each vial with 20 ml bacteriostatic water for injection to make 21 mg/ml solution. Further dilute the desired dose in 250 ml of NS (D_5W should not be used for dilution).
Administration	Infuse the initial loading dose over 90 minutes and subsequent maintenance doses over 30 minutes if the loading dose is well tolerated. Premedication, consisting of acetaminophen and diphenhydramine, should be considered before each infusion. Do not give IVP or bolus.
Storage and Stability	Store vials under refrigeration prior to reconstitution. Reconstituted solutions are stable for 28 days. After preparation, solutions diluted in D_5W in PVC or polyethylene bags are stable for up to 24 hours at room temperature or under refrigeration.
How Supplied	Available in vials containing 440 mg.
Dosage	Loading dose is 4 mg/kg followed by weekly maintenance doses of 2 mg/kg.
Compatibility Information	Trastuzumab should not be mixed with other drugs.

Contraindications/ Precautions	Trastuzumab should be used with caution in patients with hypersensitivity to trastuzumab, Chinese hamster cell proteins, or any other component of the product. Extreme caution should be exercised in treating patients with preexisting cardiac dysfunction.

Drug Interactions	**Agent**	**Effect**
	Paclitaxel	Concomitant therapy with trastuzumab resulted in a two-fold decrease in trastuzumab in a primate study and 1.5-fold increase in serum levels in clinical studies.
	Anthracyclines	Concomitant use with anthracyclines may increase incidence and severity of cardiac dysfunction.

Toxicity/Side Effects	**Acute and/or Potentially Life-Threatening:** CHF has occurred following trastuzumab therapy, and patients should have thorough baseline cardiac assessment, including history, physical exam, and one or more of the following: ECG, echocardiogram, and MUGA scan. The incidence and severity of cardiac dysfunction was high in patients who received trastuzumab in combination with anthracyclines and cyclophosphamide. Extreme caution should be exercised in treating patients with preexisting cardiac dysfunction. In addition, hypersensitivity reactions, including fatal anaphylaxis, infusion reactions, including some fatal, and pulmonary events resulting in respiratory distress syndrome and death have occurred. **Serious:** See above. **Other:** Diarrhea, infections, chills, fever, nausea, vomiting, pain, rigors, headache, dizziness, rash, and asthenia.
Special Considerations	Extreme caution should be exercised in treating patients with preexisting cardiac dysfunction.
Monitoring Parameters	Monitoring is recommended prior to initiation of therapy and at periodic intervals during therapy unless otherwise specified. • HER2/neu overexpression: Recommended prior to initiation of therapy. • Cardiac function tests: MUGA or LVEF recommended prior to initiation of therapy and at periodic intervals during therapy.
Indications	Indicated in the treatment of metastatic breast cancer tumors that overexpress the HER2 protein.
Dosage Adjustment Recommendations	None noted.
Pharmacokinetics	Dose-dependent pharmacokinetics demonstrate average half-lives of 1.7 and 12 days at the 10- and 500-mg doses, respectively.
Manufacturer	Genentech, Inc., South San Francisco, CA

Appendix A. Dosing Chemotherapeutic Agents With Hepatic Dysfunction Recommendations

Chemotherapeutic Agent	Adjustment for Hepatic Dysfunction: Percent of Full Dose to Be Administered			
	T. Bili[a] < 1.5 or SGOT[b] < 60	T. Bili = 1.5–3.0 or SGOT = 60–180	T. Bili = 3.1–5.0 or SGOT > 180	T. Bili > 5.0
Cyclophosphamide[c]	100%	100%	75%	Omit
Cytarabine	Manufacturer recommends dosage adjustment in hepatic impairment.			
Dacarbazine	Unknown; carefully monitor in hepatic impairment.			
Daunorubicin (including liposomal product)	< 1.2 mg/dl: 100%	1.2–3.0 mg/dl: 75%	> 3.0 mg/dl: 50%	Omit
Daunorubicin[c]	100%	75%	50%	Omit
Docetaxel	If t. bili > ULN[d] and SGOT and/or SGPT[e] > 1.5 x ULN + alkaline phosphatase >2.5 x ULN, hold dose.			
Doxorubicin (including liposomal product)	<1.2 mg/dl: 100%	1.2–3.0 mg/dl: 50%	> 3.0 mg/dl: 25%	Omit
Doxorubicin[c]	100%	50%	25%	Omit
Etoposide[c], etopophos	100%	50%	Omit	Omit
Fluorouracil[c]	100%	100%	100%	Omit
Floxuridine	If AST[f] 2x baseline, administer 80% dose; if AST 3x baseline, bilirubin 1.5x baseline, and/or alkaline phosphatase 1.5x baseline, administer 50% dose; hold dose if impairment greater than stated.			
Gemcitabine	Administer with caution in patients with significant hepatic impairment.			
Idarubicin[g]	100%	≥ 2.5 mg/dl: 50%	50%	Omit
Irinotecan	Metabolized in liver; use with caution in patients with hepatic impairment.			
Methotrexate (MTX[h])	100%	100%	75%	Omit
Mitoxantrone[i]	100%	50%	25%	—
Paclitaxel[h]	≤ 1.5 mg/dl: ≥ 135 mg/m²	1.6–2.9 mg/dl: ≤ 75 mg/m²	≥ 3.0 mg/dl: ≤ 50 mg/m²	—
Procarbazine	Undue toxicity may occur in patients with hepatic dysfunction.			
Topotecan	No adjustment needed if t. bili > 1.5–< 10 mg/dl.			
Vinblastine[h]	100%	50%	50%	Omit
Vinblastine	100%	> 3.0 mg/dl: 50%	—	—

(Continued on next page)

Appendix A. Dosing Chemotherapeutic Agents With Hepatic Dysfunction Recommendations (Continued)

Chemotherapeutic Agent	Adjustment for Hepatic Dysfunction: Percent of Full Dose to Be Administered			
	T. Bili[a] < 1.5 or SGOT[b] < 60	T. Bili = 1.5–3.0 or SGOT = 60–180	T. Bili = 3.1–5.0 or SGOT > 180	T. Bili > 5.0
Vincristine[h]	100%	50%	Omit	Omit
Vincristine	100%	100%	> 3.0 mg/dl:50%	—
Vinorelbine	< 2.0 mg/dl: 30 mg/m²	2.1–3.0 mg/dl: 15 mg/m²	> 3.0 mg/dl: 7.5 mg/m²	—

[a] Total bilirubin
[b] Serum glutamic oxalacetic transaminase
[c] Perry, M.C. (1992). Chemotherapeutic agents and hepatotoxicity. Seminars in Oncology, 19, 551–561.
[d] Upper limit of normal
[e] Serum glutamic-pyruvic transaminase
[f] Aspartate aminotransferase
[g] Dorr, R.T., & Von Hoff, D.D. (Eds.). (1994). Cancer chemotherapy handbook (2nd ed.). Norwalk, CT: Appleton & Lange.
[h] Venook, A.P., Egorin, M., Brown, T.D., Batist, G., Budman, D.R., & Rosner, G.L. (1994). Paclitaxel (Taxol) in patients with liver dysfunction (CALGB 9264) [Abstract 350]. Program/ Proceedings of the American Society of Clinical Oncology Thirtieth Annual Meeting (May 14–17, Dallas, TX), 13, 139.
[i] Weiss, R.B. (1989). Mitoxantrone: Its development and role in clinical practice. Oncology, 3(6), 135–141.

Note. All other information is per product inserts.

THIS INFORMATION SERVES ONLY AS DOSAGE MODIFICATION RECOMMENDATIONS. PLEASE USE CLINICAL JUDGMENT AND CURRENT LITERATURE WHEN FORMULATING DOSAGE MODIFICATIONS.

Appendix B. Dosing Chemotherapeutic Agents With Renal Failure Recommendations

Chemotherapeutic Agent	Adjustment for Renal Failure Percent of Full Dose to Be Administered Based on CrCl[a] (ml/minute)			
	46–60 ml/minute	31–45 ml/minute	10–30 ml/minute	<10 ml/minute
Bleomycin	70%	60%	50%	NR[b]
Carboplatin[c] (if not AUC[d] dosing)	41–59 ml/minute: 250 mg/m^2	16–40 ml/minute: 200 mg/m^2	< 15 ml/minute: No data available.	
Cisplatin Cisplatin[e]	75% > 60 ml/minute: 100%	50% 30–60 ml/minute: 50%	NR < 30 ml/minute: Avoid	NR Avoid
Cyclophosphamide	100%	100%	100%	50%
Cytarabine (1–3 gm/m^2)	60%	50%	NR	NR
Dacarbazine	80%	75%	70%	70%
Daunorubicin (including liposomal product)[c]	If SCr[f] > 3 mg/dl: 50% dose reduction.			
Doxorubicin (including liposomal product)[c]	100%	100%	100%	25%
Etoposide	85%	80%	75%	50%
Etopophos	If CrCl > 50 ml/minute: 100%	If CrCl 15–50 ml/minute: 75%	Consider further dose reduction if CrCl < 15 ml/minute.	
Floxuridine	Use with caution in renal impairment; lower doses recommended.			
Fludarabine	80%	75%	< 30 ml/minute: 65%	
Gemcitabine[c]	Use with caution in marked renal impairment.			
Hydroxyurea	85%	75%	50%	20%
Idarubicin[c]	Consider dose adjustment if SCr elevated; SCr ≥ 2 mg/dl: Reduce dose by 25%.			
Ifosfamide	80%	75%	70%	50–70%
Irinotecan[c]	No data available; not evaluated per manufacturer.			
Melphalan (IV)	85%	75%	70%	50%
Melphalan[c]	50% decrease if BUN[h] ≥ 30 mg/dl			
Mercaptopurine	No recommendation, but reduce dosage if marked renal impairment.			
Methotrexate	65%	50%	Avoid	Avoid
Mitomycin[g]	100%	100%	75%	75%

(Continued on next page)

Appendix B. Dosing Chemotherapeutic Agents With Renal Failure Recommendations (Continued)

	Adjustment for Renal Failure Percent of Full Dose to Be Administered Based on CrCl[a] (ml/minute)			
Chemotherapeutic Agent	46–60 ml/minute	31–45 ml/minute	10–30 ml/minute	< 10 ml/minute
Nitrosoureas (BCNU[i], CCNU[j], semustine)	75%	70%	NR	NR
Plicamycin	100%	75%	50%	50%
Procarbazine	No recommendation; closely monitor in renal failure.			
Streptozocin	100%	75%	50%	NR
Thiotepa	No recommendation; closely monitor 85% renally eliminated.			
Topotecan	80%	75%	70%	< 20 ml/minute: Insufficient data available to make recommendation.
Topotecan[c]	40–60 ml/minute: No adjustment necessary.	20–39 ml/minute: 0.75 mg/m²		

[a]Creatinine clearance
[b]Not recommended
[c]Per package insert
[d]Area under the concentration curve
[e]Perry, M.C. (Ed.). (1992). *The chemotherapy source book*. Baltimore: Williams & Wilkins.
[f]Serum creatinine
[g]Manufacturer recommends the drug not to be used in patients with SCr > 1.7 mg/dl.
[h]Blood urea nitrogen
[i]Bischloroethylnitrosourea
[j]Chloroethylcyclohexylnitrosourea (lomustine)

Note. With all of these agents, extreme caution should be used when administering other nephrotoxic drugs (e.g., aminoglycosides, amphotericin B).

Based on information from Kintzel, P., & Dorr, R. (1995). Anticancer drug renal toxicity and elimination: Dosing guidelines for altered renal function. *Cancer Treatment Reviews, 21*(1), 33–64.

THE ABOVE INFORMATION SERVES ONLY AS DOSAGE MODIFICATION RECOMMENDATIONS. PLEASE USE CLINICAL JUDGMENT AND CURRENT LITERATURE WHEN FORMULATING DOSAGE MODIFICATIONS.

References

Abramowicz, M. (Ed.). (1993). Drugs of choice for cancer chemotherapy. *The Medical Letter, 35*(897), 43–50.

Alberts, D.S., & Garcia, D.J. (1997). Safety aspects of pegylated liposomal doxorubicin in patients with cancer. *Drugs, 54*(4), 30–35.

Balmer, C., & Valley, A.W. (1997). Basic principles of cancer treatment and cancer chemotherapy. In J.T. DiPiro, R.L. Talbert, G.C. Yee, G.R. Matzke, B.G. Weels, & L.M. Posey (Eds.) *Pharmacotherapy: A pathophysiologic approach* (pp. 2403–2465). Stamford, CT: Appleton & Lange.

Berkery, R., Cleri, L., Baltzer, L., & Skarin, A. (Eds.). (1997). *Oncology pocket guide to chemotherapy*. St. Louis, MO: Mosby-Wolfe.

Buggia, I., Locatelli, F., Regazzi, M., & Zecca, M. (1994). Busulfan. *Annals of Pharmacotherapy, 28,* 1055–1061.

DeVita, V.T. (1978). The evaluation of therapeutic research in cancer. *New England Journal of Medicine, 298,* 907.

DeVita, V.T., Hellman, S., & Rosenberg, S.A. (Eds.). (1997). *Cancer: Principles and practice of oncology*. Philadelphia: Lippincott-Raven.

Dorr, R.T., & Von Hoff, D.D. (Eds.). (1994). *Cancer chemotherapy handbook* (2nd ed.). Norwalk, CT: Appleton & Lange.

Fischer, D.S., Knobf, M.T., & Durivage, H.J. (Eds.). (1993). *The cancer chemotherapy handbook*. St. Louis, MO: Mosby.

Gabizon, A., & Martin, F. (1997). Polyethylene glycol-coated (pegylated) liposomal doxorubicin: Rationale for use in solid tumors. *Drugs, 54*(4), 15–21.

Goodin, S. (1996). Overview of the topoisomerase I inhibitors. *Highlights in Oncology Practice, 14*(3), 69–73.

Gullatte, M.M., & Graves, T. (1990). Advances in antineoplastic therapy. *Oncology Nursing Forum, 17,* 867–876.

Hersh, S.M. (Ed.). (1968). *Chemical and biologic warfare: America's hidden arsenal*. New York: Bobb's Merrill.

Jordan, V.C. (Ed.). (1997). Antiestrogens: Past, present, and future. *Oncology, 11*(2, Suppl. 1), 1–64.

Lacy, C., Armstrong, L.L., Ingrim, N.B., & Lance, L.L. (Eds.). (1997–98). *Drug information handbook*. Hudson, OH: Lexi-Comp Inc.

Lam, Y.W., Chan, C.Y., & Kuhn, J.G. (1997). Pharmacokinetics and pharmacodynamics of the taxanes. *Journal of Oncology Pharmacy Practice, 3*(2), 76–93.

Medical Economics Company, Inc. (1999). *Physicians' desk reference*. Montvale, NJ: Author.

Miller, L.J., Chandler, S., & Ippoliti, C.M. (1994). Treatment of cyclophosphamide-induced hemorrhagic cystitis with prostagladins. *Annals of Pharmacotherapy, 28,* 590–594.

Morgan, A. (1996). Recently approved antineoplastic agents. *Highlights in Oncology Practice, 14*(3), 74–78.

Perry, M.C. (Ed.). (1992). *The chemotherapy source book*. Baltimore: Williams & Wilkins.

Reddy, P., & DeFusco, P. (1998). The role of antiestrogens in the treatment and prevention of breast cancer. *Formulary, 33,* 744–768.

Relais, V., & Skirvin, J.A. (1997). Topoisomerase I inhibitors: 1. Topotecan. *Journal of Oncology Pharmacy Practice, 3*(4), 173–185.

Scheife, R.T., & Kearns, C.M. (Eds.). (1997). Current issues in chemotherapy: The taxanes, platinum compounds, and oxazaphosphorines. *Pharmacotherapy, 17*(5, Part 2), 93S–158S.

Skeel, R.T., & Lachant, N.A. (Eds.). (1995). *Handbook of cancer chemotherapy.* Boston: Little, Brown & Co.

Skirvin, J.A., & Relias, V. (1998). Topoisomerase I inhibitors: 2. Irinotecan. *Journal of Oncology Pharmacy Practice, 4*(2), 103–116.

Solimando, D.A., Jr. (1998a). Cancer chemotherapy update: Capecitabine and floxuridine. *Hospital Pharmacy, 33,* 935–937.

Solimando, D.A., Jr. (1998b). Cancer chemotherapy update: Carmustine and lomustine. *Hospital Pharmacy, 33,* 812–818.

Solimando, D.A., Jr. (1998c). Cancer chemotherapy update: Mechlorethamine and procarbazine. *Hospital Pharmacy, 33,* 1300–1304, 1319.

Solimando, D.A., Jr. (1998d). Cancer chemotherapy update: Mercaptopurine and thioguanine. *Hospital Pharmacy, 33,* 1476–1487.

Solimando, D.A., Jr. (1999a). Cancer chemotherapy update: Altretamine and trastuzumab. *Hospital Pharmacy, 34,* 404–406.

Solimando, D.A., Jr. (1999b). Cancer chemotherapy update: Aminoglutethimide and megestrol. *Hospital Pharmacy, 34,* 271–276.

Trissel, L.A. (2001). *Handbook on injectable drugs* (11th ed.). Bethesda, MD: American Society of Health-System Pharmacists.

USPDI. (1998–1999). *Oncology drug information.* Taunton, MA: World Color Book Services.

van Meerten, E., Verweij, J., & Schellens, J.H.M. (1995). Antineoplastic agents: Drug interactions of clinical significance. *Drug Safety, 12*(3), 168–182.

Williams, G., & Jeffrey, A.M. (1997). Safety assessment of tamoxifen and toremifene. *Oncology, 11*(5, Suppl. 4), 41–51.

CHAPTER 6

Legal Issues in Chemotherapy Administration

Marilyn Frank-Stromborg, EdD, JD, ANP, FAAN
Anjeanette Christensen, BA, JD

With an increase in the number of lawsuits that name nurses as defendants, being educated about the law can be a nurse's most valuable asset. Cancer malpractice cases are more frequent and more costly than ever. Million-dollar awards are not uncommon in these suits. Nurses involved in the care and treatment of patients with cancer must follow exacting standards to provide quality care and avoid malpractice liability. Nurses should not only possess general knowledge of the law but also should maintain an understanding and familiarity with the issues that are increasingly and substantially affecting their nursing role.

A basic understanding of the legal process begins with knowing the origin of different sources of law. Nurses who are familiar with and understand the different sources of law are better able to determine how these laws affect their practice and, in turn, can make the laws work for them instead of against them. Four types of laws in the United States directly affect healthcare providers and their practices: constitutional law, statutory law, administrative law, and judicial law. These laws affect nurses and their practice in different ways. For example, constitutional amendments that guarantee freedom of speech may affect nurses personally, whereas other laws, such as administrative laws, may regulate the nurse's professional acts (Aiken & Catalano, 1994).

Source of Laws

Constitutional Law

The Constitution of the United States, or "the supreme law of the land," guarantees individuals certain fundamental rights and freedoms (Aiken &

Catalano, 1994). The Constitution grants power from the states to the federal government but puts certain limitations on these powers, such as the first 10 amendments, or the Bill of Rights (Trandel-Korenchuk & Trandel-Korenchuk, 1997). These amendments guarantee such rights as an individual's right to privacy, equal protection, and freedom of speech and religion (Aiken & Catalano). Although very little constitutional law affects health care and nursing practice directly, the personal rights protected by the Bill of Rights do not just belong to every nurse but to every patient, as well.

Statutory Law

Statutory laws, or statutes, are formal, written laws enacted by federal, state, and local legislative branches of government that declare, command, or prohibit something (Black, 1990). Legislative bodies officially enact statutes by voting on and passing them and compiling them into codes, collections of statutes, or city ordinances (Guido, 2001). State legislatures have enacted a variety of provisions to deal with a multiplicity of health-related issues and concerns. For example, nurse practice acts are specific statutes passed by the legislature to define and regulate the practice of nursing within each state (Aiken & Catalano, 1994). In addition to nurse practice acts, other statutory laws that affect the practice of nursing include statutes of limitations, protective and reporting laws, natural death acts, and privacy and informed consent laws (Guido).

Administrative Law

Administrative, or regulatory, law is the body of law created by administrative agencies by way of rules, regulations, orders, and decisions. An administrative, or regulatory, agency is defined as a government body responsible for control and supervision of a particular activity or area of public interest (Black, 1990). Once the legislature creates a statute or law, such as the state nurse practice acts, it then delegates authority to an administrative agency, the state boards of nursing, which the acts created, to implement and enforce the acts. The administrative agency may carry out its authority by writing rules and regulations for the enforcement of the statutory law and by conducting investigations and hearings to ensure the law's proper enforcement (Guido, 2001). A few of the federal agencies with which nurses should be familiar are the U.S. Department of Health and Human Services (DHHS), the U.S. Food and Drug Administration (FDA), and the U.S. Occupational Safety and Health Administration (OSHA). Some of the state agencies include the department of public health and the board of nursing or other bodies that regulate professions and occupations in the state (Brent, 1997).

Judicial Law

Judicial law is probably the source of law that is familiar to most people. Judicial laws, or decisional laws, are created by the court's interpretation of legal issues that are in dispute. Depending on the level of court in which the case is being heard, the judicial law may be made by a single justice, with or without the assistance of a jury, or by a panel of justices. In deciding cases, the courts will render a decision based on their interpretation of statutes and regulations or may decide which of two conflicting statutes or regulations apply to the given fact situation. For example, nurses who question the authority of the state board of nursing may file a claim, or a court action, if they have cause to believe that there has been a legal or procedural error on the part of the board's action against them (Guido, 2001).

Nursing Liability

Central to nurses' understanding of the different sources of law is their awareness of the possibility of malpractice or negligence claims being filed against them and knowledge about the different theories under which these claims can be filed. Although legal actions against medical practitioners have a long history in English law, both the number of claims against them and the size of resulting awards have risen dramatically over the past decade (Korgaonkar & Tribe, 1995). Professionals from all fields are being held liable for damages resulting from their actions and decisions, and, today, nurses are facing the same level of scrutiny (Howard, Steiert, Deason, & Godkin, 1997). For example, in 747 cases filed from 1988–1993, nursing negligence in hospitals was found to have caused or contributed to 219 deaths (Miller-Slade, 1997). Legal issues are involved in any healthcare setting, and all nurses should be aware of them. The constantly evolving field of nursing practice has brought increased responsibility and, along with it, increased exposure to liability. With the expanding role of the nurse comes a greater possibility for lawsuits. Nurses must stay informed about changing laws, regulations, and public policies (Aiken & Catalano, 1994). A nurse who is knowledgeable about the law and its relation to the practice of nursing will be more aware of the potential for problems that could lead to a lawsuit and will be better able to take the necessary steps to avoid committing malpractice.

Negligence

Negligence is a general term that means failing to exercise due care. Thus, negligence is similar to carelessness, or a deviation from the standard of care that a reasonable person would use in a particular set of circumstances. Negligence also may include conducting an activity that a reasonable and prudent person would not (Guido, 2001).

Malpractice: Malpractice is a specific type of negligence that occurs when the standard of care that is reasonably expected from professionals, such as physicians or nurses, is not met. For a negligent act to be considered malpractice, the person committing the act must be a professional. To be liable for malpractice, the nurse must fail to act as other reasonable and prudent nurses who have the same knowledge and education would have acted under similar situations (Aiken & Catalano, 1994).

Over the years, several cases have been brought against nurses and their employers for professional malpractice. In any medical malpractice suit brought against a nurse, a patient (the plaintiff) must prove four elements of negligence: (1) that the nurse owed a duty of care to the patient, (2) that the nurse breached that duty with conduct that violated a standard of care recognized in the profession, (3) that the breach of the duty was the cause of the suffering or injury, and (4) that the patient suffered damages as a result (Aiken & Catalano, 1994).

Duty: The first element that must be proved in any action alleging negligence is the existence of a duty on the part of the caregiver. First, it must be proved that a duty was owed to the patient who was harmed. The duty that exists evolves out of the relationship between the nurse and the patient. This is a relationship of reliance, wherein one person depends on another for quality, competent care (Guido, 2001). If the nurse holds himself or herself out as possessing special skills and knowledge, and the patient relies on the nurse as possessing such, then the nurse owes a duty to that patient (Pennels, 1997). A nurse owes a duty to any patient he or she treats at a healthcare facility (Korgaonkar & Tribe, 1995).

Second, the scope of that duty, sometimes called the standard of care, must be proved. The standard of care for nurses is the degree of care that would be exercised by a "reasonably prudent nurse" acting under similar circumstances. A judge or jury will make this determination based on expert testimony, published standards, and common sense (Guido, 2001).

Breach of duty: Once the duty is proved, the second element that must be proved is that the duty was breached. The nurse-patient relationship includes a duty to conform to certain minimally acceptable standards of care. The nurse would be judged according to the skills, knowledge, and care that is reasonably possessed and used by members of his or her profession. A nurse whose conduct falls below this standard of care is breaching the duty that he or she owes to the patient. The patient could then bring a negligence action against the nurse because of the nurse's failure to do what a reasonably skilled and competent nurse would do in the same or similar situation.

Litigators often will try to establish a nursing negligence case in the same way they would a case against a doctor. The appropriate specialty is identified, and a nurse of that specialty is located to testify and provide information about the standard of care and any deviation from it (Sweeney, 1991). For example, in a case brought against an oncology nurse for his or her negligence in treating a patient, another oncology nurse may be asked to testify to what the standard of care is in that kind of nursing setting. The nursing record also could be used to prove a breach of the duty owed (Trandel-Korenchuk & Trandel-Korenchuk, 1997).

Causation: The third element that the patient has to prove to claim that the nurse was negligent is causation. It must be legally proven that the breach of the duty caused the injury (Guido, 2001). Establishing causation involves two separate analyses. First, causation itself must be established, called "causation in fact." The basic test for this is the "but for" test: proving that the injury would not have occurred "but for" the nurse's act (Trandel-Korenchuk & Trandel-Korenchuk, 1997).

Establishing causation in fact, however, is not the end of the analysis. Often, there are intervening forces that contribute to or increase the injury, thereby requiring a determination that the negligence of the nurse was the "cause in law," or the proximate cause of the injury (Trandel-Korenchuk & Trandel-Korenchuk, 1997). A proximate cause is that which, in natural and continuous sequence and unbroken by any new, independent cause, produces a reasonably foreseeable injury; without it, the injury would not have occurred (Black, 1990). Proximate cause must be established by showing that there is a "reasonably close" causal connection between the nurse's act and the resulting harm.

Damages: To bring a claim of negligence, the patient must have suffered some sort of compensable injury or damages. The person making the claim must demonstrate physical, financial, or emotional injury resulting from the breach of duty (Trandel-Korenchuk & Trandel-Korenchuk, 1997). The basic purpose of awarding damages is compensatory, which means the court will attempt to restore the injured party to his or her original position to the extent financially possible. The purpose of awarding damages to the plaintiff is not to punish the defendants but rather to assist the injured party (Guido, 2001).

Liability Issues for Nurses

Independence of thought, decision making, action, and concern for personal dignity and human relationships are all very important basic human rights that become even more important in the healthcare setting. During illness, the presence or absence of human rights becomes a necessary deciding factor in survival, recovery, and restoration. It is especially important for oncology nurses to be aware of patients' rights, such as privacy rights, confidentiality rights, and the right to informed consent. A prime responsibility for nurses is to ensure that these rights are preserved for patients (O'Keefe, 2001).

Tort

A nurse can be held liable for violating patient rights by committing a tort, which is a private or civil wrong or injury committed by one person against another person or a property (Aiken & Catalano, 1994). An intentional tort involves a volitional or willful act by the defendant, intending to bring about, or cause, the consequences of the act. Examples of intentional torts include assault, battery, false imprisonment, and intentional infliction of emotional distress. A quasi-intentional tort is a volitional action and involves direct causation, but intent is lacking (Guido, 2001). A nurse who violates a patient's privacy or releases a patient's confidential information without consent is committing a quasi-intentional tort against the patient. The patient's right to privacy and confidentiality is a key concept in the American Nurses Association Code for Nurses, as well as the nurse practice acts in each state. Patients have a right to expect that nurses will not divulge information to those not directly involved in their care (O'Keefe, 2001). Nurses must be knowledgeable about and respect their patients' rights to avoid committing a tort.

Patient Privacy

A patient's right to protection against unreasonable and unwarranted interferences with his or her solitude is well recognized in the law. This includes the protection of personality as well as the protection against interference with one's right to be left alone (Guido, 2001). An invasion of this right by a healthcare provider can lead to a lawsuit for invasion of privacy, a quasi-intentional tort, which can take one or more of three basic forms. The first of these occurs when the nurse, for his or her own benefit, appropriates or uses the plaintiff's name or likeness. In the second form of invasion of privacy, the nurse makes an unreasonable and extremely offensive intrusion upon the patient or his or her personal affairs. In the third type of invasion of privacy, the nurse places the patient in a false light in the public eye (O'Keefe, 2001).

Claims for invasion of privacy can arise from the unauthorized release of information regarding a patient (Trandel-Korenchuk & Trandel-Korenchuk, 1997). Information concerning patients is confidential and may not be disclosed without authorization. Authorization may be by a patient waiver or pursuant to a valid reporting statute (Guido, 2001).

Release of information regarding the medical condition or medical record of a patient must be approached with caution and must only occur in compliance with applicable state and federal laws (Aiken & Catalano, 1994). Most hospitals and institutions have policies and guidelines regarding to whom and under what circumstances information may be released (Guido, 2001).

Patient Confidentiality

Confidentiality respects patient privacy in that individuals should feel comfortable seeking medical and nursing assistance with the expectation that any care and treatment they receive will not be made known to the public (Trandel-Korenchuk & Trandel-Korenchuk, 1997). It is well known that hospitals and their employees have a duty to protect patients' medical records. However, patient information must be safeguarded even if it is not in the written form of a medical record (O'Keefe, 2001). The primary reason for confidentiality of medical records is to promote candor between patients and healthcare providers so that an optimal level of medical and nursing care will be provided (Guido, 2001). The wrongful disclosure of a patient's private information without his or her authorization is considered to be a breach of confidentiality.

This tort protects patients so that they can share information with healthcare providers without fear that the information will be released to those not involved in their care (Brent, 1997). Many cases deal with healthcare workers' wrongful disclosure of verbal information, such as a patient's diagnosis or even the fact that the patient is in the hospital. A patient with cancer or another serious condition may not want to share the diagnosis with others (Fiesta, 1994).

To gain a perspective on how the public views nurses' legal accountability, citizens who had served on juries that heard liability cases were asked whether RNs should be held liable for personal injury resulting from negligence inflicted while following acceptable practices and procedures and for violation of patient confidentiality. Results revealed that 72.3% of respondents believe that RNs should be held liable for violation of patient confidentiality (Howard et al., 1997).

To avoid liability, nurses should operate only on a need-to-know standard. If a nurse is involved in the care of a patient, then that nurse should be given the appropriate information; however, if the nurse is not involved in the care, the information should not be shared (Fiesta, 1994). Institutional policies concerning confidentiality must be followed.

Confidentiality and privacy are essential rights that a patient must be afforded when under the care of a healthcare professional. All nurse-patient relationships are based on fidelity (e.g., promise-keeping, trust), respect for the individual, and restraint from causing harm, oncology nurses must be especially cautious not to undermine the relationships they have with patients. Patient surveys indicate that oncology nurses maintain a vital role in patient well-being. Oncology nurses have in-depth, day-to-day patient contact and often serve as liaisons between physician-specialists and patients. Patients with cancer often view their oncology nurses as professionals to whom they can turn for advice and support on a variety of medical and quality-of-life topics (Houston, 1997). A breach in patient's privacy or confidentiality could have a detrimental impact on the delicate and unique relationship that the nurse maintains with his or her patients, and could, in turn, negatively affect a patient's overall treatment and recovery.

Informed Consent

Much like a patient's rights of confidentiality and privacy, the process of obtaining informed consent, if not carried out properly, can be detrimental to both the patient with cancer and the oncology nurse. Informed consent requires physicians or healthcare providers to inform patients of the benefits, risks, options, and alternatives to medical treatment (Calfee, 1996). For a patient's consent to treatment to be legally effective, the consent must be what the law considers "informed consent." This means that the physician or healthcare provider has given enough information regarding the risks and benefits of the proposed treatment and its alternatives to enable the patient to make an intelligent or informed decision (Aiken & Catalano, 1994; Gullatte, 1998). Additionally, the consent is limited to the specific test or treatment for which it was obtained. For instance, consent to a breast biopsy does not permit a surgeon to go further and perform a mastectomy, regardless of the findings.

There are two types of informed consent: express and implied. Express consent is given by an oral declaration concerning a particular treatment or by a written document that the patient signs. In health care, the written consent form is used most frequently. Except in certain situations, such as in research settings, written consent for health care is not a requirement. Rather, it helps the patient to understand to what he or she is consenting. The other type of informed consent, implied consent, is consent that an individual gives through conduct or actions rather than verbally or in writing. For example, when a nurse tells a patient that he or she is going to take the patient's blood pressure and the patient extends an arm to the nurse, the patient has given implied consent (Brent, 1997).

Treatment or attempts to treat without such consent may result in a lawsuit in which the patient claims that the healthcare provider is liable for assault and/or battery, both of which are intentional torts (Aiken & Catalano, 1994). Healthcare providers who fail to obtain informed consent open themselves to potential lawsuits for negligence (Guido, 2001). The written document indicating consent for treatment can reliably prove that consent was obtained in the event that a lawsuit is filed (Brent, 1997).

Regardless of the setting, the nurse who is in contact with patients will likely be involved in some way with obtaining informed consent. This does not mean that nurses obtain written consent each time they give an injection or take vital signs. Most nursing interventions rely on oral expressed or implied consent that may be inferred from a patient's actions. The doctrine of informed consent means that nurses must continually communicate with a patient, explaining procedures and obtaining the patient's permission (Guido, 2001).

Nurses often will be actively involved in obtaining signatures on consent forms (Calfee, 1996). Sometimes, under hospital policy, nurses are asked to witness the document. If this is the hospital policy, the nurse should actually witness the physician obtaining the patient's signature on the form (Fiesta, 1994). The doctrine of informed consent also means that the patient's refusal to allow a certain procedure must be respected. Nurses play an important role if patients subsequently wish to revoke their prior consent or if it becomes obvious that a patient's already-signed informed consent form does not meet the standards of informed consent. In such a case, nurses should contact their immediate supervisor and the responsible physician (Guido, 2001).

A very real concern for nurses lies in obtaining consent for the nursing aspects of medical procedures in which another practitioner performs, in whole or in part, the primary or entire medical procedure. Physicians may legally delegate the responsibility of obtaining informed consent to the nurse, but they do so at their own risk because most practice acts hold the physician responsible for obtaining informed consent. Thus, any deficiencies in the nurse's procedure of obtaining informed consent may be imputed back to the responsible physician. The delegated nurse acts in the role of the physician and must ensure that all information is given to patients in language that they can understand. Therefore, the nurse, as well as the delegating physician, may incur liability for the patient's informed consent (Guido, 2001).

Each state's law of informed consent differs, and, therefore, it is necessary to consult each state's statute for specific information. Along with state case law and statutory law, healthcare practitioners also should ensure that they comply with the rules of the appropriate regulatory and accrediting agencies (Aiken & Catalano, 1994).

Clinical Trials

Oncology nurses who work in the research setting often are involved in obtaining informed consent from clinical trial participants. To avoid legal repercussions, informed consent is a necessary part of patient participation in clinical trials. Nurses are in the position to evaluate patients' understanding of study and to determine that the decision to participate has been voluntary (Jenkins & Curt, 1996). Once a consent form is read and explained to a patient participating in the clinical trial, the nurse must clarify the consent to ensure that the patient is knowingly consenting to medical treatment.

The person who conducts the consent interview should be knowledgeable about the study and able to answer questions. The FDA does not specify who this individual should be. Some sponsors and some institutional review boards (IRBs) require the clinical investigator to personally conduct the consent interview. However, if someone other than the clinical investigator conducts the interview and obtains consent, such as a nurse, the clinical investigator should formally delegate this responsibility, and the person delegated should have appropriate training to perform this activity (FDA, 1998). Chapter 8 provides additional information on clinical trials.

Oncology nurses also are responsible for monitoring patients during the study. All nurses should be monitoring patients for how well they fit the study's eligibility criteria. The nurse's role may include preparing the patient for studies required to document protocol eligibility and ensure protocol compliance. The staff nurse usually is the first to notice unusual or expected symptoms and should report them to the research nurse or the principal investigator (Jenkins & Curt, 1996).

One of the most critical roles the research nurse performs is the documentation and data management of the patient's chart for the evaluation of treatment. All patients who participate in clinical trials must have documentation of what types of procedures have been performed, the types and amounts of medications that have been administered, and the dates, times, and effects of the procedures and medications. This documentation must remain accurate and up-to-date.

The role of the oncology nurse in cancer clinical trials is multifaceted, which creates a great deal of responsibility for the nurses involved. An oncology nurse in the research setting who does not ensure that informed consent has been received, who fails to sufficiently monitor a patient, or who does not properly document a record can cause serious harm to the patient, cause error in the studies, and create legal repercussions for himself or herself.

Liability Regarding Chemotherapy Administration

The role of the oncology nurse is very different from that of any other hospital personnel. Oncology nurses play an important role in chemotherapy administration. In addition to infusing chemotherapy, oncology nurses are responsible for verifying the dose and schedule of the agents administered during the preparatory stage of chemotherapy administration (Schulmeister, 1997).

Chemotherapy administration is a complex procedure involving the use of drugs that can lead to fatal consequences if not administered correctly. Unlike many other medications that have standardized dose and schedule guidelines, antineoplastic agents are administered in a wide array of doses using a variety of schedules, and, even under the best of circumstances, cancer chemotherapy is toxic to some degree (Fischer, Alfano, Knobf, Donovan, & Beaulieu, 1996). As with any other medication, the nurse is responsible for the safe administration of chemotherapy and is accountable for his or her actions (Schulmeister, 1997).

Medication Errors

The administration of medication on the part of the oncology nurse has resulted in a number of lawsuits based on a nurse's failure to follow the acceptable standard of care. Since the discovery of several fatal errors at a reputable cancer center in New England in 1995, reducing medication errors in chemotherapy administration has been a national priority. Edgar, Lee, and Cousins (1994) reported a summary of 568 actual or potential medication errors to a national medication error database from August 1991 to April 1994. Of the 43 reported incidents that resulted in death, 11 involved chemotherapy overdoses (Schulmeister, 1997).

For example, patient X was admitted to the oncology unit for initiation of chemotherapy as part of her treatment for breast cancer. During clinical rounds, the primary oncologist ordered stat blood work before the administration of the initial dose of chemotherapy and also ordered Coumadin® (Dupont Pharmaceuticals Company, Wilmington, DE) 1.0 mg PO daily. The medication order for the Coumadin was faxed to the pharmacy while the unit secretary transcribed the information to the medication administration record. In her transcribing, she overlooked the decimal point and recorded it as "Coumadin 10 mg PO QD." As the nurse was preparing to administer the drug, she noticed the contradiction between the 1 mg of Coumadin she was about to administer and the amount on the medication administration record (MAR). She checked the physician's order and found the transcription error. Fortunately for the patient, the error was caught, but this is not always the case. Nurses working in the oncology setting must be extremely careful when recording and administering drugs because the legal ramifications of a medication error are severe. In the case cited, the nurse greatly decreased her chances of becoming involved in a lawsuit because she correctly verified the medication order before administering it (Lilley & Guanci, 1997).

Failure to Follow Standard of Care

In addition to verifying the drug and dosage, nurses must also verify that they are administering the drug to the correct patient. As obvious as this may sound, there have been several instances where patients have received another patient's drug. For example, a seven-year-old boy who was admitted for a fever to the same hospital where he received treatment for cancer was given 30–50 times the normal dosage of the chemotherapy drug (cytosine arabinoside) meant for someone else. The child suffered serious effects from this drug mixup but was expected to recover (Cook & Zarek, 1998).

A case like this is considered to be a failure of the standard of care, and the person who administers the chemotherapy drug, usually an oncology nurse, is the one at fault. The nurse is responsible for the safe administration of chemotherapy, even when another healthcare provider orders an excessive dose or the wrong medication (Schulmeister, 1997).

Lack of Knowledge About Medication and Administration

Oncology nurses who have correctly followed the acceptable standard of care by verifying the drug, dosage, and patient can still be held liable for their knowledge about the drugs they administer. For example, patient Y, who had been diagnosed with advanced head and neck cancer six months earlier, was discharged from his local hospital's oncology unit to convalesce at home after receiving his last series of chemotherapy and radiation treatments. Patient Y's homecare nurse was to continue to administer his IV medication and assess his tolerance to two medications and his progress daily. On the third day at home, the patient reported increasing difficulty in swallowing solids, and he could no longer swallow the oxycodone tablets he was taking for his pain. The nurse found that he could swallow liquids and soft foods, so she decided to crush the oxycodone tablet and mix the powder with fruit juice to maintain analgesia. About 90 minutes after drinking the juice, the patient experienced clinical signs of respiratory depression as a result of the nurse's lack of knowledge about a major warning associated with OxyContin® (Purdue Pharma, Inc., Norwalk, CT), the patient's pain medication: the medication should be swallowed whole, and tablets should never be broken, chewed, or crushed (Lilley & Guanci, 1996).

Because of the toxicity of chemotherapy agents, nurses must understand the sensitivity of the agents they administer and must be aware of the effect of any changes. Most chemotherapy doses are based on a certain amount of drug to be administered per body surface area (BSA) or square meter (Schulmeister, 1997). Doses computed using BSA vary from protocol to protocol and may be adjusted individually to prevent or minimize chemotherapy-related toxicities (Schulmeister). In addition, the scheduling of chemotherapy also varies by protocol (Schulmeister). A nurse who makes chemotherapy dose and scheduling changes should be very familiar with the chemotherapy medications administered and should follow established protocols and institutional policies and procedures. Before administering a medication to a patient, a nurse should always know the drug's dosage range, possible adverse effects, toxicity levels, indications, and contraindications (Eskreis, 1998).

Insufficient Patient Monitoring

Failure to monitor patients is another common cause of malpractice suits. In Grandi v. Shah (1994), a patient brought an action against his physician, a nurse, and others involved in his care. The plaintiff underwent surgery to have a cancerous tumor removed from his stomach. On February 10, 1983, the plaintiff went to the hospital, where the physician treated him intravenously with three chemotherapy drugs. The physician first administered Adriamycin® (Pharmacia & UpJohn, Peapack, NJ) and Oncovin® (Eli Lilly and Company, Indianapolis, IN), which are known as vesicants because they cause burning sensations and destroy tissue if they extravasate the vein. At the trial, the plaintiff testified that the defendant doctor left him alone in the treatment room after administering the vesicants, and, about 20 seconds later, he experienced burning sensations in his left wrist and called for help. Thereafter, the defendant doctor returned to the treatment room and stated that the needle came out of the patient's vein and that the nurse should have stayed with the patient. A settlement agreement was reached prior to trial between the nurse and the patient regarding the nurse's negligent involvement in the case.

Lack of Patient Preparation

In the 1991 case of Latham v. Southwest Detroit Hospital and Jane Doe, a patient, age 63, was receiving chemotherapy and had a subcutaneous (SC) infiltration that necessitated multiple plastic surgeries. She alleged that the defendant nurse was negligent in allowing the needle to go SC. The nurse contended that she checked for good blood flow before administering the chemicals and that the patient reached for the telephone during the administration of the drugs, causing the needle to move. According to the nurse, nothing could have been done to alter the outcome, but the jury must have thought otherwise because it returned a $500,000 verdict against the nurse (Fiesta, 1994).

In this case, the oncology nurse more than likely could have avoided this lawsuit if she had properly informed the patient about the procedure and what the patient should or should not do during the administration of the drugs, hence discouraging the patient from moving her arm during the process.

Risk Reduction Ideas and Practices

Fortunately, oncology nurses can take actions to avoid these and other types of danger associated with the administration of chemotherapy. Recommendations specifically for the prevention of medication errors in cancer chemotherapy include

- Educate healthcare providers about the various drugs that are used, especially when new ones are introduced, and the effect they have on individual patients; infusion guidelines and dosage requirements; adverse side effects; and methods to reduce medication errors.
- Verify the dose.
- Establish dosage limits.
- Standardize the prescribing vocabulary by using full generic names of drugs instead of abbreviations, brand names, and common drug classes; expressing all drug doses in milligrams or units; dating all drug orders; using a leading zero in orders when the dose is less than a whole unit; refraining from using a trailing zero in drug orders; and including the current BSA with the order.
- Work with drug manufacturers by reporting errors to the Medication Errors Reporting Program (operated by United States Pharmacopoeia in cooperation with the Institution for Safe Medication Practices), and eliminate ambiguous dosing information from educational resources.
- Educate patients about the agent, therapeutic indications, and possible adverse effects; instruct patients on how to protect themselves from medication errors; and listen carefully to what patients are saying.

- Improve communication regarding medication errors and potential problems and solutions (Cohen et al., 1996).

More specifically, nurses should make the following suggestions an integral part of their daily performance of these different tasks.

- Prescribing
  - Chemotherapy orders must be written or faxed and signed by the attending physician prior to the pharmacy admixing the chemotherapy.
- Administering
  - The receiving nurse must check doses against the original physician's order by complying with whatever drug order verification procedures are in place at the facility (e.g., initialing the pharmacy patient profile).
  - Each time a nurse administers chemotherapy to a patient, he or she is required to ensure proper transcription of the original order onto the chemotherapy MAR.
  - Two oncology professionals are required to verify chemotherapy prior to administration for correct patient, chemotherapy drug, dose, day, route, and duration. This is done by checking the chemotherapy drug labels against the original physician's order and chemotherapy MAR; two oncology professionals must initial the MAR.
  - A nurse is required to assess blood return every 1–2 hours for continuous infusion of vesicants and irritants administered via a central line.
- Monitoring and education
  - Nurses must be certified for IV chemotherapy administration and recertified annually.
  - Bimonthly, nurses should attend in-services provided by pharmacists for oncology nursing staff, covering topics such as new chemotherapy agents, protocols, and orders.
  - Nurses should be involved in providing chemotherapy information to all patients receiving chemotherapy (Gilmore & Suresky, 1998).

In addition, oncology nurses should inform other healthcare providers about how to improve in these areas and should be active in incorporating the afore mentioned suggestions into formal guidelines that every oncology nurse in the facility must follow.

Summary

The nurse's expanding role in patient care and an increase in specialization inevitably will be accompanied by a continued increase in legal liability for nurses. Liability can arise for oncology nurses for violations of patient's rights, such as the patient's expectations of privacy and confidentiality. Obtaining informed consent in clinical trials and other types of settings and administering chemotherapy also can potentially put nurses in the position of being named defendants in medical malpractice suits. Oncology nurses must guard against liability by keeping up-to-date on every aspect of their practice, identifying risk factors, and implementing risk-reduction practices and following them until they become second nature.

References

Aiken, T., & Catalano, J. (1994). *Legal, ethical, and political issues in nursing* (pp. 1–19, 96–117, 136–157). Philadelphia: F.A. Davis.

Black, H.C. (1990). *Black's law dictionary* (6th ed.). Eagan, MN: West Group Publishing.

Brent, N. (1997). *Nurses and the law.* Philadelphia: W.B. Saunders.

Calfee, B. (1996). *Nurses in the courtroom.* Houston, TX: ARC Publishing Company, Inc.

Cohen, M., Anderson, R., Attilio, R., Green, L., Muller, R., & Pruemer, J. (1996). Preventing medication errors in cancer chemotherapy. *American Journal of Health-System Pharmacy, 53,* 737–746.

Cook, S., & Zarek, C. (1998, February 5). Drug mix-up victim recovers. *The Daily Iowan,* p. 1A.

Edgar, T.A., Lee, D.S., & Cousins, D.D. (1994). Experience with a national medication error reporting program. *American Journal of Hospital Pharmacy, 51,* 1335–1338.

Eskreis, T.R. (1998). Seven common legal pitfalls in nursing. *American Journal of Nursing, 98*(4), 34–40.

Fiesta, J. (1994). *20 legal pitfalls for nurses to avoid.* Albany, NY: Delmar Publishers.

Fischer, D., Alfano, S., Knobf, M.T., Donovan, C., & Beaulieu, N. (1996). Improving the cancer chemotherapy use process. *Journal of Clinical Oncology, 14,* 3148–3155.

Gilmore, C., & Suresky, P. (1998). Development and implementation of a chemo-therapy error-prevention policy. *Hospital Pharmacy, 33,* 1214–1219.

Grandi v. Shah, 633 N.E.2d 894 (Ill, 1994).

Guido, G.W. (2001). *Legal and ethical issues in nursing* (3rd ed.). Englewood Cliffs, NJ: Prentice-Hall, Inc.

Gullatte, M.M. (1998). Legal issues influencing cancer care. In J. Itano & K. Taoka (Eds.), *Core curriculum for oncology nursing* (3rd ed.) (pp. 734–740). Philadelphia: W.B. Saunders.

Houston, D. (1997). Supportive therapies for cancer chemotherapy patients and the role of the oncology nurse. *Cancer Nursing, 20,* 409–410.

Howard, J., Steiert, A., Deason, C., & Godkin, L. (1997). Jurors rate RNs counting the costs. *Nursing Management, 28*(1), 39–40.

Jenkins, J., & Curt, G. (1996). Implementation of clinical trials. In R. McCorkle, M. Grant, M. Frank-Stromborg, & S. Baird (Eds.), *Cancer nursing: A comprehensive text-book* (pp. 470–484). Philadelphia: W.B. Saunders.

Korgaonkar, G., & Tribe, D. (1995). *Law for nurses.* London: Cavendish Publishing Limited.

Lilley, L.L., & Guanci, R. (1996). Don't overlook directions. *American Journal of Nursing, 96,*(12), 14–15.

Lilley, L.L., & Guanci, R. (1997). Careful with the zeros! *American Journal of Nursing, 97*(5), 14.

Miller-Slade, D. (1997). Liability theories in nursing negligence cases. *Trial, 33*(5), 52–54.

O'Keefe, M.E. (2001). *Nursing practice and the law.* Philadelphia: F.A. Davis.

Pennels, C.J.E. (1997). Legal issues. Nursing and the law. *Professional Nurse, 13*(1), 49–53.

Schulmeister, L. (1997). Preventing chemotherapy dose and schedule errors. *Clinical Journal of Oncology Nursing, 1,* 79–85.

Sweeney, P. (1991). Proving nursing negligence. *Trial, 27*(5), 34–40.

Trandel-Korenchuk, D.M., & Trandel-Korenchuk, K.M. (1997). *Nursing and the law* (5th ed.). Gaithersburg, MD: Aspen Publishers Inc.

U.S. Food and Drug Administration. (1998, September). *Information Sheets: Guidance for institutional review boards and clinical investigators.* Retrieved November 16, 2000 from the World Wide Web: www.fda.gov/oc/ohrt/irbs/faqs.html#Informed%20 Consent%20/process

CHAPTER 7

Symptom Management

Joyce Alexander, RN, MSN, AOCN®

The experience of symptoms related to cancer treatment affects the quality of life of the person diagnosed with cancer. The adequacy of symptom management also may affect the decision to continue with treatment. Ultimately, the management of symptoms sometimes determines life or death.

Nurses have the opportunity, as well as the responsibility, to assist in managing symptoms produced by disease and treatment. Patient education prior to chemotherapy treatment not only includes the purpose, actions, and side effects of the drugs but also focuses on strategies for symptom management that the person with cancer and the family can implement. During any patient stay in the inpatient or outpatient area, the nurse assists the patient with managing symptoms by demonstrating effective strategies. Information is reinforced upon discharge from the clinic or hospital. The outpatient nurse often is called upon to triage phone calls, and specific questions about symptoms are included in the phone assessment. Based on that assessment, the nurse makes suggestions for symptom management or asks the patient to come to the office or go to an emergency facility.

Common symptoms related to antineoplastic therapy include nausea and vomiting, mucositis, fatigue, pain, and pancytopenia caused by bone marrow suppression. Oncology nurses are aware of risk factors and utilize assessment skills to determine the presence, severity, and sequelae of side effects and symptoms. Strategies for prevention and management are used in both care and teaching of the individual experiencing cancer treatment.

Nausea and Vomiting

The first question new patients often ask about chemotherapy is, "Will I be sick?" Many people associate mental images of prolonged and intractable nausea and vomiting with cancer treatment. Chemotherapy does cause nausea and vomiting, and some drugs have a greater emetic potential than others. However, nurses can assure patients that this side effect can be controlled. The recent advent of improved control of the emetic effects of chemotherapy has significantly changed the experience of receiving chemotherapy.

Nausea is an unpleasant, subjective symptom mediated by the autonomic nervous system. Objective symptoms accompanying nausea often include pallor, perspiration, and tachycardia. Nausea may precede chemotherapy-induced vomiting or may occur separately.

Vomiting, expulsion of stomach contents through the mouth, requires the coordinated activity of muscles of the gastrointestinal (GI) and respiratory system. Vomiting is believed to be coordinated through a region of the dorsolateral reticular formation referred to as the vomiting center (see Figure 7-1).

Figure 7-1. The Vomiting Center

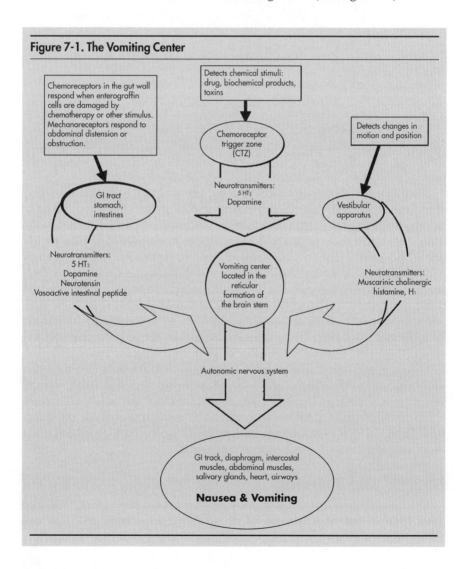

A variety of neurotransmitters conduct impulses to the vomiting center from the chemoreceptor trigger zone (CTZ), the GI system, the vestibular apparatus, and the cerebral cortex. The CTZ, located between the medulla oblongata and the fourth ventricle, responds to the presence of drug or cellular byproducts in the blood or to neurotransmitters, especially serotonin. The GI system stimulates the vomiting center through activation of vagal and visceral afferent pathways as well as by serotonin released by damaged or irritated cells. Motion sickness results from transmission of impulses from the vestibular apparatus. Visual images, taste, smell, and memory contribute to nausea and vomiting through impulses transmitted from the cerebral cortex to the vomiting center. Although many neurotransmitters are present in the area of the vomiting center, dopamine, serotonin, histamine, and cholinergic receptors mediate the majority of transmissions.

Risk Factors for Nausea and Vomiting

The risk of nausea and vomiting varies with the emetic potential of the chemotherapeutic agent. Antiemetic regimens often are tested using the chemotherapy agent cisplatin (Platinol-AQ®, Bristol-Myers Squibb Oncology/ Immunology Division, Princeton, NJ) because of the high emetic potential of the drug. Figure 7-2 lists certain commonly used chemotherapeutic drugs by emetic potential. In regimens with multiple drugs, the emetic potential is combined, and, thus, is higher than that of any one drug alone. In addition, higher doses of chemotherapeutic agents have a higher emetic potential.

Figure 7-2. Potential of Common Chemotherapeutic Agents to Cause Nausea and Vomiting

Drugs Highly Likely to Cause Nausea and Vomiting
• Cisplatin
• Dacarbazine
• Streptozocin
• Mechlorethamine
• Cytarabine (high-dose)
• Cyclophosphamide (high-dose)
• Melphalan (high-dose)
• Dactinomycin
• Procarbazine
• Amifostine (chemoprotectant drug)

Drugs Moderately Likely to Cause Nausea and Vomiting
• Carboplatin
• Ifosfamide
• Daunorubicin
• Doxorubicin
• Mitomycin-C

• Etoposide
• Methotrexate (high-dose)
• Idarubicin
• Pentostatin
• Topotecan
• Mitoxantrone

Drugs Less Likely to Cause Nausea and Vomiting
• Busulfan
• Bleomycin
• Fluorouracil
• Fludarabine
• Hydroxyurea
• Chlorambucil
• Methotrexate (lower-dose)
• Melphalan (lower-dose)
• Paclitaxel
• Docetaxel
• Chlorodeoxyadenosine

Note. Based on information from Berger & Clark-Snow, 1997; Camp-Sorrell, 1997; National Cancer Institute, 1999.

Patients with a history of motion sickness or severe morning sickness are more likely to experience nausea and vomiting with chemotherapy, as are patients who suffered severe nausea and vomiting with a previous course of treatment. Anxiety increases risk, and women are more likely than men to have nausea and vomiting. Patients who have a roommate who is vomiting are more likely to experience emesis. Chronic alcohol users tend to experience less nausea and vomiting (Berger & Clark-Snow, 1997).

Nausea and vomiting also are caused by factors other than chemotherapy. Often, the healthcare team must sort out whether nausea and vomiting are caused by chemotherapy or by disease processes or other treatments. Risk factors related to disease include GI obstruction, tumor of the central nervous system (CNS), and increased intracranial pressure. Medications that cause nausea include digitalis, antibiotics, iron, vitamins, and opioid drugs. Electrolyte disturbances, including hypercalcemia, hyperglycemia, and hyponatremia, also increase risk (Berendt, 1998). Finally, patients receiving chemotherapy are susceptible to infectious agents producing GI symptoms.

Patterns of Nausea and Vomiting With Chemotherapy

Three types of nausea and vomiting are described in association with chemotherapy. Anticipatory nausea and vomiting occur before the patient receives the chemotherapeutic agent. Often associated with olfactory or visual cues, anticipatory nausea is a conditioned response demonstrating the cerebral connection to the vomiting center. Acute nausea and vomiting occur during or within a few hours following chemotherapy administration. Delayed nausea and vomiting occur more than 24 hours after the drugs are given and may persist for several days. Just as the emetic potential varies among drugs, the onset and duration of nausea and vomiting tend to vary among drugs but occur in patterns with specific drugs (Berger & Clark-Snow, 1997).

Assessment

Prior to treatment, the nurse assesses the patient for risk of nausea and vomiting and intervenes with prophylactic therapy when that risk is high. Following treatment, assessment includes the patient's subjective impression of nausea, as well as the frequency, volume, and character of emesis. The presence of blood in emesis requires immediate notification of the physician. The nurse also assesses the pattern and relation of nausea and vomiting to treatment and other factors.

Weight, fluids and electrolytes, and nutritional status are assessed when nausea and vomiting are protracted. Frequent vomiting results in GI loss of potassium, causing hypokalemia. Nursing assessment includes cardiac rhythm, mental status, reflexes, strength, and blood pressure, as well as potassium levels (obtained through a lab report). Evidence of dehydration includes weight loss, decreased skin turgor, weakness, thirst, orthostatic hypotension, and concentrated urine with decreased output. The nurse must consider risk factors for vomiting other than chemotherapy, including GI obstruction, increased intracranial pressure, and metastasis of disease to the brain. An assumption that symptoms are produced solely by treatment prevents recognition of serious complications.

Pharmacologic Management of Nausea and Vomiting

Drugs used in the treatment of nausea and vomiting interfere with the transmission of impulses by various pathways to the vomiting center. The first drugs used as antiemetics act by blocking dopamine transmission.

Phenothiazines: The phenothiazines, including prochlorperazine (Compazine®, SmithKline Beecham Pharmaceuticals), promethazine (Phenergan®, Wyeth-Ayerst, Philadelphia, PA), and chlorpromazine (Thorazine®, SmithKline Beecham Pharmaceuticals), act by inhibition of dopamine. Phenothiazines are effective in treating or preventing nausea and vomiting associated with drugs with low to moderate emetic potential and often are used for delayed nausea and vomiting. Prochlorperazine and promethazine are the most commonly used phenothiazines. The usual oral dose of prochlorperazine is 5–10 mg given every 4–6 hours, with the long-acting form given every 10–12 hours. Prochlorperazine is available in a tablet or controlled-release oral form, as well as in parenteral and rectal formulations. The parenteral dosage of 5–10 mg may be given intramuscularly or as a slow IV injection or infusion. Bolus injection should not be used (Medical Economics Company, Inc., 2000). Promethazine doses range from 12.5–25 mg and may be given orally, intramuscularly, intravenously, or rectally every four to six hours. Side effects of the phenothiazines include sedation, orthostatic hypotension, dizziness, drowsiness, motor restlessness, dystonias, and other extrapyramidal effects.

Butyrophenones: Droperidol (Inapsine®, Johnson & Johnson Corporation, New Brunswick, NJ) and haloperidol (Haldol®, Ortho-McNeil Pharmaceuticals, Raritan, NJ) also act as dopaminergic receptor antagonists and have antiemetic activity. The usual dose is 0.5–1 mg. Adverse effects include sedation, tachycardia, hypotension, rash, and extrapyramidal symptoms. Butyrophenones should not be used in patients with Parkinson's disease (Medical Economics Company, Inc., 2000).

Metoclopramide: Metoclopramide (Reglan®, A.H. Robins Company, Richmond, VA) given in 5- to 10-mg doses increases gastric emptying. At higher doses (0.5–3 mg/kg given intravenously), metoclopramide has been shown to be an effective antiemetic, even for agents with a high emetic potential. Metoclopramide once was thought to act strictly as a dopamine antagonist, but effectiveness of the drug has now been attributed to an additional weak serotonin antagonism. Side effects of high-dose metoclopramide, however, include dystonic extrapyramidal effects and akathisia. The extrapyramidal system controls gross motor movements. Therefore, extrapyramidal side effects include tremor, cogwheeling rigidity, jerking repetitive movement of extremities or the head and neck, and hyperactive reflexes. Akathisia is described as a sense of restlessness or inability to sit still. Diphenhydramine (Benadryl®, Parke-Davis, Morris Plains, NJ) may be given with metoclopramide to counter side effects.

5-HT$_3$ antagonists: The most effective drugs against acute chemotherapy-associated nausea and vomiting are the serotonin receptor (5-HT$_3$) antagonists. Three 5-HT$_3$ antagonists currently used in the United States are ondansetron (Zofran®, Glaxo Wellcome Inc., Research Triangle Park, NC), granisetron (Kytril®, SmithKline Beecham Pharmaceuticals), and dolasetron (Anzemet®,

Hoechst Marion Roussel, Kansas City, MO). The current IV dosage recommendation for ondansetron is for a single 32-mg dose prior to chemotherapy (Glaxo Wellcome Inc., 1999). Ondansetron also may be given orally as tablets, solution, or an orally disintegrating tablet. The recommended oral dose is 8 mg given twice daily beginning 30 minutes before chemotherapy (Anastasia, 2000). Granisetron may be given as a single IV dose of 10 mcg/kg 30 minutes before chemotherapy or as a 1-mg oral dose given before chemotherapy and repeated in 12 hours. Dolasetron is given as a single IV dose of 1.8 mg/kg 15 minutes prior to chemotherapy or a single oral dose of 100 mg one hour prior to chemotherapy. Side effects of serotonin antagonists include headache, constipation or diarrhea, fatigue, and dry mouth. Product literature for dolasetron urges caution in patients with existing or potential prolongation of cardiac conduction intervals (Medical Economics Company, Inc., 2000). A number of studies have compared the 5-HT$_3$ antagonists. Among these, Fox-Geiman et al. (1999) found oral ondansetron or granisetron to be effective in patients undergoing stem cell transplant and to be more cost-effective than IV ondansetron. Studies comparing ondansetron and granisetron have not shown one to be superior to the other (Fox-Geiman et al.; Nakamura, Taira, & Kodaira, 1999). A combination of serotonin antagonist drugs with dexamethasone has been shown to be more effective than the serotonin antagonists alone (Hesketh et al., 2000; The Italian Group for Antiemetic Research, 2000). The 5-HT$_3$ antagonists are effective but expensive drugs. Use of oral administration rather than IV is one way of decreasing cost (Anastasia). Many institutions use algorithms or prescribing guidelines suggesting other antiemetics for chemotherapy regimens of low emetogenic potential to limit the institutional cost of antiemetics. Serotonin antagonists should not be used for anticipatory or delayed nausea and vomiting, for which they have not been shown to be effective. Nor should the dose be increased, as studies have shown that dose escalation does not increase effectiveness (Fauser et al., 1999).

Steroids: Dexamethasone (Decadron®, Merck & Company, West Point, PA) and methylprednisolone (Solu-Medrol®, Pharmacia & Upjohn, Peapack, NJ) often are included in antiemetic combinations and are sometimes used alone with chemotherapeutic agents having low or moderate emetic potential. The mechanism of action for the antiemetic effect of steroids is poorly understood but may be related to an effect on prostaglandin activity in the brain.

Cannabinoids: Although a politically popular topic, the cannabinoids have not proven to be especially useful as antiemetics for most patients (Berger & Clark-Snow, 1997; National Cancer Institute [NCI], 1999). Dronabinol (Marinol®, Roxane Laboratories, Columbus, OH), a form of cannabinoid currently available for medical use, affects the CNS. Dronabinol is useful in selected patients. Usual dosage is 5 mg/m^2 begun one to three hours before chemotherapy, then every two to four hours up to six doses/day. Dosage may be gradually increased in 2.5-mg increments if needed, if the patient has no side effects, to a maximum of 15 mg/m^2 (Medical Economics Company, 2000). Side effects include euphoria or dysphoria, depression, anxiety, paranoia, panic, and other CNS symptoms, as well as tachycardia, vasodilation, and orthostatic hypotension.

Benzodiazepines: The benzodiazepines lorazepam (Ativan®, Wyeth-Ayerst Company, Philadelphia, PA), midazolam (Versed®, Roche Laboratories, Nutley, NJ), and alprazolam (Xanax®, Pharmacia & Upjohn) may be used in antiemetic combinations. The benzodiazepines function as antiemetics through an effect on the CNS and are more likely to be effective adjuncts to other antiemetics than to be effective alone. Lorazepam, however, is sometimes effective against anticipatory nausea and vomiting, especially when combined with behavioral interventions.

Combinations: A number of combinations have been used as antiemetic prophylaxis and treatment and have proven more effective than any single agent. The combination of serotonin antagonists with dexamethasone or methylprednisolone is the most effective prophylactic regimen currently available for acute nausea and vomiting. This regimen is commonly used for drugs with high emetic potential and should be followed with an additional drug, most commonly prochlorperazine or promethazine, for prevention of delayed nausea and vomiting.

Prior to the introduction of serotonin antagonists, combinations using high-dose metoclopramide were common. Such combinations continue to provide a lower-cost option in certain settings. Diphenhydramine is included to prevent extrapyramidal and akinetic side effects; lorazepam adds an anxiolytic, as well as amnesic, effect; and dexamethasone potentiates the antiemetic effect. Nurses administering this regimen must, however, monitor for extrapyramidal and akinetic side effects and be mindful of patient safety. Sedation, especially in patients receiving hydration, can lead to falls or injury.

Nonpharmacologic Strategies

What nurse has not at some time applied a cool, damp cloth to a patient's forehead, washed the patient's face, provided a cool-water mouth rinse, or simply comforted the patient or family member who is feeling nauseous? Such measures are nonpharmacologic nursing strategies, that may not eliminate nausea but probably increase patient comfort. Like many nursing interventions, these simple actions have not been studied and are not reported in the nursing literature on chemotherapy-related nausea and vomiting. Reported nonpharmacologic strategies include behavioral and dietary interventions, acupressure, and music therapy.

Behavioral interventions include progressive muscle relaxation, guided imagery, self-hypnosis, biofeedback, distraction, and systematic desensitization. Often, these interventions are combined. Depending on patient preference and interest, most studies have shown benefit when behavioral interventions with elements of relaxation are used as adjuncts to pharmacologic interventions. Although time-consuming when implemented by the nurse, interested patients can learn and self-administer interventions using audiotapes. Behavioral interventions have been most frequently studied in the treatment of anticipatory nausea and vomiting, for which medications (other than lorazepam) have been largely ineffective. Systematic desensitization has been most effective in treatment of the conditioned response of anticipatory nausea and vomiting.

Music therapy, when combined with pharmacologic interventions, has been shown to be effective in hematopoietic cell transplant (HCT) patients receiving high-dose therapy. In one study, music therapy involved simply listening to self-selected music at times when nausea was most likely to develop (Ezzone, Baker, Rosselet, & Terepka, 1998).

Acupressure for nausea and vomiting involves pressure applied at specific pressure points associated with relieving nausea. Dibble, Chapman, Mack, and Shih (2000) reported on a study in which finger pressure on the P6 (Nei-Guan) pressure point located in the wrist reduced the daily experience of nausea in a small sample of patients. Elastic bands on the wrist also have been designed for this purpose. Transcutaneous electrical nerve stimulation (TENS) in the form of a wrist band reduced the severity of delayed nausea when used as an adjunct to a pharmacologic antiemetic protocol (Pearl, Fischer, McCauley, Valea, & Chalas, 1999). Additional research with larger sample sizes is needed to validate this intriguing mode of treatment.

In a study of self-care actions, one-fourth to one-half of the patients surveyed used dietary manipulation to control nausea and vomiting. Patients reported that the following actions were mildly effective: eating cold or room-temperature foods, avoiding cooking odors and foods with high fat content, eating smaller amounts more frequently, eating crackers, and sipping clear liquids (Foltz, Gaines, & Gullatte, 1996).

Mucositis

Chemotherapy often results in direct or indirect damage to the mucous membranes lining the mouth, pharynx, and esophagus. New cells produced in the basal cell layer of the mucosa move upward to become squamous cells near the surface. The squamous epithelium regenerates every 7–14 days. Chemotherapeutic agents interfere with the replication and division of all rapidly dividing cells, including basal cells of the oral mucosa. The resulting inflammation, mucosal atrophy, and ulceration are direct effects of chemotherapy. The term *mucositis* refers to an inflammatory and ulcerative response of mucous membranes. *Stomatitis* refers to this response in the mucous membranes of the mouth and oropharynx. Infection of the oral cavity is an indirect effect, resulting from bone marrow suppression and destruction of the protective barrier of the mucous membrane.

Certain drugs cause mucositis more frequently than others. The antimetabolites, including fluorouracil, methotrexate, and cytosine arabinoside (cytarabine, ARA-C, Cytosar-U®, Pharmacia & Upjohn, Peapack, NJ) are most notorious for this effect. The antitumor antibiotics and plant alkaloids also are frequent culprits. High or ablative doses of many other chemotherapeutic agents, such as those given in blood and marrow transplant settings, also cause severe mucositis. Patients receiving concurrent treatment with chemotherapy and radiation therapy to the head and neck are at extremely high risk for mucositis.

Patterns of mucositis vary with the chemotherapeutic agents and the individual. Mucositis may begin as early as 2 days following treatment or as late as

14 days. Most commonly, symptoms are seen 7–14 days and resolve 14–21 days following treatment. Pain may precede visible evidence of mucositis. White patches, which are areas of dead or dying cells, often are seen prior to ulceration. Salivary glands also often are affected, producing thick, ropy saliva and xerostomia (i.e., dry mouth).

Mucositis Prevention

Prevention begins with good oral hygiene and regular prophylactic dental care long before chemotherapy is begun. Assessment of the oral cavity prior to beginning chemotherapy should include the condition of the teeth and gums and oral hygiene habits. The National Oral Health Information Clearinghouse (NOHIC) recommends a dental evaluation prior to chemotherapy treatment. The dentist identifies and treats any existing infections, eliminates potential sites of infection, evaluates dentures for proper fit, and instructs patients on oral hygiene (NOHIC, 1999b).

During chemotherapy administration, cryotherapy has been used to reduce mucositis in patients receiving short infusions of drugs, such as fluorouracil or melphalan. The patient sucks on ice chips or ice pops from 5 minutes before to 30 minutes after chemotherapy infusion. The reduction in temperature protects the cells by decreasing drug exposure through vasoconstriction (Biron et al., 2000). Additional measures to prevent mucositis or decrease its severity are currently being studied. Administration of the cytoprotective agent amifostine (Ethyol®, Alza Pharmaceuticals, Palo Alto, CA) prior to radiation and chemotherapy has been shown to provide mucosal protection (Taylor, Briggs, Epner, & List, 1999; Trog, Fuller, & Wendt, 1999). Growth factors, including granulocyte-colony-stimulating factor (G-CSF) and granulocyte-macrophage-colony-stimulating factor (GM-CSF) and more specific epithelial growth factors (e.g., keratinocyte growth factor), also are being studied for mucositis prevention (Biron et al., 2000).

During treatment, the patient is advised to keep the mouth moist and clean. Drinking fluids, sucking ice chips or sugar-free hard candy, chewing sugarless gum, and swishing a saliva substitute are recommended to provide moisture. NOHIC (1999a) advises patients to keep the mouth clean by brushing teeth, gums, and tongue with a soft toothbrush and fluoride toothpaste after every meal and at bedtime. Daily flossing is recommended, avoiding any areas that bleed or are painful. A frequent rinse with a solution of ¼ teaspoon baking soda and ⅛ teaspoon salt followed with plain water also is recommended. Patient teaching and professional materials on preventive oral hygiene may be obtained through NOHIC on the Internet at www.aerie.com/nohicweb. Other experts advise differentiating between patients with prior good oral hygiene habits, who can safely continue good oral hygiene as described here, from those for whom previous poor oral hygiene increases the risk of bleeding and infection. In the latter group of patients, cautious cleaning with sponge-head swabs may be advisable (Biron et al., 2000).

Other methods that have been trialed as prophylaxis for mucositis include nutrition supplements, antibacterial mouth rinses, and the helium-neon laser.

Glutamine is an important fuel for mucosal cells of the gut, as well as other rapidly dividing cells. Researchers at the University of Minnesota have shown that low-dose oral glutamine supplementation reduced severity of mucositis in patients undergoing high-dose conventional chemotherapy and autologous HCT. Glutamine was administered as a $1\text{-}g/m^2$ suspension, which patients swished and swallowed four times a day (Anderson et al., 1998). Other studies, however, have not shown a benefit for glutamine (Coghlin-Dickson et al., 2000). The use of chlorhexidine mouth rinse, an agent with antimicrobial activity, as a preventive for chemotherapy-induced mucositis is controversial. Although early studies indicated some benefit in reduction of mucositis, a randomized clinical trial involving 222 patients treated in outpatient and office settings indicated no benefit over rinsing with water (Dodd et al., 1996). A low-energy helium-neon laser treatment has been used to delay onset and reduce severity of mucositis in patients being treated with HCT as well as with radiation therapy (Bensadoun et al., 1999; Biron et al., 2000).

Oral Assessment

Regular and thorough assessment of the oral cavity is an important aspect of care for all patients receiving cytotoxic therapy. Assessment includes evaluating the voice, swallowing ability, taste, and pain, as well as visible evidence of mucositis. The first step in assessment is to ask the patient about pain, taste, and swallowing and to assess the voice for hoarseness or difficulty forming words. The nurse should then inspect the oral cavity using a light, tongue blade, and gloved hand. Include the lips, tongue, teeth or dentures, gingiva, buccal cavity, oropharynx, and uvula in the inspection. Observe for moisture, color, cleanliness, bleeding, and tissue integrity in each of these areas. Note evidence of infection by viral or fungal organisms, including blisters, ulcers, or white coating. Scoring systems frequently are used to quantify the severity of mucositis but vary between facilities and research groups.

Interventions

Maintaining oral hygiene becomes even more important as breakdown of the oral mucosa occurs. Patients should continue to brush the teeth using a very soft toothbrush, which may be further softened by rinsing with warm water. Spongehead swabs may be used for patients with severe mucositis when brushing is painful or causes bleeding. Mouth rinses should be increased in frequency to at least every two hours during the day and every four hours at night. Commercial mouthwashes containing alcohol should be avoided. A number of agents have been used in practice for treatment of mucositis. Plain water, normal saline, or a mixture of salt and sodium bicarbonate in water are effective and will not cause harm. Hydrogen peroxide in a dilute solution has been used but may harm delicate healing tissue. Chlorhexidine is used in many centers but is controversial and also may damage healing tissue and increase resistant organisms. One commercially available mouthwash containing naturally occurring antibacterial salivary enzymes (Biotene®, Laclede Research Laboratories, Gardena, CA) has been recommended but has not been tested in a randomized trial.

Prophylactic antifungal agents include swish-and-swallow solutions, troches, and systemic medications. When local agents are used, the healthcare team must be alert to the possibility of esophageal fungal infection occurring without oral symptoms. Antiviral agents are recommended for patients with positive herpes titers who will receive regimens likely to cause neutropenia or mucositis.

Management of pain associated with mucositis varies depending on the extent of involvement. Local anesthetics (e.g., viscous lidocaine, 20% benzocaine) and products containing local anesthetics are effective when used for localized lesions. The patient must, however, use caution in self-medication, as anesthetic agents can dull the gag-and-cough reflex, resulting in aspiration. Substances that provide a protective coating also may be used on localized lesions. When mucositis is extensive or involves areas not accessible to local products, systemic pain management is required. Effective pain control is achieved with analgesics given on a scheduled, around-the-clock basis. Short-acting drugs are scheduled to reach peak effectiveness at meal times. When long-acting drugs are used, breakthrough medication is given prior to meals. For severe mucositis, IV patient-controlled analgesia (PCA) may be required.

Teach the patient to avoid foods that may further irritate the mucosa. Chips and other foods with sharp edges and highly spiced, hot, and very salty foods may be irritating. Some patients report that even cold foods and drinks containing caffeine increase pain. A diet of bland, soft foods is better tolerated. Patients with severe mucositis require nutritional supplements or hyperalimentation to maintain nutritional status.

Taste Changes

Taste changes are another frequently reported side effect of chemotherapy and can have a significant impact on nutritional status. A large, multisite study examined patients' perceptions of taste changes (Wickham et al., 1999). Sixty-eight percent of patients reported taste changes, including lack of taste, metallic taste, or difference in taste of specific foods. Two drugs most commonly associated with moderate to major taste changes and more distress from taste changes were doxorubicin and cisplatin. Wickham et al. also examined patient reports of self-care behaviors and professional suggestions for management of taste changes. The most helpful self-care behavior reported was increasing seasonings. Nurses most frequently recommended eating candy, chewing gum, eating cold foods, and increasing seasonings. Further research is needed to describe and validate effective interventions.

Fatigue

Fatigue, an overwhelming sensation of weariness or tiredness, is reported by more than 90% of people undergoing treatment for cancer (Gaston-Johansson, Fall-Dickson, Bakos, & Kennedy, 1999; Gregory et al., 1999). Fatigue affects the daily life of the individual–the ability to continue with work or home responsibilities, the ability to interact and maintain relationships within the family and community, and the ability to concentrate, learn, and pay attention. Yet, fatigue has been infrequently assessed, and research on fatigue in patients with cancer is just now entering an exciting phase of development which, in a few years, will yield an expansive knowledge base and proven nursing interventions.

Fatigue experienced by individuals with cancer is different from the tiredness experienced by healthy people following activity, exercise, or a long day at work. In the healthy individual, fatigue serves as a warning, an indication of the need to rest. Cancer-related fatigue may occur without excessive activity, may be constantly present, or may occur suddenly and be unrelieved by sleep or rest. Patients with cancer have described fatigue as tiredness, weakness, lack of energy, exhaustion, lethargy, depression, inability to concentrate, malaise, asthenia, boredom, sleepiness, lack of motivation, and decreased mental status (Winningham et al., 1994). Like pain, fatigue is a subjective phenomenon experienced by the patient and described in terms of the patient's experience.

Fatigue Risk Factors

A diagnosis of cancer alone places the individual at risk for cancer-related fatigue. Treating cancer with radiation therapy, chemotherapy, hormonal therapy, or biological response modifiers (BRMs) increases the risk of fatigue, with combination treatment compounding the effect. The presence of other side effects of disease or treatment, including anemia, nausea, pain, dehydration, or malnutrition, further increases the risk.

Etiology of Fatigue

Cancer-related fatigue is multidimensional—it is affected by and subsequently affects all areas of the individual's life. Physiologic mechanisms of fatigue are poorly understood. However, the balance between energy production and expenditure can affect fatigue. Energy is produced and consumed in the body at the cellular level. For energy to be produced, fuel and oxygen must be available and must be transported to the cells. The rates at which fuel and oxygen are utilized, as well as the rate at which energy is consumed, are controlled by factors affecting the metabolism. Increased demand for energy expenditure without increased production of energy produces a deficit.

Consider the availability of fuel for the production of energy. Many people undergoing cancer treatment experience nausea, vomiting, or anorexia. These symptoms affect the individual's ability to take in adequate nutrition. Mucositis, enteritis, intestinal obstruction, liver disease, and other factors may affect absorption of food. Inadequate nutrition and weight loss place the individual at high risk for fatigue. Deficits of specific vitamins, minerals, and other nutrients also may affect cellular function, increasing fatigue risk.

Oxygen also is necessary for cellular metabolism. Disease affecting the respiratory system, decreasing the availability of oxygen, increases fatigue risk. Hemoglobin in the red blood cells (RBCs) is necessary for oxygen transport. Low hemoglobin and hematocrit levels (i.e., anemia) often are caused by bone marrow suppression associated with chemotherapy. Patients with anemia commonly experience shortness of breath (SOB) and fatigue.

The transport of nutrition and oxygen also is affected by cardiovascular changes. Dehydration and hypotension impede the flow of oxygen and nutrition within the circulatory system, as does cardiovascular disease. In addition, deconditioning occurs when activity is decreased as a result of disease or treatment (Winningham et al., 1994). Deconditioning results in changes in the cardiovascular, respiratory, and musculoskeletal systems, all of which affect transport within the blood stream.

Changes in the rate at which energy is produced and consumed within the body result from a number of factors. Fever and infection increase heart rate and respirations, with subsequent increased oxygen demand. Cytokines produced following chemotherapy or radiation may affect metabolic rates. Treatment with BRMs may likewise cause fatigue through cytokine-induced metabolic changes. Deconditioning related to immobility slows the metabolism, decreasing the production of energy. Stress also contributes to the development of cancer-related fatigue, as do sleep disturbances.

Patterns of Fatigue in Patients Undergoing Chemotherapy

Patients receiving chemotherapy commonly experience a peak of fatigue within the first three to four days following treatment and sometimes report another increase coinciding with the nadir of the blood counts, followed by a decline in fatigue until the next treatment. In clinical experience, patients often report feeling their best the week before a scheduled treatment. Several recent studies have addressed patterns of fatigue. Patients with breast cancer receiving chemotherapy on 21- or 28-day cycles experienced a peak in fatigue 24–48 hours following chemotherapy (Berger, 1998). Fatigue was consistently low at mid-cycle and did not increase beyond the original peak with subsequent courses of treatment. Schwartz et al. (2000) likewise showed a peak in fatigue in the days following chemotherapy, with a gradual decline over time. Severity of fatigue peaked at similar levels after initial and subsequent chemotherapy courses in patients receiving four cycles of treatment (Morrow, Lindke, Hickok, & Moore, 1999). Patients receiving combination treatment, either radiation and chemotherapy or hormones and chemotherapy, experienced more fatigue than patients receiving any of these three treatments alone (Woo, Dibble, Piper, Keating, & Weiss, 1998).

Fatigue Assessment

Fatigue, like pain, is a subjective symptom assessed in terms of the individual's experience. Cultural influences also affect the individual's perception and description of fatigue. In the clinical setting, a verbal scale of 0–10, with 0 being no fatigue and 10 being the worst fatigue, or a 0–5 scale may be used to rate fatigue. It also is important to assess the person's definition and understanding of fatigue, patterns of fatigue, factors that make fatigue better and worse, and the extent to which fatigue is interfering with daily activities (Winningham et al., 1994). Assessment of potential contributing factors, including sleep patterns, nutritional status, hemoglobin/hematocrit, and fluid and electrolyte status, also is important. A fatigue diary is a useful tool. The patient lists levels of fatigue at different times, interventions, and what seemed to make fatigue better and worse. The nurse reviews the diary with the patient, using it as a starting point for interventions. Finally, fatigue and depression have been shown to correlate to one another, as well as to pain and a poor total health status (Gaston-Johansson et al., 1999). Patients with fatigue should be assessed to differentiate symptoms of depression. Patients who exhibit symptoms of clinical depression require referral for further assessment.

Interventions

Interventions for fatigue include correction of known causes, such as anemia, sepsis, or hypoxia, and teaching strategies for energy conservation and restoration. The anemia associated with cancer treatment is not generally caused by deficiencies in iron or vitamin B_{12} and does not respond to replacement of these substances. Transfusion of RBCs provides temporary relief. Erythropoietin is a RBC growth factor normally produced by the kidneys. In patients with cancer receiving chemotherapy, serum erythropoietin may be less than optimal for replacement of RBCs (Glaspy et al., 1997). Epoetin alfa (Procrit®, Ortho Biotech Inc., Raritan, NJ) is a form of erythropoietin currently available for subcutaneous (SC) administration. Epoetin alfa has been shown to increase hemoglobin, activity levels, and quality of life and to reduce transfusion requirements in patients with cancer who are anemic and receiving chemotherapy. The recommended dose of epoetin alfa is 150 units/kg, given subcutaneously three times a week (Rieger & Lynch, 1999). A single weekly dose of 40,000 units recently has been recommended (Gabrilove et al., 2001).

Self-care strategies that balance restorative activities with energy conservation are key in the management of fatigue. Energy conservation strategies are best taught using concrete, simple suggestions and including the patient in discussion. Suggestions include sitting to shower, prepare meals, wash dishes, or do other light chores; using assistive devices, such as a shower brush or long-handled shoe horn; organizing activities prior to beginning; and using simplified methods for accomplishing tasks (Clark, 1999). Prioritization and delegation are additional strategies that allow the individual to make the best use of available energy.

The normal response to fatigue in healthy individuals is to rest. Although the patient with cancer experiencing fatigue needs rest, rest must be balanced by activity. Too much time spent sleeping or in bed contributes to deconditioning and exacerbates fatigue. Exercise and activity may decrease fatigue. Schwartz (2000) described patterns of fatigue in women who did and did not exercise while receiving adjuvant chemotherapy. Women who exercised experienced fewer days of high fatigue levels than those who did not. In a previous study of patients who had exercised regularly prior to beginning cancer treatment, Schwartz (1998) showed that 76% used moderate exercise as an intervention to reduce fatigue. Exercise is a restorative strategy.

Sleep also is restorative, and the interaction among quality of sleep, exercise, and fatigue is complex. Berger and Farr (1999) studied the influence of daytime inactivity and nighttime restlessness on cancer-related fatigue, finding that patients with breast cancer who were more active during the day and restful at night reported lower levels of cancer-related fatigue. Patients who were awake more frequently during the night experienced fatigue, took naps, and decreased activity. The authors suggested that this sedentary lifestyle may have led to deconditioning and further fatigue. Management of symptoms, such as nausea or pain, that may awaken the patient during the night is a factor in prevention of cancer-related fatigue. Strategies to improve the quality of sleep also include omitting caffeine in the evening, limiting exercise within a few hours of bedtime, and establishing a regular routine and a peaceful environment for sleep (Clark, 1999).

Maintenance of adequate nutrition also is a restorative strategy. People experiencing fatigue may lack the energy to prepare meals or to eat large meals. Suggestions for assistance include having prepared foods available, preparing meals in advance, or asking friends and family for help with food preparation. Eating more frequent, smaller meals may be easier for the fatigued individual and benefits the digestion and utilization of foods.

Attention-restoring activities decrease mental fatigue. Activities that are fascinating to the individual and allow freedom from concerns can be attention-restoring (Winningham et al., 1994). Depending on the individual's interest, gardening, walking in a park, bird watching, painting, photography, or other activities may be attention-restoring.

Pain

Cancer-related pain originates from a number of sources. It is beyond the scope of this chapter to provide a full discussion of cancer-related pain; the reader may refer to several excellent texts for a complete description. The following discussion will be limited to pain as a side effect of cancer treatment with chemotherapy.

Chemotherapeutic agents do not normally cause pain with infusion. The nurse should interpret any reports of pain or discomfort during chemotherapy administration by peripheral or central venous access as a possible indication of extravasation. The infusion should be stopped immediately and measures taken to limit tissue damage (see Chapter 3).

Painful Peripheral Neuropathy

Peripheral neuropathy is a side effect of a number of chemotherapeutic agents, most commonly cisplatin, paclitaxel (Taxol®, Bristol-Myers Squibb Oncology/Immunology Division), and the vinca alkaloids, especially vincristine (Oncovin®, Eli Lilly and Company, Indianapolis, IN). Severity of neuropathy is commonly associated with the cumulative dose of the drug. Cisplatin, and less frequently carboplatin (Paraplatin®, Bristol-Myers Squibb Oncology/Immunology Division), affect the large sensory fibers, primarily causing changes in the sense of position and vibration, occurring weeks to months after treatment and requiring up to a year to resolve (Armstrong, Rust, & Kohtz, 1997).

Patients are at risk for injury because of falls, and pain occurs as the neuropathy resolves.

Vincristine, other vinca alkaloids, and paclitaxel affect small fibers, causing loss of pain and temperature sensation, occurring within hours or days after treatment (Armstrong et al., 1997). Although normal pain sensation may be decreased, damaged nerves, conversely, cause a pain syndrome. Patients report a burning or tingling pain, primarily in the hands and feet, which is worsened by normal stimuli (Goldstein, 1999). In extreme cases, patients are unable to tolerate walking or standing, which may be accompanied by weakness and loss of motor reflexes. Patients must be cautioned to use a thermometer to test water temperature before touching and to otherwise protect hands and feet from extreme temperatures.

Neuropathy of the cranial nerves also has been reported with vincristine, vinorelbine (Navelbine®, Glaxo Wellcome Inc.), and other vinca alkaloids. Cranial nerve neuropathy results in headache and pain in the jaw, pharynx, and parotid glands, as well as paresis, paralysis, or palsies of facial muscles.

Amifostine has been shown to have a protective effect in preventing cisplatin- and paclitaxel-induced neuropathy. Current studies are examining the potential of amifostine for the treatment of established neuropathy (Ndubisi, Guthrie, Benrubi, & Nuss, 1999). Other areas of study include nerve growth factor (DeSantis et al., 2000) and glutamate (Boyle, Wheeler, & Shenfield, 1999).

Pain related to neuropathies often is resistant to treatment with analgesics alone. The addition of adjuvants, such as antidepressants, anticonvulsants, clonidine, or benzodiazepines, may be helpful in treating neuropathic pain (Goldstein, 1999).

Myalgia and Arthralgia

Paclitaxel more commonly produces transient myalgia and arthralgia, beginning within two to three days of treatment and resolving within four to six days (Medical Economics Company, Inc., 2000). Myalgia also occurs occasionally with docetaxel, vincristine, vinorelbine, and other vinca alkaloids. Arthralgia and headaches have been reported with topotecan (Hycamtin®, SmithKline Beecham), and back pain and headache reported with irinotecan (Camptosar®, Pharmacia & Upjohn) (Medical Economics Company, Inc.). Patients experiencing myalgia and arthralgia complain of aching in legs and joints. Myalgia generally is amenable to treatment with acetaminophen or nonsteroidal anti-inflammatory agents or to mild opioid combinations.

Acral Erythema

Pain also may be caused by cutaneous toxicity of chemotherapeutic agents. Acral erythema, also called "hand-foot syndrome," is a painful syndrome involving the skin of the hands and feet. This syndrome is seen primarily in individuals receiving high-dose chemotherapy with cytarabine, methotrexate, hydroxyurea (Hydrea®, Bristol-Myers Squibb Oncology/Immunology Division), fluorouracil, or etoposide (VP-16, VePesid®, Bristol-Myers Squibb Oncology/Immunology Division) (Armstrong et al., 1997). Patients report burning, tingling, swelling, and erythema of the hands and feet within 24 hours to three weeks following chemotherapy (Armstrong et al., 1997). As the syndrome progresses, the hands become dark red, and bullae form. Eventually, desquamation of the palms and soles occurs. The hands and feet remain painful until desquamation and swelling resolve and healing occurs. Pain is increased with infusion of cyclosporine in patients undergoing HCT.

Treatment for acral erythema often includes pyridoxine or PCA with a basal rate. Nursing interventions include elevation of the extremities, cold compresses, cold-water soaks, and measures taken to prevent infection (Armstrong et al., 1997).

Bone Marrow Suppression

Cells of the hematopoietic system within the bone marrow are the most rapidly dividing normal cells in the body. Rapidly proliferating cells are most vulnerable to the effects of chemotherapy. Therefore, the bone marrow is suppressed by most chemotherapeutic agents, with alkylating agents and nitrosoureas having the greatest potential for myelosuppression (Camp-Sorrell, 1998). Other drugs likely to cause myelosuppression include docetaxel, paclitaxel, vinorelbine, gemcitabine, and carboplatin. Any drugs given in combination or in higher doses have the potential for myelosuppression. Autologous HCT utilizes marrow-ablative doses of chemotherapeutic agents while providing rescue for the bone marrow. Suppression of the bone marrow includes all cell lines of the hematopoietic system, causing neutropenia, thrombocytopenia, and anemia.

Neutropenia

Granulocytes have a short life span in the circulation and are rapidly replaced by the marrow. For this reason, neutropenia is the most common effect of marrow suppression. The point in time at which granulocytes are at the lowest level is called the nadir and, for most drugs, occurs at 7–14 days after chemotherapy administration. A low granulocyte count places the patient at high risk for infection. Most laboratories report granulocytes as a percentage of the total white count. The nurse must calculate the absolute granulocyte count (AGC) or absolute neutrophil count (ANC) based on the reported percentages. See Figure 7-2 for calculation of the ANC or AGC. For patients receiving repeating cycles of chemotherapy, blood counts must recover prior to giving the next cycle. Therefore, chemotherapy is held if the ANC is less than an established level (usually 1,500). An exception to this rule is the patient being treated for leukemia. Chemotherapy is not withheld because of a low neutrophil count in a patient with leukemia. The patient is considered neutropenic when the ANC is < 1,000 and profoundly neutropenic when the ANC is < 500.

Colony-stimulating factors (CSFs) are a group of naturally occurring glycoproteins that function to regulate the growth and proliferation of the hematopoietic cells. Specific CSFs act at points on specific cell lines to stimulate growth and maturation of that cell line. Two CSFs are known to stimulate the maturation and proliferation of granulocytes: G-CSF (filgrastim [Neupogen®, Amgen

---

Figure 7-2. Calculation of the Absolute Neutrophil Count or Absolute Granulocyte Count

---

Absolute neutrophil count (ANC)/absolute granulocyte count (AGC) = % neutrophils times number of white blood cells (WBCs).

WBC count: Most laboratories report in thousands, with the notation "K" or "th." Convert to an actual number; this is the total WBC count.

% neutrophils: Refer to the differential blood count. Add segmented neutrophils (segs or polys) and bands. (% segs + % bands) = % neutrophils (or granulocytes)

Multiply the % neutrophils by the total WBC count.

(Remember to take two decimal spaces for the %.)

The result is the total or ANC/AGC.

Inc., Thousand Oaks, CA]) and GM-CSF (sargramostim [Leukine®, Immunex Corporation, Seattle, WA]). These substances have been manufactured using genetic recombinant techniques and are given to decrease the time and impact of neutropenia. Neupogen is indicated for patients who are receiving a repeat course of chemotherapy after having experienced prolonged neutropenia in a previous course, for patients on a treatment where more than 40% of patients can be expected to develop neutropenia, for patients with clinically deteriorating febrile neutropenia, and for patients undergoing autologous HCT (Shaffer, 1997). The usual dose of Neupogen is 5 mg/kg/day, rounded to either 300 mg or 480 mg, given subcutaneously or intravenously. Neupogen administration begins no earlier than 24 hours after chemotherapy is completed. Patients receiving Neupogen often experience bone pain as the counts recover. For most patients, acetaminophen or a combination oxycodone/acetaminophen product effectively manages bone pain. Leukine stimulates growth and proliferation of a somewhat broader range of white cells. GM-CSF is used primarily in patients with leukemia and in transplant settings.

The risk of infection increases with the severity and duration of neutropenia. Patient education prior to chemotherapy includes simple preventive measures, such as frequent hand washing and avoiding crowds during periods of neutropenia. Many centers recommend that patients avoid gardening, caring for pets (especially changing bird cages or cat litter), having live flowers or plants in the house or hospital room, and eating salads and other raw fruits and vegetables. Patients often are advised to wear masks outside the home, although no data are available proving that masks actually decrease infections.

Care of the patient with neutropenia includes good hand washing by all members of the healthcare team. Because of the risk of infection, invasive procedures are avoided whenever possible. Rectal temperatures, enemas, suppositories, and intramuscular (IM) injections are contraindicated.

Neutropenic patients are not only at higher risk of infection but also at higher risk of fatal outcome. Without the protective function of granulocytes, infections progress rapidly. Septic shock can develop within hours. Early recognition of symptoms of infection is vital. Patient education includes monitoring temperatures at home and calling the healthcare provider at the first evidence of fever or other symptom of infection. In patients with neutropenia, a temperature of 100.5°F is significant.

Nursing assessment of the patient with neutropenia includes taking the patient's temperature and inspecting potential sites of infection. Inquire about symptoms, such as cough, sore throat, frequency of or burning with urination, diarrhea, anal or perineal discomfort, and any sore or tender areas. Inspect the skin, venous access sites, and sites of any invasive procedure for areas of redness or discomfort. Patients with neutropenia will not produce pus, which is comprised primarily of neutrophils. Inspect the lips and oral cavity for blisters, redness, ulcers, or white patches. Listen to lung sounds. The patient also should be assessed for symptoms of developing septic shock, including a rapid heart rate, mottled or splotchy skin color, changes in mental status, and widening pulse pressure. When the patient with neutropenia exhibits a fever or other symptoms of infection, cultures are obtained and antibiotics started immediately. Broad-spectrum antibiotics are started empirically. If necessary, antibiotics are changed when culture results are reported. Patients developing symptoms of septic shock must be monitored closely, antibiotics started promptly, and the blood pressure maintained with fluids and dopamine if necessary.

Thrombocytopenia

Suppression of megakaryocyte, and, subsequently, platelet production occurs in many patients receiving chemotherapy. Patients most at risk for thrombocytopenia are those being treated for hematologic malignancies and those receiving high-dose chemotherapy for HCT. Carboplatin, alkylating agents, and other myelosuppressive chemotherapeutic agents also may cause thrombocytopenia. Normal platelet counts range from $150,000–400,000/mm^3$. When the level is below 50,000, patients are at risk for bleeding with invasive procedures. A level of 20,000 places the patient at risk for bleeding with normal activity; a level $< 10,000$ poses a risk for spontaneous bleeding (Camp-Sorrell, 1998).

Patient education includes the potential for thrombocytopenia, and patients are encouraged to monitor for bleeding, bruising, and petechiae. Platelet counts are monitored on a regular basis for regimens expected to produce thrombocytopenia and at the first evidence of bleeding, bruising, or petechiae in patients receiving other chemotherapy.

Oprelvekin (IL 11, Neumega®, Genetics Institute, Cambridge, MA) is a growth factor that stimulates the proliferation and maturation of megakaryocytes (Rust, Wood, & Battiato, 1999). Oprelvekin is given to prevent development of thrombocytopenia in patients with a nonhematologic malignancy who are receiving a chemotherapeutic agent likely to cause thrombocytopenia. The drug is given subcutaneously at a recommended dose of 50 mcg/kg/day starting 6–24 hours after chemotherapy is completed. Doses are calculated using the patient's actual weight, require accurate measurement, and are not rounded off (Rust et al.). Side effects of oprelvekin are related to a shift in plasma volume and may include weight gain, atrial arrhythmias, and transient anemia. Some patients also experience visual problems or redness and dryness of the eyes. Patients with a history of atrial arrhythmias or who are at risk for congestive heart failure require careful consideration prior to use of oprelvekin and close monitoring if the drug is used. All patients receiving oprelvekin are monitored for weight, fluid status, SOB, dyspnea, fatigue, and eye irritation or discomfort.

In assessing the patient who is thrombocytopenic, the nurse must look for any evidence of bleeding. Bruising, conjunctival bleeding, petechiae, bleeding of gums, epistaxis, and prolonged bleeding from sites of procedures may indicate a falling platelet count. Stools, urine, and emesis should be assessed for blood. Headache; change in sensation, movement, or strength of extremities; or change in level of consciousness may signal intracranial bleeding. Abdominal pain and rigidity may indicate an abdominal bleed. Vital signs should be monitored.

Interventions for thrombocytopenia include administration of platelet transfusions. Administration of platelets for counts between 10,000–20,000 is controversial. However, platelet administration for counts < 10,000 is a nursing priority. When invasive procedures are scheduled, it is usual practice to infuse platelets to increase the count up to 50,000 or to infuse platelets during the procedure. If a patient experiences a fall or injury when platelet counts are < 50,000, immediate platelet transfusion may be indicated. Platelet products for infusion may include single-donor platelets, collected by apheresis; random-donor platelets, separated from six to eight whole blood donations; human lymphocyte antigen- (HLA-) matched platelets; and cross-matched platelets. Platelets may be leukocyte-depleted (WBCs removed) at the time of apheresis collection or by using a leukocyte removal filter at the time of administration. Alloimmunization, causing platelet counts to fail to increase in response to platelet transfusions, is reduced by giving leukocyte-depleted or HLA-matched platelets.

Nursing measures include bleeding precautions. Caution patient against activities that may lead to bruising or injury. Encourage patients to use a soft toothbrush and an electric razor and to exercise caution when handling sharp objects. Assist patients who may be unstable. Keep a light on at night to prevent falls. Avoid invasive procedures, including rectal temperatures, suppositories, enemas, bladder catheterization, IM injections, deep suctioning, and nasogastric tubes. When venipuncture or other invasive procedures are required, apply firm, direct pressure to the site for at least five minutes. When SC injection is required, use the smallest needle possible and apply ice immediately. Initiate a bowel program, including regular assessment, stool softeners, and laxatives as needed, to prevent constipation. Interventions to stop bleeding include ice packs, pressure, administration of platelets, and use of topical thrombin products.

Anemia

RBCs have a longer life in the circulation. Therefore, anemia often develops later than neutropenia or thrombocytopenia. Risk is greatest in patients receiving myelosuppressive drugs (i.e., those which produce neutropenia and thrombocy-topenia.) and in patients who have received multiple cycles of chemotherapy. Nephrotoxic drugs also increase risk for anemia because of decreased production of erythropoietin in the kidneys.

Anemia is one cause of cancer-related fatigue, as discussed previously. Patients are taught to report symptoms of anemia, including fatigue and SOB or palpitations on exertion. Nursing assessment includes levels of fatigue, skin color, heart rate, respiratory rate, and presence of SOB. Laboratory values should be assessed in patients at risk. Hemoglobin < 11 g/dl is rated Grade I anemia in NCI studies; < 8 g/dl is rated Grade III (Rieger & Lynch, 1999).

Treatment of anemia caused by myelosuppressive chemotherapy was previously limited to transfusion of RBCs. Although transfusion is helpful and necessary when hemoglobin levels are very low, there are associated risks. Concerns about disease transmission, suppression of immune competence, and development of autoimmune responses have decreased willingness to transfuse donor blood. The CSF erythropoietin, normally produced in the kidneys, stimulates proliferation and maturation of RBCs. Recombinant erythropoietin (Epogen®, Amgen Inc. and Procrit) is available and is indicated for anemic patients with nonmyeloid malignancies receiving chemotherapy. The usual dose is 150 units/kg given subcutaneously three times a week (Rieger & Lynch, 1999). Erythropoietin is continued until the hemoglobin is > 13 g/dl or until completion of chemotherapy and resolution of anemia (Rieger & Lynch).

Summary

The greatest challenge to the oncology nurse is not in the administration of chemotherapy but in the support of the patient who has received treatment. Assessment for side effects and sequelae is essential. As managed care and cost consciousness increasingly moves oncology care to the outpatient setting, teaching self-care strategies to manage side effects becomes more critical.

References

Anastasia, P.J. (2000). Effectiveness of oral 5-HT$_3$ receptor antagonists for emetogenic chemotherapy. *Oncology Nursing Forum, 27*, 483–493.

Anderson, P.M., Ramsay, N.K.C., Shu, X.O., Rydholm, N., Rogosheske, J., Nicklow, R., Weisdorf, D.J., & Skubitz, K.M. (1998). Effect of low-dose oral glutamine on painful stomatitis during bone marrow transplantation. *Bone Marrow Transplantation, 22*, 339–344.

Armstrong, T., Rust, D., & Kohtz, J.R. (1997). Neurologic, pulmonary, and cutaneous toxicities of high-dose chemotherapy. *Oncology Nursing Forum, 24*(Suppl. 1), 23–33.

Bensadoun, R.J., Franquin, J.C., Ciais, G., Darcourt, V., Shubert, M.M., Viot, M., Dejou, J., Tardieu, C., Benezery, K., Nguyen, T.D., Laudoyer, Y., Dassonville, O., Poissonnet, G., Vallicioni, J., Thyss, A., Hamdi, M., Chauvel, P., & Demard, F. (1999). Low-energy He/Ne laser in the prevention of radiation-induced mucositis.

A multicenter phase III randomized trial in patients with head and neck cancer. *Supportive Care in Cancer, 7*(4), 244–252.

Berendt, M.C. (1998). Alterations in nutrition. In J.K. Itano & K.N. Taoka (Eds.), *Core curriculum for oncology nursing* (3rd ed.) (pp. 223–258). Philadelphia: W.B. Saunders.

Berger, A. (1998). Patterns of fatigue and activity and rest during adjuvant breast cancer chemotherapy. *Oncology Nursing Forum, 25,* 51–62.

Berger, A., & Clark-Snow, R.A. (1997). Adverse effects of treatment: Nausea and vomiting. In V.T. DeVita, Jr., S. Hellman, & S.A. Rosenberg, (Eds.), *Cancer: Principles and practice of oncology* (5th ed.) (pp. 2705–2714). Philadelphia: Lippincott-Raven.

Berger, A., & Farr, L. (1999). The influence of daytime inactivity and nighttime restlessness on cancer-related fatigue. *Oncology Nursing Forum, 26,* 1663–1671.

Biron, P., Sebban, C., Gourmet, R., Chvetzoff, G., Philip, I., & Blay, J.Y. (2000). Research controversies in management of oral mucositis. *Supportive Care in Cancer, 8*(1), 68–71.

Boyle, F.M., Wheeler, H.R., & Shenfield, G.M. (1999). Amelioration of experimental cisplatin and paclitaxel neuropathy with glutamate. *Journal of Neuro-Oncology, 41*(2), 107–116.

Camp-Sorrell, D. (1997). Chemotherapy: Toxicity management. In S.L. Groenwald, M.H. Frogge, M. Goodman, & C.H. Yarbro (Eds.), *Cancer nursing: Principles and practice* (4th ed.) (pp. 385–425). Boston: Jones and Bartlett.

Camp-Sorrell, D. (1998). Myelosuppression. In J.K. Itano & K.N. Taoka (Eds.), *Core curriculum for oncology nursing* (3rd ed.) (pp. 207–219). Philadelphia: W.B. Saunders.

Clark, J. (1999). *Strength for living: Managing cancer-related fatigue* [Slide presentation kit]. Pittsburgh: Oncology Education Services, Inc.

Coghlin-Dickson, T.M., Wong, R.M., Offrin, R.S., Shizuru, J.A., Johnston, L.J., Hu, W.W., Blume, K.G., & Stockerl-Goldstein, K.E. (2000). Effect of oral glutamine supplementation during bone marrow transplantation. *Journal of Parenteral Enteral Nutrition, 24*(2), 61–66.

DeSantis, S., Pace, A., Bove, L., Cognetti, F., Properzi, F., Fiore, M., Triaca, V., Savarese, A., Simone, M., Jandolo, B., Manzione, L., & Aloe, L. (2000). Patients treated with antitumor drugs displaying neurological deficits are characterized by a low circulating level of nerve growth factor. *Clinical Cancer Research, 6*(1), 90–95.

Dibble, S., Chapman, J., Mack, K., & Shih, A. (2000). Acupressure for nausea: Results of a pilot study. *Oncology Nursing Forum, 27,* 41–47.

Dodd, M., Larson, P., Dinnle, S., Miaskowski, C., Greenspan, D., MacPhail, L., Hauck, W., Paul, S.M., Ignoffo, R., & Shiba, G. (1996). Randomized clinical trial of chlorhexidine versus placebo for prevention of oral mucositis in patients receiving chemotherapy. *Oncology Nursing Forum, 23,* 921–927.

Ezzone, S., Baker, C., Rosselet, R., & Terepka, E. (1998). Music as an adjunct to antiemetic therapy. *Oncology Nursing Forum, 25,* 1551–1556.

Fauser, A.A., Fellhauer, M., Hoffman, M., Link, H., Schlimok, G., & Gralla, R.J. (1999). Guidelines for anti-emetic therapy: Acute emesis. *European Journal of Cancer, 35,* 361–370.

Foltz, A.T., Gaines, G., & Gullatte, M. (1996). Recalled side effects and self-care actions of patients receiving inpatient chemotherapy. *Oncology Nursing Forum, 23,* 679–683.

Fox-Geiman, M., Fisher, S.G., Kiley, K., McLean, M., Fletcher-Gonzalez, D., Roczniak, L., Porter, N., Balhotra, D., Harrison, J., & Stiff, P. (1999). Double-blind randomized comparison of oral granisetron, oral ondansetron and IV ondansetron for regimen-related nausea and vomiting in patients undergoing stem cell transplants. *Proceedings of the Annual Meeting of the American Society of Clinical Oncologists, 18,* A2288.

Gabrilove, J.L., Cleeland, C.S., Livingston, R.B., Sarokhan, B., Winer, E., & Einhorn, L.N. (2001). Clinical evaluation of once-weekly dosing of epoetin alfa in chemotherapy patients: Improvements in hemoglobin and quality of life are similar to three-times weekly dosing. *Journal of Clinical Oncology, 19,* 2875–2882.

Gaston-Johansson, F., Fall-Dickson, J.M., Bakos, A.B., & Kennedy, M.J. (1999). Fatigue, pain, and depression in pre-autotransplant breast cancer patients. *Cancer Practice, 7*(5), 240–247.

Glaspy, J., Bukowski, R., Steinberg, D., Taylor, C., Tchekmedyian, S., & Vadhan, R.S. (1997). Impact of therapy with epoetin alfa on clinical outcomes in patients with nonmyeloid malignancies during cancer chemotherapy in community oncology practice. *Journal of Clinical Oncology, 15,* 1218 1234.

Glaxo Wellcome Inc. (1999). *Zofran, ondansetron HCl injection/tablets/oral solution* (Product literature, Publication #ZOD003RO). Philadelphia: Author.

Goldstein, M.L. (1999). Cancer-related pain. In M. MacCaffery & C. Pasero (Eds.), *Pain: Clinical manual* (2nd ed.) (pp. 537–539). St. Louis, MO: Mosby.

Gregory, C., Breitbart, W., Cella, D., Groopman, J., Horning, S., Itri, L., Johnson, D., Miaskowski, C., Portenoy, R., Scherr, S., & Vogelzang, N. (1999). Impact of cancer-related fatigue on the lives of patients. *Proceedings of the Annual Meeting of the American Society of Clinical Oncologists, 18,* A2214.

Hesketh, P.J., Roman, A., Hesketh, A.M., Perez, E.A., Edelman, M., & Gandara, D.R. (2000). Control of high-dose-cisplatin-induced emesis with an all-oral three-drug antiemetic regimen. *Supportive Care in Cancer, 8*(1), 46–48.

The Italian Group for Antiemetic Research. (2000). Dexamethasone alone or in combination with ondansetron for the prevention of delayed nausea and vomiting induced by chemotherapy. *New England Journal of Medicine, 342,* 1554–1559.

Medical Economics Company, Inc. (2000). *Physicians' desk reference* (54th ed.). Montvale, NJ: Author.

Miller, A., & Leslie, R. (1994). The area postrema and vomiting. *Frontiers in Neuroendocrinology, 15,* 301–320.

Morrow, G.R., Lindke, J.T., Hickok, J., & Moore, D.F.J. (1999). Longitudinal assessment of fatigue in consecutive chemotherapy patients: A URCC CCOP study. *Proceedings of the Annual Meeting of the American Society of Clinical Oncologists, 18,* A2293.

Nakamura, H., Taira, O., & Kodaira, S. (1999). A multicenter randomized parallel comparison of granisetron injection with ondansetron injection in the acute emesis induced by emetogenic chemotherapy. *Proceedings of the Annual Meeting of the American Society of Clinical Oncologists, 18,* A2324.

National Cancer Institute. (1999). Nausea and vomiting. *PDQ, supportive care, health professionals.* Bethesda, MD: Author. Retrieved March 16, 1999, from the World Wide Web: http://cancernet.nci.nih.gov

National Oral Health Information Clearinghouse. (1999a). *Chemotherapy and your mouth.* (Publication No. 99–4361). Baltimore: U.S. Department of Health and Human

Services, National Institutes of Health.

National Oral Health Information Clearinghouse. (1999b). *What the oncology team can do* (Publication No. 99–4360). Baltimore: U.S. Department of Health and Human Services, National Institutes of Health.

Ndubisi, B., Guthrie, T., Benrubi, G., & Nuss, R. (1999). A phase II open-label study to evaluate the use of amifostine (Ethyol®) in reversing chemotherapy-induced peripheral neuropathy in cancer patients–Preliminary findings. *Proceedings of the Annual Meeting of the Society of Clinical Oncologists, 18,* A2326.

Pearl, M.L., Fischer, M., McCauley, D.L., Valea, F.A., & Chalas, E. (1999). Transcutaneous electrical nerve stimulation as an adjunct for controlling chemotherapy-induced nausea and vomiting in gynecologic oncology patients. *Cancer Nursing, 22,* 307–311.

Rieger, P.T., & Lynch, M.P. (1999). *Anemia and the advanced practice nurse.* [Slide presentation kit]. Pittsburgh: Oncology Education Services, Inc.

Rust, D., Wood, L.S., & Battiato, L.A. (1999). Oprelvekin: An alternative treatment for thrombocytopenia. *Clinical Journal of Oncology Nursing, 3,* 57–62.

Schwartz, A. (1998). Patterns of exercise and fatigue in physically active cancer survivors. *Oncology Nursing Forum, 25,* 485–491.

Schwartz, A. (2000). Daily fatigue patterns and effect of exercise in women with breast cancer. *Cancer Practice, 8*(1), 16–24.

Schwartz, A., Nail, L., Chen, S., Meek, P., Barsevick, A.M., King, M.E., & Jones, L.S. (2000). Fatigue patterns observed in patients receiving chemotherapy and radiotherapy. *Cancer Investigations, 18*(1), 11–19.

Shaffer, S. (1997). Protective mechanisms. In S. Otto (Ed.), *Oncology nursing* (3rd ed.) (pp. 792–815). St. Louis, MO: Mosby.

Taylor, C., Briggs, A., Epner, E., & List, A. (1999). Amifostine cytoprotection in an outpatient high dose chemotherapy regimen for breast cancer. *Proceedings of the Annual Meeting of the American Society of Clinical Oncologists, 18,* A525.

Trog, D., Fuller, J., & Wendt, T. (1999). Clinical experience with the cytoprotective agent amifostine after 742 applications at different tumor entities during radiochemotherapy. *Proceedings of the Annual Meeting of the American Society of Clinical Oncologists, 18,* A2344.

Wickham, R.S., Rehwaldt, M., Kefer, C., Shott, S., Abbas, K., Glynn-Tucker, E., Potter, C., & Blendowski, C. (1999). Taste changes experienced by patients receiving chemotherapy. *Oncology Nursing Forum, 26,* 697–709.

Winningham, M.L., Nail, L.M., Barton Burke, M., Brophy, L., Cimprich, B., Jones, L.S., Pickard-Holley, S., Rhodes, V., St. Pierre, B., Beck, S., Glass, E.C., Mock, V.L., Mooney, K.H., & Piper, B. (1994). Fatigue and the cancer experience: The state of the knowledge. *Oncology Nursing Forum, 21,* 23–36.

Woo, B., Dibble, S.L., Piper, B.F., Keating, S.B., & Weiss, M.C. (1998). Differences in fatigue by treatment methods in women with breast cancer. *Oncology Nursing Forum, 25,* 915–920.

CHAPTER 8

Clinical Trials

Judith Ann Kostka, RN, MS, MBA
Mary Magee Gullatte, RN, MN, ANP, AOCN®, FAAMA

The importance of clinical trials in cancer care cannot be overstated. A clinical trial involves prospective clinical evaluation of a new intervention against disease in people (National Cancer Institute [NCI], 1999). Clinical trials have played an important role in decreasing cancer morbidity and mortality. Clinical studies promote the discovery of new methodologies for cancer prevention, detection, and treatment and improve the quality of life for cancer survivors. The benefits derived from cancer-related clinical trials include the discovery of new treatments, new indications for existing medications, alternative dosing parameters, and routes and schedules of administration. Many patients base their decision to undergo or continue cancer treatment on the anticipated severity of treatment side effects. Hence, numerous clinical trials are focused on supportive care. These trials may examine the role of growth factors in managing hematologic side effects of chemotherapy or more effective antiemetic and analgesic regimens. In practical terms, clinical trials have a broad-based applicability across the cancer-care continuum.

Clinical trials involving drugs or invasive procedures are categorized by phases (see Table 8-1). In the clinical arena, clinicians most often are involved in the first three trial phases. Phase I trials usually involve a limited number of subjects, whereas Phase III trials typically involve a large number of patients enrolled at various treatment sites throughout the country. The Phase III trials are generally randomized and double-blind and compare a new treatment to the standard of care. Phase III studies are typically targeted to a site-specific cancer previously established during Phase II studies.

Funding for clinical trials comes from a variety of sources. Common sponsors are pharmaceutical companies, NCI, and the American Cancer Society (ACS). Cancer trials are conducted by cooperative groups, cancer and academic medical centers, and private oncology practice groups. Trials conducted through

Table 8-1. Categories of Clinical Trials

Phase	Activities
I	Establish drug treatment, safety, feasibility, dosing, and administration
II	Evaluate treatment efficacy, safety, and benefit; focus is on a specific cancer type.
III	Compare new treatment effectiveness to current standard therapy.
IV	Postmarketing surveillance; new drug is already on the market and approved by the U.S. Food and Drug Administration.

cooperative groups collectively enter about 20,000 new patients on treatment trials each year. Since 1976, the Cooperative Group Outreach Program (CGOP) through NCI has enabled community physicians to provide their patients with access to cooperative group trials (Breslin, 2000).

Institutional Review Boards

Before launching a clinical trial, approval must be obtained from an institutional review board (IRB). The main functions of the IRB in clinical research are to (a) review the proposed research and determine whether the potential benefits outweigh the risks to the participants, (b) ensure that the rights of study subjects are protected, including both the fairness of the selection procedure and proper study management, and (c) ensure that appropriate steps are in place for the potential subject to be adequately "informed" during the consenting process (Barnett International, 1993). These review boards usually consist of physicians, researchers, clergy, attorneys, patient advocates, nurses, and other healthcare providers as appropriate. IRBs may be local, such as those established within hospitals, or central, including those that oversee studies conducted at multiple nationwide centers. NCI will be piloting the use of a central IRB for multicenter trials covering a broad geographical area.

Drug Development Process

The drug development process typically consists of preclinical drug design and discovery, in vitro testing for efficacy, animal pharmacokinetics and toxicology, and human clinical research and development. Clinical research is divided into Phase I, Phase II, Phase III, and Phase IV studies. The development of a medication can represent as much as a $400 million investment that can evolve over a 12-year interval.

Phase I Studies

Phase I trials are based on new treatments or interventions and test primarily for safety in humans. Phase I trials typically last for six to eight months and involve a small number of patients, usually in specialized centers. These studies are generated from promising preclinical data obtained from in vitro cytotoxicology profiles of tumor cell lines and animal models demonstrating safe administration of the compound with a reproducible anticancer effect (Leventhal & Graham, 1988). The study drug may be given as a single agent or administered in combination with other standard agents. To be eligible for Phase I trials, the patient must have a confirmed malignancy for which no effective standard treatment exists. Study subjects need not have a specific cancer to participate in a Phase I trial; however, if the drug used has decided activity against a particular cancer, then it will be confined to that cancer. Participants usually must meet medical criteria for inclusion in a study based on the patient's overall physical performance or overall body system function (i.e., cardiac, renal, pulmonary) and ability to tolerate expected drug toxicities.

The maximum tolerated dose of a drug also is defined in the Phase I studies. Various dose escalation schema are used, with rapid escalation at lower, more tolerable doses and higher doses at successively smaller increases. Phase I studies also may be designed to determine if there is benefit to be obtained by shortening or extending an infusion or dose cycle or by using an alternate route of administration.

Close clinical monitoring of study subjects is obtained in Phase I trials via serum testing and other objective measures that monitor the treatment's effects on body systems. Pharmacodynamic monitoring also occurs as part of this process. Measurements of a medicine's half-life, peak and trough levels, and associated side effects on body systems are integral to evaluating drug effectiveness and toxicity profiles.

Phase II Studies

Phase II studies address the efficacy and short-term safety of new antineoplastic agents, new combination therapies, or new modalities of therapy. This phase of drug testing can last up to four years, utilizing hundreds of patients. Based on dosage and administration specifications obtained during Phase I, this new treatment is administered to the "healthiest of the sick" subjects with the indicated cancer. In most cases, treatment efficacy has been determined in preclinical animal models. These protocols are designed to evaluate efficacy in limited populations of patients and establish minimum/maximum effective dose ranges (Friedman, 1995). In Phase II studies, a medication is used the first time to prevent, diagnose, or treat the disease or condition for which it is intended. While evaluating efficacy, the clinical researcher observes any new or existing toxicities of the treatment. To be eligible for a Phase II study, a subject must have quantifiable disease and satisfactory performance status and be free of significant concomitant disease.

To evaluate the response of subjects to treatment, there must be a reliable measure of the disease. Disease may be objectified indirectly, as in the visualization of nodules and/or masses on a chest radiograph or MRI examinations, or by the direct measurement of a subcutaneous lymph node or mass. Tumor response is referred to as complete, partial, or stable. A complete response indicates the disappearance of all known sites of disease without the observance of any new disease for at least one month. A partial response is at least a 50% decrease in the sum total of the measurable disease and no evidence of new disease for at least one month. Stable response means no change (increase or decrease) in the measurable disease for at least one month (Grossman & Burch, 1988). Outcomes in a Phase II study are measured by the disease response to treatment (i.e., recurrence of disease, disease progression, patient survival). Patients may continue to receive the new agent as long as the tumor responds or remains stable.

As in Phase I trials, patients in Phase II studies also must be clinically monitored (though not continuously) by serial laboratory and radiographic evaluations to detect organ damage. Phase II agents that demonstrate a partial response may be considered for further testing or may be combined with other agents of proven efficacy (Grossman & Burch, 1988). New agents are discarded if serious toxicity is noted in Phase II studies. However, if the new agent is favorably reviewed, it advances to Phase III trial testing, where it is compared to the current treatment standard.

Phase III Studies

Phase III studies are designed to compare and contrast the new treatment to one or more therapies of proven efficacy. These protocols enroll the "sickest of the sick" and test the new therapy in clinical situations resembling those of fully approved medications. The outcome of the Phase III study will yield a new drug or drug combination, which is judged inferior, equivalent, or superior to the current standard. As in all trial phases, there must be clinically quantifiable disease, good performance status, and acceptable organ function for a patient to qualify for enrollment (Gullatte & Otto, 2001).

Patients are randomly selected to receive the new and the established treatment options to ensure an unbiased comparison of the new agent. A large sample of patients adds statistical power. Study patients should number 100–1,000 or more, with accrual often taking more than five years (Freireich, 1979; Moon, 1979). The dosages, schedules, and routes of administration of the agent are based on the results of the Phase II trials. Patient population criteria for Phase III trials are broader than earlier phases in that they include patients receiving concomitant therapies and having unrelated diseases. End points of all Phase III clinical trials include measures of disease-free survival, a toxicity profile, cancer response rates, patterns of recurrence, and the quality of life for the patient. New drug applications are submitted to the U.S. Food and Drug Administration (FDA) if effectiveness and safety is demonstrated during Phase III testing. New drug approvals take an average of three years.

Occasionally, a clinical trial may be discontinued. Reasons for stopping a study include (a) discovery of a dangerous adverse effect, (b) determination that a medication lacks significant beneficial effect or is less advantageous than an existing therapy, (c) determination that a drug has a significant effect that is not enough to warrant the risk associated with its use, or (d) clear evidence that the drug is safe and effective, warranting an expeditious review and approval by the FDA.

Phase IV Studies

Phase IV trials provide continued study of a drug's safety and efficacy following FDA approval. Along with postmarketing surveillance, Phase IV studies provide more data on drug-related adverse events and information that may point to a competitive advantage of the product. These trials often last from several months to several years and involve 2,000–2,500 patients. Phase IV trials are typically of a larger scale than are premarketing studies, involve different patient populations, and collect data on pharmacoeconomic and treatment algorithms. Comparison with other medicines can occur during this phase of development, as can evaluations of different formulations, dosages, durations of treatment, and drug interactions.

Informed Consent

Any patient entering a research study or clinical trial must be counseled in detail about his or her rights as a study participant. "Informed consent is the freely given agreement on the part of a competent person in full possession of all available pertinent information to participate as a subject in a research experiment" (Barnett International, 1993, p. 21). Prior to consenting to participate in a clinical trial, patients must be informed of their prognosis and the availability of other investigational or standard therapies, potential risks associated with participation in a clinical trial, and the obligations of the sponsor and researcher in the event of injury that occurs as a direct result of participation (NCI, 1999). The investigator or designee reviews with the patient the purpose of the research, any known side effects of the new agent, confidentiality of records, and who to contact with questions or in the event of injury. Patients should be realistically advised about the potential benefit and risk associated with the new agent. Furthermore, patients should be informed about compensation and the limits of financial support for supportive care and diagnostic tests that will be supplied by the sponsor. Patients also must be told about required diagnostic monitoring during the study.

Patients must know their rights, including their right to refuse to participate in the trial or to withdraw if they choose without compromising their care. Sufficient time must be provided for patients to consider participation, the consent document must be in lay language, and the patient must be given a copy of the consent form. Mentally competent adults must sign for themselves. To maintain the ethical integrity of any research investigation using human subjects, administering and obtaining informed consent must be the foundation of clinical research.

Patients must not be coerced to participate in a study. Full disclosure and ethical research principles apply in all phases of clinical investigation. The race to develop new breakthrough treatments raises concerns about whether current policies provide adequate protection of human subjects in particularly vulnerable populations. Another hot issue is researchers' financial arrangements that may influence their enrollment decisions. Increased scrutiny of research methods and policies can be expected as the IRBs and FDA wrestle with these mounting challenges (Wechsler, 2000).

Educational Resources

Many advocacy groups provide a strong voice supporting research and have established important resources for consumers. Consumers are credited with achieving increased budgets for research and for influencing policy at local and national levels. However, in the wake of healthcare restructuring, many health plans and insurance policies specifically exclude access to "investigational" therapy. The focus has been on reducing cost rather than on enhancing treatment quality using cutting-edge, well-designed clinical trials. This shifting priority will threaten progress in treating life-threatening diseases like cancer.

Healthcare professionals and consumers have several sources available to them for cancer-related research information. These include the following.

- http://cancertrials.nci.nih.gov/
  NCI's comprehensive clinical trials information center for patients, health professionals, and the public. Includes information on understanding clinical trials, deciding whether to participate in trials, finding specific trials, research news, and other resources.
- http://cancernet.nci.nih.gov/pdq.htm
  Comprehensive, informative, user-friendly clinical trials information system.
- http://ctep.info.nih.gov/coopgroup/ctep_accomplishments_main.htm
  Lists major achievements of NCI's Clinical Trials Cooperative Groups over the past 10 years.
- http://ctep.info.nih.gov
  Provides reports from the Cancer Clinical Trial Review Group and the Clinical Trials Implementation Group on NCI's reassessment and action plan. CTEP coordinates all aspects of clinical trials relative to cancer treatment agents.

Summary

Future advances in cancer care will arise from clinical trials conducted today. Nurses are uniquely positioned to advise and support patients as they consider enrollment in research studies. Through public education, nurses have the opportunity to have a positive impact on public perception of cancer research. Nurses also are directly involved in the conduct of clinical trials as clinical research coordinators and are promoting clinical research in a variety of settings and roles.

References

Barnett International. (1993). *Barnett International self-instructional study site curriculum #3: IRBs and informed consent.* Berlin, Germany: Barnett International Clinical Training Group, Parexel International Corp.

Breslin, S. (2000). History and background. In A.D. Klimaszewski, J.L. Aikin, M.A. Bacon, S.A. DiStasio, H.E. Ehrenberger, & B.A. Ford (Eds.), *Manual for clinical trials nursing* (pp. 3–5). Pittsburgh: Oncology Nursing Press, Inc.

Freireich, E.J. (1979). Methods of design and evaluation of adjuvant trials. In S.E. Jones & S.E. Salmon (Eds.), *Adjuvant therapy of cancer II* (pp. 97–105). New York: Grune and Stratton.

Friedman, M.A. (1995). Clinical trials. In G.P. Murphy, W. Lawrence, & R.E. Lenhard (Eds.), *American Cancer Society textbook of clinical oncology* (2nd ed.) (pp. 194–197). Atlanta: American Cancer Society.

Grossman, S.A., & Burch, P.A. (1988). Quantitation of tumor response to anti-neoplastic therapy. *Seminars in Oncology, 15,* 441–454.

Gullatte, M.M., & Otto, S. (2001). Cancer clinical trials. In S. Otto (Ed.), *Oncology Nursing* (4th ed.) (pp. 760–784).

Leventhal, B.G., & Graham, M.L. (1988). Clinical trials in pediatric oncology. *Seminars in Oncology, 15,* 482–487.

Moon, T.E. (1979). Statistical design of adjuvant trials. In S.E. Jones & S.E. Salmon (Eds.), *Adjuvant therapy of cancer II* (pp. 87–96). New York: Grune and Stratton.

National Cancer Institute. (1999). *Clinical trials.* Bethesda, MD: National Institutes of Health.

Wechsler, J. (2000). Clinical trials face scrutiny in new year. *Applied Clinical Trials, 9,* 20–23.

CHAPTER **9**

Psychosocial Support of the Patient Receiving Chemotherapy

Barbara Johnson Farmer, MSN, MSA, RN, FNP

Social Support Theory

Pasacreta and Pickett (1998) asserted that psychosocial responses to cancer and its subsequent treatment vary widely and are influenced by many factors. They also reported that social support is one of the most important factors that influences psychosocial responses, and Holland (1989) concurred. Social support also has been associated with health behaviors, and interest in the concept of social support has dramatically increased since the 1970s because it is believed to affect health and well-being (Caplan, 1974). Theorists began using the concept of social support to explain the phenomenon of cancer, stress, and coping. These theorists also used social support to make recommendations on the types of support (e.g., emotional, instrumental, appraisal, informational) that influence outcomes (Beder, 1995; Bloom, Ross, & Burnell, 1978).

Social support is a multidimensional and diverse concept. This phenomenon has been researched in a variety of disciplines, including anthropology, architecture, environmental design, epidemiology, gerontology, psychology, health education and planning, social work, medicine, and sociology (Bruhn & Phillips, 1984; Cohen & Syme, 1985). Social support could be expressed as an embrace, information, communication, or tangible and intangible resources. To define social support, dissection of the term is helpful. The *American Heritage Dictionary* (1982) defined social as living together in communities or groups; concerning humans and their living together and dealing with one another. Support means an act or process that promotes assistance; helps, comforts, or carries the weight of; holds up something else; or gives courage or faith.

Kahn (1979) defined social support as "interpersonal transactions that include one or more of the following: the expression of positive affects of one person toward another; the affirmation or endorsement of another person's behaviors, perceptions, or expressed views; and the giving of symbolic or material aid to another. The key elements in supportive transactions are affect, affirmation, and aid" (p. 85). In explaining these concepts, Kahn used the metaphoric term "convoy" to infer that each person can be thought of as moving through life surrounded by a set of significant other people. The individual is related to a set of significant others and gives or receives social support. The individual's convoy, at any point in time, consists of people on whom he or she relies for support and, in turn, who rely on him or her for support. These subsets may overlap and may be symmetrical; one may both give and receive support.

Affective transactions are seen as expressions of liking, admiration, respect, or love (e.g., the support group facilitator respects the support group members and the support group members respect the facilitator). Transactions of affirmation are expressions of agreement with and acknowledgment of the appropriateness or rightness of some act or statement of another person. Affirmation occurs, for example, when two individuals leave a group meeting together and one asks the other for confirmation of his or her perceptions and interpretations of what really happened or was said at the meeting. Finally, aid transactions are transactions of direct aid or rendering assistance (e.g., giving of material aid, such as money, to another individual).

Norbeck, Lindsey, and Carrieri (1981) endorsed Kahn's conceptual definition in the development of the Norbeck Social Support Questionnaire. Norbeck (1988) defined social support in terms of "interpersonal transactions" yet said, "professionals provide surrogate support that is designed to replace the support that is inadequate or unavailable from a patient's support network" (p. 102). She reported that "this support may be temporary, as during a crisis, or it might be provided on an ongoing basis for socially marginal individuals" (p. 102).

Cohen and Syme (1985) reported several reasons for the increasing interest in social support, including health, well-being, and several other factors, such as (a) its possible role in the etiology of disease and illness, (b) the role social support may play in treatment and rehabilitation programs instituted following illness, and (c) its potential for aiding in the conceptual integration of the diverse literature on psychosocial factors and disease. Kaplan, Cassel, and Gore (1977) identified two types of psychosocial processes of importance in disease. The first type of psychosocial process is deleterious and termed "stressor" factors. The stressor factors enhance disease susceptibility. The second type of psychosocial process is termed "protective" factors, which buffer or cushion the organism from the effects of noxious stimuli (including psychosocial stressor factors). These protective factors are a function of or depend on the nature, strength, and availability of social supports. The joint effects of these two processes determine, to a considerable extent, the susceptibility of the organism to physicochemical disease agents, including nutritional deficiencies, microorganisms, toxins, and chemicals (Kaplan et al.).

The culmination of work done early in the 1970s by epidemiologist John Cassel and social psychiatrist Gerald Caplan contributed to the nature and public health implications of social support. Cassel's classical work of synthesizing two bodies of knowledge culminated into a proposition stating that the immediate environment is capable of altering a person's resistance to disease via the metabolic effects they trigger. He proposed the relationship between psychosocial processes and stress and believed that certain forms of social disorganization, changes in these patterns, and biologic changes could affect the individual's vulnerability to disease (Caplan, 1974).

Caplan continued to develop the work of Cassel, notably, the evidence suggesting that the harmful effects of social disorganization stems from confusing or absent feedback from the social environment. He contributed his work, called "support systems," and set himself to the task of untangling the nature of social support. According to Caplan (1976), social support is composed of objective and subjective support. Objective support is defined by observable indicators of support that can be gathered from others. Subjective support, on the other hand, is support seen from the individual's perspective and evaluation.

Social support most often has been studied from a psychological perspective after Cobb (1976) found it to act as a buffer for stress. Cobb defined social support as information leading the subject to believe that he is cared for and loved, esteemed, and a member of a network of mutual obligations. According to Cobb, social support is conceived to be information belonging to one or more of these classes. The first class, information that one is cared for and loved (i.e., emotional support), is conveyed in intimate situations involving mutual trust. The second class, information that one is valued and esteemed (i.e., esteem support), is most effectively proclaimed in public. It leads the individual to esteem himself and reaffirms his or her sense of personal worth. The final class is information that one belongs to a network of mutual obligations that must be common and shared (i.e., social networks). Information must be common in the sense that each member is aware that everyone in the network has and shares the information.

Cobb (1976) purported that adequate social support can protect individuals in crisis from a wide variety of pathological states, including during such life events as birth, death, depression, and alcoholism. He also believed that social support has beneficial effects on the bereaved following a death. Social support is an important concept in helping individuals to cope during stressful events in their lives. Receiving a cancer diagnosis and undergoing treatment with chemotherapy are viewed as stressful life events.

Support of Patient and Caregivers

Cancer as a disease does not discriminate. It affects people of all races, genders, socioeconomic status, and ages. The American Cancer Society (ACS) (2001) reported that, in the United States, an estimated one out of three women and one out of two men will develop cancer during their lifetime. An estimated 1,268,000 new cancer cases are expected to be diagnosed in the United States in 2001 (Greenlee, Hill-Harmon, Murray, & Thun, 2001). The National Cancer Institute (NCI) (1999) reported that about 8.4 million people are living with cancer in the

United States. Some of these individuals are considered cured, whereas others still have evidence of cancer and are undergoing treatment. This number reflects an increase of 200,000 cancer survivors from 1999. This increase in cancer survival is a result of early diagnosis and improved treatment. Because people are living longer, cancer has become a chronic condition.

Psychosocial issues continue to be a major factor for cancer survivors. A diagnosis of cancer is life-threatening and life-altering. The diagnosis often precipitates a major life crisis (Youssef, 1984). The individual and family are faced with mortality issues, and many individuals are not prepared for this reality. With a cancer diagnosis, the individual experiences such emotions as shock, anger, fear, hopelessness, helplessness, frustration, withdrawal, depression, denial, excessive dependency, guilt, increased anxiety, lowered self-esteem, loneliness, and uncertainty, as well as abandonment of prior life and relationships (Beder, 1995; Bloom, 1982; DeCosse & Cennerazzo, 1997; Pelusi, 1997). The diagnosis of cancer evokes images of pain, fear, and death; even if the surgical procedure is considered curative, uncertainty exists because of the fear of metastasis (Bloom).

Individuals who receive a cancer diagnosis are faced with major changes in their lives that affect both their well-being and their relationships with others (Bloom, 1982). Many treatments for the disease seriously challenge the individual's self-image and sexuality (Oktay, 1998; Youssef, 1984). The loss of a body part may affect a woman's femininity, a man's masculinity, or an individual's physical attractiveness and the way he or she views himself or herself (Bloom). The impact of cancer on the individual is multifaceted. After certain cancer surgeries, individuals are forced to change their self-image and to incorporate new information into their evaluation of themselves as a whole person. The adjustment process is dynamic and continues as new information is gained.

Family members also must learn to adjust to this life-altering diagnosis, living with the fear of their loved one dying, role changes, and uncertainty about disease recurrence. A cancer diagnosis and its treatment are major life challenges and affect both those with the diagnosis and those who care about them. Most patients with cancer and their families experience the full impact of their diagnosis and the disruptions cancer brings to their lives in both their homes and communities (Howell & Jackson, 1998). Family issues are equally important because of this impact on the family unit, including relationships with children and spouses or partners (Oktay, 1998). The development of a measure of social support for cancer survivors for use in guiding health care and assessing the effects of social support on the patient's health status is needed—specifically, with a view of providing a clinical measure of social support (Bottomley & Jones, 1997).

Northouse, Dorris, and Charron-Moore (1995) reported that a diagnosis of cancer creates emotional distress for patients as well as family members. Families must learn to balance the need of all members and adjust family roles to ensure stability. The nurse can support this balance by determining the patient's system of perceived social support.

The concept of "perceived social support" allows the nurse to assess patients' evaluation of the supportive quality of their relationships. The nurse is able to describe social networks in terms of their composition and structure (i.e., the number of people involved and the number of people who know each other). By being informed, the nurse can be aware that benefits are directly proportional to the size and range of the network and that having a relationship is equivalent to getting support. However, there is always an exception to the rule, and through trust, listening, and communication, the nurse can ascertain patient and family needs.

Berkman (1995) reported that "individuals do not live in a vacuum; rather they are enmeshed in a social environment and in a series of relationships" (p. 245). She further noted that these relationships are strong and supportive. Individuals are integrated into their communities, and these relationships are related to the health of the individual. Because individuals do not live in a vacuum, they want emotional and informational support during a cancer diagnosis and treatment (Howell & Jackson, 1998). Individuals need informational support to make informed decisions about their cancer care and emotional support to help them to get through it.

Perceived social support involves an evaluation or appraisal of whether and to what extent an interaction, a pattern of interactions, or relationships are helpful. The nurse might assess three types or functions of social support–emotional, tangible, and informational support–as they relate to the patient who will receive chemotherapy.

Emotional support includes intimacy and attachment, reassurance, and being able to confide in and rely on another. In the case of a cancer survivor receiving chemotherapeutic treatment, the nurse must provide education as well as genuine comments and care. The nurse must be supportive and offer anticipatory guidance to make the chemotherapy experience bearable. By informing the family and significant others about chemotherapy and its effects, the nurse can encourage them to be proactive in their ability to support their loved one before, during, and after treatment. Nurses have a responsibility for promoting a positive attitude and educating patients and families throughout the cancer trajectory. Caplan's (1974) conceptual model, that of social systems, focuses on continuing social aggregates that provide individuals with opportunities to learn about themselves and gain validation of their expectations about others. He believed that this validation and feedback offset deficiencies within the community context.

As Caplan (1974) noted, most people develop and maintain a sense of well-being by involving themselves in a range of relationships. These include relationships with coworkers; members of religious organizations; members of social, cultural, political, and recreational associations; neighbors; and providers of service, as well as intermittent relationships with doctors, teachers, nurses, members of the clergy, and community leaders. He proposed that social aggregates offer guidance and, thus, act as a buffer against disease.

Caplan (1974) reported three major contributions to people's well-being: that significant others help the individual to mobilize psychological resources and master emotional burdens, or emotional mastery; they share the task; and they provide extra supplies of money, tools, skills, materials, and cognitive guidance to improve handling of situations.

Tangible support involves direct aid or services and can include loans, gifts of money or goods, and provision of services (e.g., taking care of someone, doing a chore). The nurse, acting as an advocate and case manager, must first communicate with the patient to form a relationship of mutual trust if the patient is going to share his or her cancer experience. If the patient feels that the nurse is allowing him or her to be himself or herself, the patient will potentially relax and continue with open interactions. Nurses must recognize, encourage, and establish environments in which personal aspects of the relationship can develop (Bushkin, 1995). In an open system, the patient and nurse should have mutual interactions, each taking from and giving to the other.

Informational support includes giving information and advice that could help a person to solve a problem and providing feedback about how he or she is doing. Both the individual and family will need informational support. By being aware of chemotherapy's effects, the individual and family will be better able to cope. Awareness gives the family anticipatory guidance; therefore, they can develop strategies to help them through the cancer diagnosis and chemotherapy treatment. When the nurse is knowledgeable about potential survivor outcomes, the direction for oncology practice and research can be defined.

Nurses must be aware that social support is a facet of everyday life; although the need for it may be more acute in times of stress, the need never disappears.

Social support is a factor that affects cancer survivors and their families throughout their lifetimes. Nurses must develop a clear perspective on social support to guide patients through the experience of a cancer diagnosis or chemotherapy administration and the many debilitating changes that can result.

Through qualitative and quantitative analyses, dimensions of nursing phenomena (in this case, psychosocial variables of chemotherapy and social support) can be sharpened, subconcepts can be validated, and basic propositions can be tested, all adding to the substantive knowledge. Triangulation methods of research yield data that reveal an understanding of cancer survivors.

Systems Theory for Support Group Development

Fobair (1997) reported that "a key concept in the theory of social group work is the 'open systems' model based on an ecological perspective that stresses reciprocal nature of relationships among individuals and systems. The group is viewed as a system that has a defined boundary and interrelated parts, and the support group is viewed as helping participants adapt to external conditions and to characteristics of individual participants to confront the group system" (p. 67). Fobair stated that interactions between the group leader and group members are reciprocal in that they affect each other and resonate throughout the system.

The systems theory postulates that a system is an arrangement of components that are interrelated to form a whole. Bonds or relationships tie the system together, making it a functional unit. Surrounding every system is an environment that is open or closed to influences or stimuli. A cancer support group is an open system that allows individuals with common experiences to share their knowledge, support, and experiences along the cancer trajectory.

Support Groups

For many, coming to terms with the prospect of facing life alone can be bleak and unsettling. There are times when one may benefit from solitude, enhance spirituality, and make choices without considering another individual's opinion. However, when illness strikes (e.g., a cancer diagnosis), some are unable or unwilling to choose to be alone (Klein, 1999). Cancer support groups (SGs) are built on the premise that individuals with cancer can benefit by interacting with other patients with cancer (Klemm, 1998). Formal cancer SGs are thought to assist individuals with adapting to the physiological and psychosocial sequelae of cancer (Samarel et al., 1998).

Survival rates for cancer have improved with advances in medical care, and more interventions are available to assist patients with cancer in dealing with diagnosis and treatments. The goals of these interventions are to develop SGs to decrease feelings of alienation by allowing patients to talk with others in a similar situation; to lessen patients' feelings of isolation, hopelessness, helplessness, and being neglected by others; and to assist in clarifying patients' perceptions and information (Fawzy, Fawzy, Arndt, & Pasnau, 1995).

Cancer causes significant emotional distress for a considerable majority of patients, who typically receive little formal psychological intervention. SGs are necessary to help patients to manage the overwhelming emotions they experience when diagnosed with and treated for cancer. These groups provide a forum in which patients can attempt to gain help with overcoming the psychological trauma that accompanies diagnosis, subsequent treatment, and relapse. Social support can be acquired in a support group setting. As medical treatments extend the life expectancy of individuals with cancer, the issue of appropriate, professionally led psychosocial interventions becomes more urgent (George, 1998).

Individuals diagnosed with cancer are frequently prescribed chemotherapy or radiation therapy. Although anxiety and worry exist with the various treatment modalities, family and friends are the principal source of all types of support.

Hinds and Moyer (1997) conducted a qualitative study to determine patients' experiences of support while receiving radiotherapy. Data obtained from 12 patients were analyzed using the procedures and techniques of grounded theory. A substantive theory of support emerged, which showed that support is an interpersonal process embedded in an array of social exchanges that involve encountering support, recognizing support, and feeling supported. The researchers uncovered three main types of support: being there, giving help, and giving information. Social support is a multifaceted concept, and all types of support are seen as important. Actions are interpreted within the norms and expectations of a relationship and are labeled as supportive by the recipient (Hinds & Moyer).

According to Ott (1997a), "when one member of a family has cancer, the entire family experiences turmoil from the day of diagnosis throughout recovery or death" (p. 27). Many areas of one's life can be affected by the diagnosis, including family, career, and social situations. Feelings of anxiety, fear, and a sense of loss of control often accompany this experience. Studies have shown that social support can mitigate caregiver stress and enhance coping (Vrabec, 1997).

Many individuals have found discussing their concerns with others who have or are currently going through similar experiences to be extremely helpful. SGs should be available to both the patient and the family unit. Knowledge about cancer illness and treatment assists family members in developing coping strategies (Van Hammond & Deans, 1995). SGs fall into two broad categories: psychoeducational and self-help or mutual SGs.

Psychoeducational SGs (PSGs) lean toward Caplan's (1976) idea of a group providing social support. In the PSG, health professionals provide psychoeducation to participants. PSGs provide knowledge about illness and treatment and create a collaborative environment between members and professionals in which they can develop coping strategies. PSGs encourage practical problem solving and create a structured home environment in which stress is reduced. They allow family members to participate fully in programming that emphasizes the development of a partner relationship and movement toward survivor and family involvement (Van Hammond & Deans, 1995).

PSGs tend to be more structured and to focus on cognitive and behavioral techniques. The overall goal of a PSG for cancer survivors is to reduce the sense of helplessness and inadequacy caused by uncertainty and lack of knowledge. These groups provide a structured intervention and, if offered early during the course of a cancer diagnosis and treatment, may be less stigmatizing, easily integrated into a comprehensive medical plan for patients with cancer, and more readily accepted by both survivors and staff. The advantages of PSGs are that they are easy to implement and replicate, they promote important illness-related problem-solving skills, and they increase patient and family participation in decision making and active coping. Fawzy et al. (1995) advocated a short-term, structured PSG for newly diagnosed patients or patients with good prognoses because they focus on learning to live with cancer.

Devine and Westlake (1995) completed a meta-analysis of 116 intervention studies published between 1973 and 1993. They found that psychoeducational care benefited adults with cancer in relation to anxiety, depression, mood, nausea, vomiting, pain, and knowledge.

Self-help and mutual SGs are voluntary, small group structures that provide alternative support for patients and families. They provide the impetus for individuals and families to seek emotional support from others experiencing the same trauma. Self-help and mutual SGs started after World War II when ACS offered a visitor's program to patients in their homes. These groups are composed of individuals who share the mutual bond that exists only among those with cancer. Through sharing, survivors can build a foundation of mutual understanding to sustain them through the cancer illness trajectory.

Klemm (1998) reported that the four major goals of a support group are to decrease the patient's sense of alienation, misconceptions and misinformation, feelings about isolation, and anxiety about treatment. Bottomley (1997) agreed that SGs are designed to provide participants the opportunity to acknowledge their experience and express emotions to other patients. The therapeutic process of SGs allows patients to adjust to the cancer situation by sharing experiences, reducing isolation, and improving relationships through better communication, as well as giving and receiving information.

SGs are beneficial for the survivor because survivors can gain valuable information through them. For example, a breast cancer survivor with pendulous breasts shared her experience of being without a prosthesis for more than six months because, even though she had insurance, she was not aware of available resources. An African American cancer survivor shared her experience of purchasing a breast prosthesis with coloration for a white woman and feeling embarrassed every time she put on the prosthesis.

Spiegel, Bloom, and Yalom (1981) conducted a one-year randomized study of SGs for women with metastatic breast cancer. One-hundred and nine women participated in the intervention, which consisted of a 90-minute weekly outpatient group meeting attended by 6–10 survivors. A psychiatrist and social worker cofacilitated the meetings, which covered issues such as treatment, illness, death, and family problems in an unstructured manner. At the end of the study, they found that 34 women in the treatment group demonstrated significantly better coping styles, fewer phobias, and less confusion and fatigue than the 24 women in the control group. This study reported no significant differences in the levels of depression, self-esteem, anxiety, or denial between the two groups.

Group interventions started in the late 1970s, and, in the new millennium, cancer SGs have taken on new looks. SGs are now available via the Internet, telephone, use of a coach, and teleconferencing (Heine, Darr-Hope, & Howell, 1999; Samarel, Fawcett & Tulman, 1993). The primary purpose of nontraditional SGs is for cancer survivors to have accessible support and anonymity within their own environment. These nontraditional support modalities help cancer survivors without benefit of a traditional support group to overcome geographic constraints, decrease isolation, and maintain privacy (Klemm, 1998). See Table 9.1 for a listing of national organizations that offer support services.

Cancer Survivorship Issues

Human response to a cancer diagnosis and subsequent treatment manifests biopsychophysiological, sociocultural, and spiritual reactions resulting from internal and external environmental stimuli. The human response to cancer survivorship must be explored because psychosocial variables exhibited by behaviors or cues could potentially affect outcomes. Therefore, nurses must understand the behavior and the values underlying the behavior to design and implement interventions. Cancer survivorship in the United States has proliferated in recent years, as NCI, ACS, and the National Coalition of Cancer Survivorship have developed programs to meet the needs of survivors. Although spectacular gains recently have been made in prolonging patients' lives, physicians and other healthcare professionals are learning about other physical and psychological problems that cancer survivors and their families may have to face (Bloom et al., 1978).

Table 9-1. National Organizations Providing Support Group Services

Organization	Address	Type of Service Provided	Telephone/Web Site
American Cancer Society (ACS)	1599 Clinton Rd. NE Atlanta, GA 30329-4251	Provides information on cancer programs and events, guidelines, publications, and support groups (SGs).	800-ACS-2345 www.cancer.org
Alliance for Lung Cancer Advocacy, Support, and Education (ALCASE)	1601 Lincoln Ave. Vancouver, WA 98660	Provides programs to improve quality of life (QOL) for people with lung cancer and their families.	360-696-2436 800-298-2436 www.alcase.org
American Brain Tumor Association (ABTA)	Suite 146 2720 River Rd. Des Plaines, IL 60018	Provides patient information, printed materials, and listings of physicians, treatment facilities, and SGs.	847-827-9910 800-886-ABTA (800-886-2282) www.abta.org
American Foundation for Urologic Disease (AFUD)	1128 N. Charles St. Baltimore, MD 21201	Provides education and support services for those who may be at risk and prostate cancer SGs.	410-468-1800 800-242-2383 www.afud.org
American Institute for Cancer Research (AICR)	1759 R St., NW Washington, DC 20009	Provides cancer prevention information, particularly on diet and nutrition, and offers a pen pal support network.	202-328-7744 800-843-8114 www.aicr.org
Cancer Care, Inc.	2nd Floor 1180 Avenue of the Americas New York, NY 10036	Provides free professional assistance to people with any type of cancer; offers one-on-one counseling, specialized SGs, referrals, and financial assistance (some information available in Spanish).	212-302-2400 800-813-HOPE (800-813-4673) www.cancercare.org
Cancer Hope Network	Suite A Two North Rd. Chester, NJ 07930	Provides individual support with matched trained cancer survivors (information available in Spanish).	877-HOPENET (877-467-3638) www.cancerhopenetwork.org

(Continued on next page)

Table 9-1. National Organizations Providing Support Group Services (Continued)

Organization	Address	Type of Service Provided	Telephone/Web Site
US TOO International, Inc.	Suite 50 930 N. York Rd. Hinsdale, IL 60521	Prostate cancer support group provides information, counseling, and educational meetings to assist men with prostate disease in making decisions about their treatment with confidence and support (located throughout the United States; call the toll-free hot line).	630-323-1002 800-80-US TOO (800-808-7866) www.ustoo.com
Sisters Network, Inc.	National Headquarters Suite 4206 8787 Woodway Dr. Houston, TX 77063	Provides support for African American breast cancer survivors.	713-781-0255 http://sistersnetworkinc.org
Y-Me National Breast Cancer Organization, Inc.	212 W. Van Buren St. Chicago, IL 60607-3908	Committed to providing information and support to those who have been touched by breast cancer; serves women with breast cancer and their families and friends through a national hot line, early detection workshops, and local chapters.	312-986-9505 800-221-2141 Spanish hot line: 800-986-9505 www.y-me.org
Cure for Lymphoma Foundation (CFL)	215 Lexington Ave. New York, NY 10016-6023	Provides education on Hodgkin's disease and non-Hodgkin's lymphoma; offers SGs and patient-to-patient telephone network, newsletters, and educational information.	212-213-9595 www.cfl.org
Encore	YWCA of the USA Office of Women's Health Initiative 3rd Floor 624 Ninth St., NW Washington DC 20001	Provides discussion and exercise program for patients undergoing breast cancer surgery (at local Young Women's Christian Association. (YWCA).	202-628-3636 800-95E-PLUS (800-953-7587) www.ywca.org

(Continued on next page)

Table 9-1. National Organizations Providing Support Group Services (Continued)

Organization	Address	Type of Service Provided	Telephone/Web Site
Gilda's Club, Inc.	195 W. Houston St. New York, NY 10014	Provides social and emotional support to individuals with cancer and their families; offers SGs, networking groups, workshops, and lectures.	212-686-9898 www.gildasclub.org
Hospice Link	Hospice Education Institute 190 Westbrook Rd. Essex, CT 06426-1510	Helps patients to find support services in their communities.	860-767-1620 Alaska and Connecticut: 800-331-1620 www.hospiceworld.org
International Myeloma Foundation (IMF)	2129 Stanley Hills Dr. Los Angeles, CA 90046	Does not sponsor an SG; however, can tell patients where groups are located and how to start an SG.	323-654-3023 800-452-CURE (800-452-2873) www.myeloma.org
Kidney Cancer Association (KCA)	Suite 203 1234 Sherman Ave. Evanston, IL 60202	Sponsors SGs and provides physician referrals.	874-332-1051 800-850-9132 www.nkca.org
Leukemia and Lymphoma Society, Inc.	1311 Mamaronek Ave. White Plains, NY 10605	Concerned with leukemia, lymphoma, and related diseases; offers financial assistance.	914-949-5123 800-955-4572 www.leukemia.org
Lymphoma Research Foundation of America (LRFA)	Suite 207 8800 Venice Blvd. Los Angeles, CA 90034	Provides educational information on lymphoma; offers a referral service to oncologists, clinical trials, and SGs.	310-204-7040 (800-500-9976) www.lymphoma.org
National Alliance of Breast Cancer Organizations (NABCO)	10th Floor 9 E. 37th St. New York, NY 10016	Maintains a list of organizations by state; offers phone numbers for SGs.	212-889-0606 888-80-NABCO (888-806-2226) www.nabco.org

(Continued on next page)

Table 9-1. National Organizations Providing Support Group Services (Continued)

Organization	Address	Type of Service Provided	Telephone/Web Site
Native American Breast Cancer Survivors' Support Network	3022 S. Nova Rd. Pine, CO 80470-7830	Improves QOL after breast cancer diagnosis for Native Americans and their loved ones.	303-838-9359 members.aol.com/natamcan
National Asian Women's Health Organization (NAWHO)	Suite 410 250 Montgomery St. San Francisco, CA 94104	Works to improve the health status of Asian women and families (resources available in Cantonese, Laotian, Vietnamese, and Korean).	414-989-9747 www.nawho.org
National Brain Tumor Foundation (NBTF)	Suite 1600 785 Market St. San Francisco, CA 94103	Provides information to patients and families coping with brain tumors; provides access to a national network of patient SGs.	800-934-CURE (800-934-2873) www.braintumor.org
National Coalition for Cancer Survivorship (NCCS)	Suite 505 1010 Wayne Ave. Silver Spring, MD 20910	Network of groups and individuals that offer support to cancer survivors and their loved ones; provides information and resources on cancer support, advocacy, and QOL issues.	301-650-8868 800-650-9127 www.cancersearch.org
National Hospice Organization (NHO)	Suite 901 1901 N. Moore St. Arlington, VA 22209	Offers information on how to find a hospice; provides hospice care.	703-243-5900 800-658-8898 www.nho.org
National Lymphedema Network (NLN)	Suite 404 2211 Post St. San Francisco, CA 94115-3457	Provides a toll-free support hot line, a referral service to lymphedema treatment centers, SGs, pen pals, educational courses, and a computer database.	415-921-3106 800-541-3259 www.lymphnet.org
National Marrow Donor Program (NMDP)	Suite 500 3433 Broadway St. NE Minneapolis, MN 55413	Provides information on bone marrow transplantation; keeps a registry of potential bone marrow donors.	612-627-5800 800-MARROW-2 (800-627-7692) www.marrow.org

(Continued on next page)

Table 9-1. National Organizations Providing Support Group Services (Continued)

Organization	Address	Type of Service Provided	Telephone/Web Site
National Ovarian Cancer Coalition (NOCC)	Suite 401 2335 E. Atlantic Blvd. Pompano, FL 33062	Promotes awareness, referral, and education; provides information, referrals, support, education, and SGs.	954-781-3500 888-OVARIAN (888-682-7426) www.ovarian.org
Patient Advocate Foundation (PAF)	Suite 100-C 780 Pilot House Dr. Newport News, VA 23606-1993	Provides education, legal counseling, and referrals concerning managed care, insurance, financial issues, job discrimination, and crisis debt matters.	757-873-6668 800-532-5274 www.patientadvocate.org
R.A. Bloch Cancer Foundation, Inc.	Suite 500 440 Main St. Kansas City, MO 64111	Matches newly diagnosed patients with cancer with trained home-based volunteers who have been treated for cancer. Provides information and has a multidisciplinary list of institutions that offer second opinions.	816-932-8453 800-433-0464 www.blochcancer.org
Support for People with Oral Head and Neck Cancer (SPOHNC)	P.O. Box 53 Locust Valley, NY 11560-0053	Patient-directed nonprofit organization dedicated to meeting the needs of patients with oral, head, and neck cancer; informs and supports patients seeking a better understanding of their illness and its impact on their lives.	516-759-5333 www.spohnc.org
Skin Cancer Foundation	Suite 1403 245 Fifth Ave. New York, NY 10016	Provides education on and awareness of the importance of protective measures; conducts public and medical education programs.	212-725-5176 800-SKIN-490 (800-754-6490) 949-660-8624
United Ostomy Association, Inc. (UOA)	Suite 19772 MacArthur Blvd. Irvine, CA 92612-2405	Helps ostomy patients through mutual aid and emotional support.	800-826-0826 (7:30 am–4:30 pm Pacific Time) www.uoa.org

Note. This list was adapted from *Cancer Facts* with permission of the Cancer Information Services of the National Cancer Institute, National Institutes of Health. A more complete list that includes pediatrics groups can be obtained by calling 800-4CANCER and requesting Cancer Facts National Organizations. Additions have been made to this list.

Cancer survivors are faced with many unique issues that individuals with other disease processes do not experience. These major challenges include physical, psychological, financial, employment, insurance, sexuality, spiritual, and cultural issues. The cancer survivor's quality of life (QOL) may be affected by these challenges. Survivors interpret their feelings of well-being using expectations, perceptions, experiences, and religious or community beliefs (Bland, 1997). Survivors' perceptions of their QOL may vary based on their life experiences and may depend on their attitude after the therapeutic intervention. Each challenge will be briefly discussed.

Physical and Psychosocial Issues

Few words can evoke such immediate, adverse, and life-changing reactions as the words "you have cancer." People with cancer can describe, in vivid detail, the day that they were told they had cancer, as well as how this news instantly changed their lives (Grassman, 1993). For an individual living with cancer, life becomes an unplanned journey, and many individuals experience a fear of the unknown. The individual is faced with many detours, yield signs, hazards, and even stop signs (Bushkin, 1995). On this journey, the individual needs to cope with body changes. Cycles of chemotherapy can be debilitating for some individuals. In addition, chemotherapy can cause nausea, vomiting, pain, stomatitis or painful sores in the mouth, loss of appetite, thinning of hair or alopecia of the entire body, depression, and severe fatigue. The survivor may need special tools to overcome a disability or discomfort. Skin changes might occur with these therapies, and problems with intimacy may be experienced. The individual sometimes is forced to give up the nurturing or breadwinner's role. This journey may last as short as a few weeks to years to indefinitely.

The individual with a cancer diagnosis faces a myriad of physical and psychosocial challenges, such as urinary and sexual dysfunction, anticipatory nausea or vomiting, psychological distress, relational and social dysfunction, fatalism, passive acceptance, avoidance, feelings of loss of control, short- and long-term disability, changes in perception of body image, infertility, skin irritation, fatigue, pain, odor with a colostomy, weight gain, menopausal symptoms, peripheral neuropathy, reestablishment of autonomy, lymphedema, limited arm movement, and survival (Anderson & Lutgendorf, 1997; Bland, 1997; DeCosse & Cennerazzo, 1997; Ott, 1997b; Powe, 1995). Antineoplastic agents may be associated with anemia, neutropenia, diarrhea, vomiting, and anorexia (DeCosse & Cennerazzo). The family or caregiver also is affected by the cancer trajectory.

Financial Challenges

Financial issues can become paramount when an individual is faced with a cancer diagnosis. Monetary issues are important to the cancer survivor, both in day-to-day existence and in planning and securing the future (Pelusi, 1997). Healthcare costs can be enormous and never-ending. Financial costs of cancer are great to the individual, family, and society. NCI (1999) estimated the overall annual cost for cancer is at $107 billion. Of this cost, $37 billion is spent on all health expenditures; more than half of this amount is spent on breast, lung, and prostate cancers. NCI also revealed that $11 billion is spent for lost productivity resulting from illness (indirect morbidity cost), and $59 billion is spent for lost productivity because of premature deaths (indirect mortality cost). However, few studies have placed a dollar amount on human suffering or the actual cost of the cancer trajectory to the individual or family.

A study done by Moore (1998) revealed that the per diem "out of pocket cost for the five major cost categories (i.e., clinic visits, support assistance, symptoms and side effects, QOL, and administrative) ranged from $12–$3,130, with a mean of $741 per month" (p. 1619). Moore further reported that the cost to the individual in terms of support and QOL was $40 and $913 per month, respectively.

Survivors may find that they are unable to secure mortgages or loans because of a cancer history. A cancer survivor's inability to obtain additional resources can affect other family members' educational and career goals, as well as day-to-day finances.

Survivors might find it difficult or impossible to obtain life, health, or disability insurance following a cancer diagnosis. Some insurance companies do not pay claims, as their policies require, or, on the other hand, premiums are so costly that survivors cannot afford the policy. Many managed care and insurance companies have not kept pace with advances in cancer care and may not cover suggested treatment modalities because they are considered experimental. Clinical trials may not be covered because of the nature of the treatment, even though it might be the individuals's only option. Some states offer coverage for cancer survivors that are unable to obtain health insurance (NCI, 1994).

Many cancer survivors incur additional costs based on their type of cancer and cancer treatment. For instance, colorectal cancer survivors must be cognizant of stoma management, as Medicare reimbursement is restricted and provisions for these supplies are limited (DeCosse & Cennerazzo, 1997).

Employability and Legality Issues

Those living with a cancer diagnosis often experience work-related problems, and the diagnosis may affect whether a person is hired. If the survivor is working in a position without the potential for advancement, he or she might be afraid to leave because of insurance and benefits issues and may feel trapped in a dead-end, unpleasant, or restrictive job. This phenomenon is termed "job-lock" (Andrews, 1997; NCI, 1999; Welch-McCaffrey, Hoffman, Leigh, Loescher, & Meyskens, 1989).

Work-related problems experienced by cancer survivors include demotion, dismissal, and reduction or elimination of work-related benefits. Many coworkers may feel that cancer is contagious or is a death sentence and avoid or pity the survivor, which further promotes a sense of alienation.

A review of the literature reveals episodes of employment discrimination against cancer survivors. One article reported on a cancer survivor who filed a lawsuit and was awarded compensation because she lost her job following a cancer diagnosis (Chambliss, 1996).

The Americans with Disabilities Act (ADA) of 1990, the Family Medical Leave Act (FMLA) of 1993, and the Consolidated Omnibus Budget Reconciliation Act (COBRA) of 1986 are well-known legal issues that were implemented to protect society. However, as with many laws, loopholes exist. For instance, for an employee to be eligible for ADA, the company must employ 15 or more employees; otherwise, the company does not have to offer ADA to protect their employees. The FMLA has similar circumstances, except the company must employ 50 or more employees or no coverage is available. COBRA will extend benefits after leaving employment for 12 months, but the cost can be excessive. In addition, the ADA and FMLA do not protect an employee whose illness creates an undue hardship for the employer. The definition of undue hardships is obscure and creates yet another loophole through which employers can avoid mandates of the law.

Insurance Challenges

A cancer diagnosis can affect the individual's way of life, health insurance, and ability to obtain life insurance. The individual can be faced with challenges, including cancellation of policies without job change, extended waiting periods, increased premiums with decreased amounts of coverage, exceeding maximum coverage limits, and exclusion of future cancer-related expenses (Andrews, 1997). As one survivor said, "My health insurance after cancer treatment is like my car insurance: after an accident, my rates went up" (B. Johnson, personal communication, April 4, 1999). Some cancer survivors have no insurance, nor do they qualify for reduced life insurance, and others have no life insurance for at least five years following a cancer diagnosis. Existing and anticipated insurance problems cause stress, anxiety about job security, economic instability, resistance to job change, lowered self-esteem, and anger over being denied insurance for statistically unsound reasons (Anderson & Lutengendorf, 1997; Moore, 1998). Even though many chemotherapeutic agents cause alopecia, some insurance policies do not cover wigs because they are considered cosmetic. The individual may be limited in the amount of surgically related garments that may be purchased. For example, some insurance companies only allow mastectomy survivors to purchase four bras per year and a prosthesis every few years.

If the survivor's spouse is the insurance carrier and changes jobs, the spouse may be unable to get a family policy because of the survivor's cancer history. If the survivor does not have insurance, he or she might not always receive quality services. Cancer survivors who do not have group health insurance are most vulnerable to insurance problems (Welch-McCaffrey et al., 1989). Results of a study by Ayanian, Kohler, Abe, and Epstein (1993) showed that women who were uninsured or covered by Medicaid presented with more advanced disease at the time of diagnosis and had a 40% higher risk of mortality than women who were privately insured.

The Health Insurance Portability and Accountability Act (HIPAA) of 1996 was designed to prevent loss of health insurance with job change or family illness. The HIPAA limits exclusion based on preexisting conditions to a lifetime aggregate total of 12 months. It also prevents loss of coverage for health reasons in small group plans.

Sexuality Challenges

Cancer and cancer treatment may affect sexual relationships. Some surgical procedures cause changes in body image. Chemotherapy can cause sexual dysfunction. The survivor may face such changes as vaginal dryness, weight gain, pain, and alopecia (Ferrell, Dow, Leigh, Ly, & Gulasekaram, 1995). Some survivors may be devastated because of loss of fertility. The individual and his or her partner need to understand the sexual problems and be informed about various interventions to deal with them, such as lubricants or hormonal therapy. The healthcare provider should discuss treatment modalities and guide the survivor and significant other in these discussions.

Men may face sexual dysfunction after prostate cancer surgery, and a male survivor and his significant other must feel that the healthcare provider can discuss different treatment modalities or refer them to a consultant. Therapies such as androgen-depleting hormones used for prostate cancer survivors can cause feminizing characteristics in men; therefore, the individual may be self-conscious in masculine roles (Clay, 1999).

When faced with the possibility of sexual dysfunction, both partners need help when cancer is diagnosed. Helping couples to mourn the loss of pretreatment sexuality is a crucial first step toward sexual healing (Clay, 1999). The nurse must be aware of these delicate issues and be willing to address them and intervene to support the couple. The nurse should refer the couple to follow-up care or educate or counsel them, depending on his or her knowledge base and comfort level (Andrews, 1997).

Spiritual Alterations

Ferrell et al. (1995) described spiritual well-being as "the ability to maintain hope and derive meaning from the cancer experience that is characterized by uncertainty. Spiritual well-being involves issues of transcendence and is enhanced by one's religion and other sources of spiritual support" (p. 913). Ott (1997c) reported that having a sick body does not prevent a person from growing spiritually or finding meaning in contributing and connecting to others.

Ferrell, Grant, Funk, Otis-Green, and Garcia (1998) reported that uncertainty about the future causes the greatest disruption to cancer survivors' spiritual well-being. They further reported that cancer survivors have positive outcomes in the area of spiritual well-being because they express a sense of purpose or reason for being alive. A diagnosis of cancer and chemotherapy treatment can cause spiritual distress. The individual may experience loneliness, anger at God, loss of faith, fatalism, despair, grief, loss over the future, an inability to find meaning and purpose along the cancer trajectory, and the notion that cancer is a punishment (Ferrell et al., 1995; NCI, 1999).

The cancer experience allows the individual and family to reexamine life for its true significance. The individual begins to live each day as though it were the last, and life takes on a greater meaning. Survivors have a new view and perspective of the lived experience, and their faith often is renewed or enhanced after a cancer experience. Many survivors become active in the cancer movement by supporting and educating others. The survivor learns that maintaining "hope and trust in the face of uncertainty is a daily challenge" (Ott, 1997c, p. 34).

Cultural Issues

Although extensive research and anecdotal reports document the emotional and psychological impact of breast cancer and mastectomy (Bloom, 1982; Carroll, 1998), the studies do not factor race and social class into their formulation (Beder, 1995). In ethnic minority and medically underserved populations that face numerous cultural, socioeconomic, and institutional barriers to cancer treatment, survivors often are painfully aware of the lack of services and information that might assist them and their social network to cope with a cancer diagnosis and the effects of chemotherapy (Haynes & Smedley, 1999).

Many societal issues, such as race, gender, racism, class, and socioeconomic status, affect African American women (Spiegel et al., 1981). Poverty, decreased education, and minimal knowledge about cancer are believed to influence cancer fatalism (Powe, 1995). Compounding an already-burdened existence with cancer survivorship and the many psychosocial issues previously addressed must seem overwhelming to these survivors of color. Some African American cancer survivors are not aware of many of the available resources in the healthcare arena; therefore, this lack of awareness could be detrimental. Interventions should be developed to improve the QOL for the cancer survivor.

All cancer survivors are different. Interventions should not be developed with the concept of "one size fits all." Each culture has its own unique qualities and characteristics, and these differences must be accounted for. To understand cancer survivors of color, nurses must be open-minded and allow patients to teach them about their cultural perspectives and lived experiences. Nurses also must be aware of available culturally appropriate resources to better serve these clients.

Nurses must be proactive in becoming culturally competent to address needs of diverse populations. Mechanisms to improve the quality of these cancer survivors' lived experience must be identified from a cultural perspective. If nursing does not fulfill its obligation to identify the domains of cancer survivorship in African American women, the opportunity to increase the knowledge base of the discipline will be waived. Social support can provide an avenue through which research can help African American women.

Summary

Nursing interventions can be developed through identifying psychosocial variables of cancer survivors, which can lead to measurable outcomes. Outcomes are the foundation of professional accountability and represent an appealing concept that has tremendous potential to translate into powerful healthcare decisions. The nurse researcher must be able to incorporate outcomes (i.e., the results or consequences of care) with process (i.e., how care is delivered) and structure (i.e., resources in the healthcare setting, such as qualifications of staff) (Jennings & Staggers, 1998) to improve all cancer survivors' QOL. Finally, to mobilize social support, interventions must be developed from a culture-specific perspective.

References

American Cancer Society. (2001). *Cancer facts and figures, 2001.* Atlanta: Author.

American heritage dictionary (2nd ed.). (1982). Boston: Houghton Mifflin Co.

Anderson, B., & Lutgendorf, S. (1997). Quality of life of gynecologic cancer survivors. *CA: A Cancer Journal for Clinicians, 47,* 218–225.

Andrews, A. (1997). But what about work? *Nebraska Nurse, 30*(2), 33.

Ayanian, J., Kohler, B., Abe, T., & Epstein, A. (1993). The relation between health insurance coverage and clinical outcomes among women with breast cancer. *New England Journal of Medicine, 329,* 326–331.

Beder, J. (1995). Perceived support and adjustment to mastectomy in socioeconomically disadvantaged black women. *Social Work in Health Care, 22*(2), 55–71.

Berkman, L. (1995). The role of social relations in health promotion. *Psychosomatic Medicine, 57,* 245–254.

Bland, K. (1997). Quality-of-life management for cancer patients. *CA: A Cancer Journal for Clinicians, 47,* 194–197.

Bloom, J.R. (1982). Social support systems and cancer: A conceptual overview. In J. Cohen, J.W. Cullen, & R.L. Martin (Eds.), *Psychosocial aspects of cancer* (pp. 129–149). New York: Raven Press.

Bloom, J.R., Ross, R.D., & Burnell, G. (1978). The effect of social support on patient adjustment after breast surgery. *Patient Counseling and Health Education, 1*(2), 50–59.

Bottomley, A. (1997). Cancer support groups: Are they effective? *European Journal of Cancer Care, 6*(1), 11–17.

Bottomley, A., & Jones, L. (1997). Social support and the cancer patient—A need for clarity. *European Journal of Cancer Care, 6*(1), 72–77.

Bruhn, J., & Phillips, B. (1984). Measuring social support: A synthesis of current approaches. *Journal of Behavioral Medicine, 7*(2), 151–169.

Bushkin, E. (1995). Signposts of survivorship. *Oncology Nursing Forum, 22,* 537–543.

Caplan, G. (1974). Support systems. In G. Caplan (Ed.), *Support systems and community mental health* (pp. 1–40). New York: Basic Books, Inc.

Caplan, G. (1976). *Support systems and mutual help: Multidisciplinary explorations.* New York: Grune & Stratton.

Carroll, S. (1998). Breast cancer, part 3: Psychosocial care. *Professional Nurse, 13,* 877–883.

Chambliss, L. (1996). The cancer reality gap. *Working Woman, 21*(10), 47–49.

Clay, R. (1999). Survivors are slow to seek help for social problems. *Monitor: American Psychological Association, 30*(6), 27. Retrieved November 7, 2000 from the World Wide Web: http://www.apa.org/monitor/june1999/sexual.html

Cobb, S. (1976). Social support as a moderator of stress. *Psychosomatic Medicine, 38,* 300–314.

Cohen, S., & Syme, S. (1985). *Social support and health.* Orlando, FL: Academic Press, Inc.

DeCosse J., & Cennerazzo, W. (1997). Quality-of-life management of patients with colorectal cancer. *CA: A Cancer Journal for Clinicians, 47,* 198–206.

Devine, E., & Westlake, S. (1995). The effects of psychoeducational care provided to adults with cancer: Meta-analysis of 116 studies. *Oncology Nursing Forum, 22,* 1369–1381.

Fawzy, F., Fawzy, N., Arndt, L., & Pasnau, R. (1995). Critical review of psychosocial intervention in cancer care. *Archives of General Psychiatry, 52*(2), 100–113.

Ferrell, B., Grant, M., Funk, B., Otis-Green, S., & Garcia, N. (1998). Quality of life in breast cancer survivors: Implications for developing support services. *Oncology Nursing Forum, 25,* 887–895.

Ferrell, B.R., Dow, K.H., Leigh, S., Ly, J., & Gulasekaram, P. (1995). Quality of life in long-term cancer survivors. *Oncology Nursing Forum, 22,* 915–922.

Fobair, P. (1997). Cancer support groups and group therapies, part 1: Historical and theoretical background and research effectiveness. *Journal of Psychosocial Oncology, 15*(1), 63–81.

George, D. (1998). Innovations in practice. Teleconferencing support: Women with secondary breast cancer. *International Journal of Palliative Nursing, 4*(3), 115–119.

Grassman, D. (1993). Development of inpatient oncology educational and support programs. *Oncology Nursing Forum, 20,* 669.

Greenlee, R., Hill-Harmon, M., Murray, T., & Thun, M. (2001). Cancer statistics, 2001. *CA: A Cancer Journal for Clinicians, 51,* 15–36.

Haynes, M.A., & Smedley, B.D. (1999). *The unequal burden of cancer: An assessment of NIH research and programs for ethnic minorities and the medically underserved.* Washington, DC: National Academy Press.

Heine, S.P., Darr-Hope, H., & Howell, C.D. (1999). Breast cancer: The supportive survivors. *Reflections, 25*(4), 14–16.

Hinds, G., & Moyer, A. (1997). Support as experienced by patients with cancer during radiotherapy treatments. *Journal of Advanced Nursing, 26,* 371–379.

Holland, J. (1989). Clinical course of cancer. In J. Holland & J. Rowland (Eds.), *Handbook of psycho-oncology: Psychological care of the patient with cancer* (pp. 75–100). New York: Oxford University Press.

Howell, D., & Jackson, J. (1998). Making cancer bearable: The Interlink Community Cancer Nurses model of supportive care. *Canadian Oncology Nursing Journal, 8,* 222–228.

Jennings, B., & Staggers, N. (1998). The language of outcomes. *Advances in Nursing Science, 20*(4), 72–80.

Kahn, R. (1979). Aging and social support. In M. Riley (Ed.), *Aging from birth to death: Interdisciplinary perspectives* (pp. 77–81). Boulder, CO: Westview Press, Inc.

Kaplan, B., Cassel, J., & Gore, S. (1977). Social support and health. *Medical Care, 15*(5), 47–58.

Klein, C. (1999). Failing life's most difficult challenges: Alone. *Coping, 13*(3), 52.

Klemm, P. (1998). A nontraditional cancer support group: The Internet. *Computers in Nursing, 16*(1), 31–36.

Moore, K. (1998). Out-of-pocket expenditures of outpatients receiving chemotherapy. *Oncology Nursing Forum, 25,* 1615–1622.

National Cancer Institute. (1994). *Facing forward: A guide for cancer survivors* (Publication No. 94-2424). Bethesda, MD: Author.

National Cancer Institute. (1999). *The cancer journey: Issues for survivors* (Publication No. 98-4259). Bethesda, MD: Author.

Norbeck, J. (1988). Social support. *Annual Review of Nursing Research, 6,* 85–109.

Norbeck, J.S., Lindsey, A.M., & Carrieri, V.L. (1981). The development of an instrument to measure social support. *Nursing Research, 30,* 264–269.

Northouse, L., Dorris, G., & Charron-Moore, C. (1995). Factors affecting couples' adjustment to recurrent breast cancer. *Social Science and Medicine, 41*(1), 69–76.

Oktay, J. (1998). Psychosocial aspects of breast cancer. *Lippincott's Primary Care Practice, 2*(2), 149–159.

Ott, C. (1997a). Breast cancer as a family disease. *Nebraska Nurse, 30*(2), 27.

Ott, C. (1997b). The impact of breast cancer on sexuality. *Nebraska Nurse, 30*(2), 28.

Ott, C. (1997c). Spirituality and the nurse. *Nebraska Nurse, 30*(2), 34–35.

Pasacreta J., & Pickett, M. (1998). Psychosocial aspects of palliative care. *Seminars in Oncology Nursing, 14,* 110–120.

Pelusi, J. (1997). The lived experience of surviving cancer. *Oncology Nursing Forum, 24,* 1343–1353.

Powe, B. (1995). Cancer fatalism among elderly Caucasians and African Americans. *Oncology Nursing Forum, 22,* 1355–1359.

Samarel, N., Fawcett, J., Krippendorf, K., Piacentino, J.C., Eliasof, B., Hughes, P., Kowitski, C., & Ziegler, E. (1998). Women's perceptions of group support and adaptation to breast cancer. *Journal of Advanced Nursing, 28,* 1259–1268.

Samarel, N., Fawcett, J., & Tulman, L. (1993). The effects of coaching in breast cancer support groups: A pilot study. *Oncology Nursing Forum, 20,* 795-798.

Spiegel, D., Bloom, J., & Yalom, I. (1981). Group support for patients with metastatic cancer. A randomized prospective outcome study. *Archives of General Psychiatry 38,* 527–533.

Van Hammond, T., & Deans, C. (1995). A phenomenological study of families and psychoeducation support groups. *Journal of Psychosocial Nursing and Mental Health Services, 33*(10), 7–12.

Vrabec, N. (1997). Literature review of social support and caregiver burden, 1980 to 1995. *Image: Journal of Nursing Scholarship, 29,* 383–388.

Welch-McCaffrey, D., Hoffman, B., Leigh, S.A., Loescher, L.J., & Meyskens, F.L. (1989). Surviving adult cancers. Part 2: Psychosocial implications. *Annals of Internal Medicine, 111,* 517–524.

Youssef, F. (1984). Crisis intervention: A group-therapy approach for hospitalized breast cancer patients. *Journal of Advanced Nursing, 9,* 307–313.

CHAPTER 10

Public and Professional Cancer Resources

Veronica A. Clarke-Tasker, PhD, RN, MBA

The new millennium brought with it many challenges for healthcare professionals. Higher patient acuity coupled with the need to decrease length of stay within hospitals across the nation reinforces the need for all healthcare professionals, and nurses in particular, to become familiar with available resources. Patients have access to the same information as their providers. Those who are computer literate and have Internet capabilities can download information about their disease, as well as various treatment options. Patients present with a list of questions and/or information about their disease and treatment options. However, they may not fully understand, for example, what a treatment protocol entails. They depend on their providers for guidance and support.

As patient advocates, teachers, and healthcare providers, nurses work closely with patients and their families. Their expectations of nurses are high. To better assist patients in making educated decisions about care, it is important for providers to be knowledgeable regarding available and appropriate resources.

Public Resources

American Brain Tumor Association
2720 River Road, Suite 146
Des Plaines, IL 60018
800-886-2282
847-827-9910
www.abta.org

Services of the association include brain tumor support groups, patient and professional education materials, and information on treatment protocols and facilities. Their newsletter *Message Line* is published triannually.

American Cancer Society (ACS)
1599 Clifton Road NE
Atlanta, GA 30329
800-ACS-2345
404-320-3333
404-329-5787, fax
www.cancer.org

ACS is a voluntary, community-based organization with offices at the national, local, state, and division level. Staffed by professional and lay volunteers, ACS is dedicated to preventing cancer. Education, prevention and early detection, research, advocacy, and patient services are the major programs offered. Listed below is a short list of some of the services that may be provided in your area. Contact the local ACS office (800-ACS-2345) for additional information.

CanSurmont: One-on-one support for patients and/or family members.

I Can Cope: Educational program that provides patients and their families with information about cancer, current treatments, coping strategies, and available resources.

Reach to Recovery: Trained volunteers who have had breast cancer and have resumed their activities visit breast cancer surgery patients pre- and postoperatively, with the approval of their physician.

Road to Recovery: Volunteers provide transportation to and from treatment sites for cancer patients.

Loan Closet: Patients and their families can borrow bedpans, hospital beds, walkers, wheelchairs, and other supplies. Many ACS units also supply dressings.

American Lung Association (ALA)
1740 Broadway
New York, NY 10019-4374
212-315-8700
800-586-4872
800-LUNG-USA
www.lungusa.org

ALA is a nonprofit organization that promotes lung health by sponsoring symposia, conferences, fellowships, and research grants. Pamphlets, films, posters, and other public education materials are listed in their free catalog and are available to the public. Facts about asthma, lung cancer, radon, secondhand smoke, and occupational lung cancer are some of the topics covered.

Association for Research of Childhood Cancer
P.O. Box 251
Buffalo, NY 14225-0251
716-689-8922

The association, which meets six times per year, is composed of parents whose children have died from cancer and other individuals. The group funds pediatric cancer research and publishes a quarterly newsletter.

Cancer Care, Inc. and the National Cancer Care Foundation
275 7th Avenue
New York, NY 10001
212-221-3300
800-813-HOPE
www.cancercare.org

This nonprofit organization provides psychological and financial support for patients with cancer and their families. Individual and group counseling services are available, along with community education programs.

Cancer Information Service (CIS)
NCI Office of Cancer Communications
Building 31, Room 10A 16
Bethesda, MD 20892
800-4-CANCER
www.nci.nih.gov/cis

Nineteen regional field offices supported by NCI make up this nationwide network. English and Spanish literature on specific cancers and clinical trials is available to the general public. Limited quantities of pamphlets and booklets listed in NCI's catalog are provided free of charge.

CaPCure: Association for the Cure of Cancer of the Prostate
1250 4th Street, Suite 360
Santa Monica, CA 90401
800-757-2873
www.capcure.org

Largest private source of funding for prostate cancer research and information.

Susan G. Komen Breast Cancer Foundation
5005 LBJ Freeway
Dallas, TX 75244
800-462-9273
www.komen.org

A national volunteer, nonprofit organization that provides mammography screening, education, and treatment for medically underserved women. Race for the Cure, a race held at different locations across the country, is one of its many fund-raising activities.

The Leukemia and Lymphoma Society of America
National Headquarters
1311 Mamaroneck Avenue
White Plains, NY 10605
914-949-5213
www.leukemia.org

Patient aid, community service, research, and public and professional education are programs supported by this national voluntary health agency. The agency seeks to determine the cause of as well as a cure for leukemia, lymphoma Hodgkin's disease, and myeloma.

Look Good ... Feel Better (LGFB)
The CTFA Foundation
1101 17th Street, NW, Suite 300
Washington, DC 20036
800-395-LOOK
www.lookgoodfeelbetter.org

LGFB is a partnership of the Cosmetic, Toiletry & Fragrance Association (CTFA) Foundation, the American Cancer Society (ACS), and the National Cosmetology Association (NCA).

Group sessions are held to help female patients cope with hair loss and skin changes while undergoing treatment. ACS administers the program, and volunteer cosmetologists from the NCA offer their expertise. CTFA provides complimentary makeup, videotapes, pamphlets, and other offerings.

Ronald McDonald House (RMDH)
One Kroc Drive
Oak Brook, IL 60523
630-623-7418
www.rmhc.com

Nonprofit organizations own and operate RMDHs. Families receive emotional support in a caring, loving, home-like environment. The homes usually are located close to pediatric treatment centers.

National Coalition for Cancer Survivorship (NCCS)
1010 Wayne Avenue, Suite 770
Silver Spring, MD 20910-5600
301-650-9127
877-622-7937
www.cansearch.org

Serving as an information clearinghouse, NCCS sends the message that individuals diagnosed with cancer can, and do, live productive lives. The organization promotes peer support while networking with others involved with cancer survivorship.

National Alliance of Breast Cancer Organizations
9 East 37th Street, 10th Floor
New York, NY 10016
888-806-2226
www.nabco.org

Nonprofit organization serves as a "voice" for women at risk for breast cancer and survivors. Breast cancer information, referrals, and assistance are available.

National Hospice and Palliative Care Organization
1700 Diagonal Road, Suite 300
Alexandria, VA 22314
703-837-1500
www.nhpco.org

Nonprofit organization that provides a variety of services to the terminally ill. Hospice also is a Medicare/Medicaid benefit. Contact the local office in your community for the services available.

National Marrow Donor Program (NMDP)
Coordinating Center
3001 Broadway Street NE
Minneapolis, MN 55413-1753
800-MARROW-2
www.marrow.org

NMDP is an international program that maintains a registry of unrelated bone marrow and blood stem cell donors. The program was created to improve the effectiveness of searching for donors, as well as to increase the number of transplants. Information is available free of charge to callers.

National Family Caregivers Association (NFCA)
10400 Connecticut Avenue, #500
Kensington, MD 20895-3944
800-896-3650
www.nfcacares.org

NFCA is a national charitable organization that promotes the belief that caregivers can have a happier, healthier life if they view the role of caregiver as only one facet of their lives. Provider services are aimed at minimizing disparities that exist between society and caregivers. Education and information services are available to caregivers and organizations.

Professional Resources and Organizations

American Association for Cancer Education, Inc. (AACE)
University of Texas Department of Epidemiology
M.D. Anderson Cancer Center
P.O. Box 189
1515 Holcombe Boulevard
Houston, TX 77030
800-392-1611
www.mdanderson.org

A multidisciplinary organization that has a membership consisting of basic scientists, oncology nursing educators, radiation oncologists, internists, surgeons, pediatricians, and other healthcare professionals. Provides a health professional forum for advancing cancer education, early detection, and treatment modalities.

American Association for Cancer Research (AACR)
Public Ledger Building, Suite 826
150 South Independence Mall West
Philadelphia, PA 19106-3483
215-440-9300
www.aacr.org

The association is the world's largest professional society. Its members have expertise in many fields, including immunology, pharmacology, epidemiology and prevention, virology, tumor biology, molecular biology, and carcinogenesis.

American Cancer Society (ACS)
1599 Clifton Road NE
Atlanta, GA 30329-4251
800-ACS-2345
404-320-3333

ACS is a voluntary, community-based organization with offices at the national, local, state, and/or division level. Staffed by professional and lay volunteers, ACS is dedicated to eliminating

404-329-5787, fax
www.cancer.org

cancer. Education, prevention and early detection, research, advocacy, and patient services are the major programs offered. ACS provides nursing scholarships at the master's and doctoral levels.

American College of Surgeons (ACOS)
Commission on Cancer
55 East Erie Street
Chicago, IL 60611
312-664-4040

Founded in 1913, the association has set high standards for surgical practice and education to improve the quality of care provided. Its members must undergo a vigorous evaluation process before they are admitted as fellows. Patients and their families can obtain general surgical information from The Office of Pubic Information, as well as a listing of board-certified surgeons in a variety of specialty areas.

American Institute for Cancer Research
1759 R Street NW
Washington, DC 20009
800-843-8114
www.aicr.org

Publications on cancer, nutrition and diet, education, and research programs are offered. The Institute responds to questions about cancer and related treatments via their CancerResource program.

American Pain Society (APS)
4700 W. Lake Avenue
Glenview, IL 60025
847-375-4715
877-734-8758 (toll free)
www.ampainsoc.org

APS, founded in 1978, is the national chapter of the International Association for the Study of Pain. Its membership consists of educators, researchers, and clinicians. The mission of this not-for-profit multidisciplinary organization is to serve people in pain by advancing education, research, and professional practice.

American Society of Clinical Oncology (ASCO)
1900 Duke Street, Suite 200
Alexandria, VA 22314
703-299-0150
www.asco.org

ASCO is an organization that provides a mechanism for cancer professionals to exchange information related to neoplastic diseases. It holds two conferences annually. The *Journal of Clinical Oncology* is the official publication of this organization.

Association of Community Cancer Centers (ACCC)
11600 Nebel Street, Suite 201
Rockville, MD 20852-2557
301-984-9496
www.accc-cancer.org

The mission of this national organization is to promote comprehensive, multidisciplinary, high-quality cancer care.

Association of Pediatric Oncology Nurses (APON)
4700 W. Lake Avenue
Glenview, IL 60025-1485
847-375-4724
www.apon.org

APON membership consists of RNs who are practicing or are interested in providing care to children or adolescents with cancer.

Association of Multicultural Counseling and Development
5999 Stevenson Avenue
Alexandria, VA 22304
800-347-6647
www.amcd-aca.org

The mission of the Association of Multicultural Counseling and Development (AMCD) is to provide leadership that promotes research, training/development, and competency for counseling professionals on issues of race, ethnicity, and related cultural concerns.

Intercultural Cancer Council
1720 Dryden, Suite C
Houston, TX 77030
713-798-5383
www.iccnetwork.org

The Intercultural Cancer Council (ICC) promotes policies, programs, partnerships, and research to eliminate the unequal burden of cancer among racial and ethnic minorities and medically underserved populations in the United States and its territories.

National Cancer Institute (NCI)
Cancer Information Service
Building 31, 10A-16
9000 Rockville Pike
Bethesda, MD 20892
800-422-6237
(800-4-CANCER)
www.nci.nih.gov

NCI conducts and coordinates federally funded research on the diagnosis, treatment, and prevention of cancer. Accurate, up-to-date information is provided via the toll-free number. The group also offers printed and technical assistance for community programs and media campaigns. Additional information resources are provided via e-mail.

Cancer Statistics: www-seer.ims.nci.nih.gov
CancerNet: www.nci.nih.gov (patient and physician information)
Grateful Med: http://nlm.nih.gov (search the U.S. National Library of Medicine)
National Cancer Institute's Clinical Trial Search Form: www.cancernet.nci.nih.gov/trialsrch.shtml
Physicians Data Query (PDQ): www.cancernet.nci.nih.gov/pdq.html

National Prostate Cancer Coalition
1158 15th Street, NW
Washington, DC 20005
888-245-9455
www.pcacoalition.org

This advocacy organization is made up of prostate cancer survivors and national, state, and local organizations. Its goal is to build a national grassroots movement that will "press elected officials to increase federal funding for prostate cancer research."

Office of Minority Health Resource Center, Public Health Service U.S. Department of Health and Human Services
P.O. Box 37337
Washington, DC 20013-7337
800-444-6472
www.omhrc.gov

Office offers expert free or low-cost technical assistance to community and professional organizations. Patient and professional information is available on cancer, HIV/AIDS, and other diseases.

Oncology Nursing Society (ONS)
501 Holiday Drive
Pittsburgh, PA 15220-2749
412-921-7373
www.ons.org

Education, research, and oncology nursing care guidelines are some of the many resources available from the Society. ONS is committed to excellence and hosts an annual Congress meeting in the spring, as well as the Institutes of Learning each fall. A complete listing of professional education materials and scholarships are available. The Oncology Nursing Certification Corporation offers testing for oncology nursing certification at the advanced and generalist levels.

Funding Sources

American Cancer Society (ACS)
1599 Clifton Road NE
Atlanta, GA 30329
800-227-2345
www.cancer.org

ACS provides annually for research grants, nursing scholarships, pre- and postdoctoral fellowships, and professorships. Contact the national office for application deadlines.

Avon Breast Cancer Crusade
Avon Women's Health Programs
212-282-5664
www.avon.com

The mission of Avon Breast Cancer Crusade is to provide women, particularly those who are medically underserved, with direct access to breast cancer education and early detection screening services. Funds medical research on breast cancer.

Susan G. Komen Breast Cancer Foundation
5005 LBJ Freeway, Suite 370
Dallas, TX 75244
800-462-9273
www.komen.org

The Foundation awards dissertation research, postdoctoral fellowship, and clinical and basic research grants. Award amounts and periods of funding vary. Annual application deadline is April 1.

National Cancer Institute (NCI)
Cancer Information Service
Building 31, 10A-16
9000 Rockville Pike
Bethesda, MD 20892
800-422-6237
http://deainfo.nci.nih.gov/cmbs/intro.htm

Mentored career development, career transition, research, and training grants are available. The nature and amount of each award and application deadlines vary. Contact NCI for further information.

R.A. Bloch Cancer Foundation
4435 Main Street, Suite 500
Kansas City, MO 64111
1-800-433-0464
www.blochcancer.org

Informational resources, medical second opinions, support groups, and peer counseling are provided to patients with cancer to increase their chances of cancer survival.

ONS Foundation
501 Holiday Drive
Pittsburgh, PA 15220-2749
412-921-7373
www.ons.org

Awards dissertation research, postdoctoral fellowships, clinical and basic research grants.

Patient and Professional Information Resources on the World Wide Web

Association of Cancer Online Resources (ACOR)
www.acor.org

Cancer-related disorders and electronic support groups can be accessed online by patients, families, and healthcare professionals.

The Brain Tumor Society
800-770-8287
www.tbts.org

Information for patients, their families, and healthcare professionals on brain cancer.

Cancer Education
www.cancereducation.com

Educational programs are available to the general public and healthcare professionals on a variety of cancer sites.

Cancer Information Services 800-4-CANCER www.nci.nih.gov	English and Spanish literature is available to the general public on specific cancers and clinical trials.
CANCERLIT®, NCI's International Cancer Information Center http://cnetdb.nci.nih.gov/cancerlit.html	Bibliographic database containing citations and abstracts for reports, journals, doctoral theses, and proceedings.
CanSearch www.cansearch.org	Cancer resources guide developed by the National Coalition for Cancer Survivorship.
Center for Disease Control Tobacco Use Prevention Program, U.S. Department of Health and Human Services www.cdc.gov/tobacco	Focus is on tobacco and smoking, educational programs, and information on smoking cessation for adults and children.
CenterWatch Clinical Trials Listing Service www.centerwatch.com	Clinical trials and new FDA-approved drug therapies are available to patients and health professionals.
International Cancer Alliance www.icare.org	A nonprofit organization that provides information to patients and healthcare professionals on all types of cancer.
International Society of Nurses in Genetics (ISONG) www.nursing.creighton.edu/isong	Nursing specialty organization dedicated to scientific and professional growth of nurses in human genetics.
National Breast Cancer Coalition www.natlbcc.org	The National Breast Cancer Coalition is an advocacy organization dedicated to fighting breast cancer.
The National Center for Complementary and Alternative Medicine (NCCAM) www.nccam.nih.gov	Information on complementary and alternative healing therapies are offered.
National Ovarian Cancer Coalition 888-OVARIAN www.ovarian.org	Education resources and information on ovarian cancer are offered to the public.

National Society of Genetic Counselors www.nsgc.org	Promotes genetic counseling as a part of the healthcare team and offers a network for communication as well as professional education opportunities.
Oncolink www.oncolink.upenn.edu/	Provided by the University of Pennsylvania; offers oncology information for patients, families, and health professionals.
Pharmaceutical Patient Assistance Program www.needymeds.com	Pharmaceutical companies have provided information on how to obtain treatment drugs for patients with cancer.
Social Security Administration 800-772-1213 www.ssa.gov	Information on Social Security benefits and disability can be obtained. Readers are encouraged to call or visit the office near you.
United Ostomy Association, Inc. 800-826-0826 www.uoa.org	Provides support for patients who have intestinal or urinary diversions.
What You Need to Know About Cancer™ http://cancernet.nci.nih.gov/index.html	NCI information service offers consumers a series of publications on cancer.

Cancer Statistics

SEER Program/National Cancer Institute
www-seer.ims.nci.hih.gov

National Center for Health Statistics: FASTATS A-Z
www.cdc.gov/nchawww

The letter *f* after a page number indicates a figure; the letter *t* indicates a table. Page numbers in **boldface** indicate monograph for that agent.

D

J

JCAHO. *See* Joint Commission on Accreditation of Healthcare Organizations
"job-lock," 344
Joint Commission on Accreditation of Healthcare Organizations (JCAHO), on safe handling of cytotoxic agents, 31
judicial law, 282-283

K

Kaposi's sarcoma (KS)
  alitretinoin indicated for, 76
  dactinomycin indicated for, 118
  etoposide indicated for, 142
  liposomal daunorubicin indicated for, 122
  liposomal doxorubicin indicated for, 135
  paclitaxel indicated for, 191
  vinblastine sulfate indicated for, 221
keratinocyte growth factor (KGF), 305
ketoconazole
  docetaxel interaction with, 128
  imatinib mesylate interaction with, 160
  paclitaxel interaction with, 190
  toremifene interaction with, 252
  tretinoin interaction with, 216
KGF (keratinocyte growth factor), 305
Kidney Cancer Association (KCA), 340*t*
kidney cancer, floxuridine indicated for, 146
KS. *See* Kaposi's sarcoma

L

L-asparaginase. *See* asparaginase
latex gloves, 34, 38, 41
latex sensitivity, 41
lavamisole, 5*t*
law. *See also* legal issues; liability
  sources of, 281-283
laxatives, irinotecan interaction with, 163
legal issues. *See also* law; liability
  for cancer survivors, 344-345
  in chemotherapy administration, 281-293
  regarding VAD use, 67
letrozole, 26, 36*t*, **239-240**
leucovorin, 36*t*, **166-169**
  capecitabine interaction with, 95
  as chemosensitizer, 10

fluorouracil interaction with, 148
for MTX toxicity, 24
leukemia
  acute erythroid, mitoxantrone hydrochloride indicated for, 189
  acute lymphocytic (ALL)
    asparaginase indicated for, 85
    cyclophosphamide indicated for, 109
    cytarabine indicated for, 112
    daunorubicin HCl indicated for, 120
    idarubicin indicated for, 156
    mercaptopurine indicated for, 181
    methotrexate indicated for, 186
    pegaspargase indicated for, 194
    pentostatin indicated for, 196
    teniposide indicated for, 208
  acute myelogenous (AML)
    arsenic trioxide indicated for, 83
    asparaginase indicated for, 85
    busulfan indicated for, 94
    cyclophosphamide indicated for, 109
    idarubicin indicated for, 156
    mitoxantrone hydrochloride indicated for, 189
  acute nonlymphocytic (ANLL)
    mercaptopurine indicated for, 181
    remission induction of, cytarabine indicated for, 112
    thioguanine indicated for, 212
  acute promyelocytic (APL)
    arsenic trioxide indicated for, 83
    mitoxantrone hydrochloride indicated for, 189
  chronic myelogenous (CML)
    asparaginase indicated for, 85
    busulfan indicated for, 94
    cyclophosphamide indicated for, 109
    cytarabine indicated for, 112
    hydroxyurea indicated for, 154
    imatinib mesylate indicated for, 161
    mechlorethamine indicated for, 176
    mitomycin indicated for, 188
    doxorubicin HCl indicated for, 132
    floxuridine indicated for, 146
  hairy cell
    cladribine indicated for, 107
    fludarabine phosphate indicated for, 147
    interferon alfa indicated for, 267
    pentostatin indicated for, 196

systems theory, for support group development, 334

T

tamoxifen, 26, 37*t*, **249-250**
tangible social support, 334
Targretin. *See* bexarotene
taste changes, as chemotherapy side effect, 307
taxane, 27
Taxol. *See* paclitaxel
Taxotere. *See* docetaxel
T cell lymphoma
  bexarotene indicated for, 88
  denileukin diftitox indicated for, 125
  pentostatin indicated for, 196
T cells, 3*t*, 4
telophase, of cell cycle, 2*f*, 3, 22
Temodar. *See* temozolomide
temozolomide, 37*t*, **205-207**
Tenckhoff catheter, 62
teniposide, 27, **207-208**
TENS. *See* transcutaneous electrical nerve stimulation
terfenadine, docetaxel interaction with, 128
TESPA. *See* thiotepa
testicular cancer
  bleomycin indicated for, 91
  chlorambucil indicated for, 103
  cisplatin indicated for, 105
  dactinomycin indicated for, 118
  etoposide indicated for, 142
  ifosfamide indicated for, 159
  plicamycin indicated for, 199
  vinblastine sulfate indicated for, 221
  vincristine sulfate indicated for, 223
testolactone, 36*t*
testosterone, **250-252**
testosterone cypionate. *See* testosterone
testosterone enenthate. *See* testosterone
testosterone propionate. *See* testosterone
Testred. *See* testosterone
tetracyclines, methotrexate interaction with, 184
thalidomide, **209-211**
Thalomid. *See* thalidomide
theophylline
  aminoglutethimide interaction with, 227
  nilutamide interaction with, 246

TheraCys. *See* bacillus Calmette-Guérin (BCG) vaccine
thiazide diuretics, toremifene interaction with, 252
thioguanine, 24, 37*t*, **211-212**
  busulfan interaction with, 93
Thioplex. *See* thiotepa
thiotepa, 23, 64, **212-214**
thrombocytopenia, 23, 315-316
  oprelvekin indicated for, 268
thrombolytics, plicamycin interaction with, 198
TICE BCG. *See* bacillus Calmette-Guérin (BCG) vaccine
T lymphocytes, 3*t*, 4
TNF. *See* tumor necrosis factor
Tobacco Use Prevention Program (CDC), 360
tolbutamide, teniposide interaction with, 208
topoisomerase II inhibitors, 25
topotecan
  arthralgias/headaches caused by, 312
  effective during G₂ cell phase, 2
topotecan hydrochloride, **214-215**
toremifene, 26, 37*t*, **252-253**
tort, 285
toxicity
  of alkylating agents, 23
  of antimetabolites, 24
  of biologic agents, 26
  as dose-limiting factor, 10, 25
  of hormonal agents, 26
  of plant alkaloids, 27
transcutaneous electrical nerve stimulation (TENS), for nausea/vomiting, 304
transport, of hazardous drugs, 42
tranylcypromine, altretamine interaction with, 77
trastuzumab, 5*t*, **272-273**
  daunorubicin HCl interaction with, 119
  idarubicin interaction with, 155
  liposomal daunorubicin interaction with, 121
  liposomal doxorubicin interaction with, 134
tretinoin, 37*t*, **215-218**
triazenes, 23
tricyclic antidepressants
  altretamine interaction with, 77

chlorambucil interaction with, 102
procarbazine interaction with, 201
trimethoprim, leucovorin interaction with, 167
trimethoprim toxicity, leucovorin indicated for, 168
Trisenox. *See* arsenic trioxide
troleandomycin, docetaxel interaction with, 128
trophoblastic tumors, dactinomycin indicated for, 118
tumor burden, effect on chemotherapy response, 9-10
tumor heterogeneity, effect on chemotherapy response, 10
tumor-infiltrating lymphocytes (TILs), 5*t*
tumor necrosis factor (TNF), 5*t*
tumor response criteria, 9, 323-324
tunneled apheresis catheter, 51
tunneled central venous catheters, 50*f*, 50-51, 51*f*, 56*t*
tyramine, foods containing, procarbazine interaction with, 201

U

United Ostomy Association, Inc. (UOA), 342*t*, 361
United States Pharmacopoeia (USP), 292
uric acid, mechlorethamine-induced increase in, 175
US TOO International, Inc., 339*t*

V

VADs. *See* vascular access devices
Valergen. *See* estradiol
valproic acid
plicamycin interaction with, 198
temozolomide interaction with, 205
valrubicin, **218-219**
Valstar. *See* valrubicin
vascular access devices (VADs), 38, 47-70. *See also specific catheter types*
comparison of, 56*t*-57*t*
documentation for use, 65-66
future research on, 67-68
history of, 47-48
liability issues and, 67
Velban. *See* vinblastine sulfate
VePesid. *See* etoposide
verapamil, as chemosensitizer, 10
Vesanoid. *See* tretinoin

vesicant chemotherapeutic agents, 38, 39*t*, 291-292
Viadur (leuprolide acetate implant). *See* leuprolide
vidarabine, pentostatin interaction with, 195
vinblastine, 27, 39*t*
vinblastine sulfate, **220-221**
vinca alkaloids, 39*t*
mitomycin interaction with, 187
myalgias caused by, 312
peripheral neuropathy caused by, 311-312
vincaleukoblastine sulfate. *See* vinblastine sulfate
Vincasar PFS. *See* vincristine sulfate
Vincrex. *See* vincristine sulfate
vincristine, 27, 39*t*
asparaginase interaction with, 84
myalgias caused by, 312
peripheral neuropathy caused by, 311-312
vincristine sulfate, **221-223**
vindesine, 39*t*
vinorelbine, 39*t*
cranial nerve neuropathy caused by, 312
myalgias caused by, 312
myelosuppression caused by, 313
vinorelbine tartrate, **223-225**
Virilon. *See* testosterone
vitamin D, plicamycin interaction with, 198
VM-26. *See* teniposide
vomiting center, 298*f*, 298-299
vomiting/nausea, 297-304, 298*f*, 299*t*
assessment, 300
nonpharmacologic strategies for, 303-304
patterns of, 300
pharmacologic management of, 301-303
risk factors for, 299*t*, 299-300
VP-16. *See* etoposide
Vumon. *See* teniposide

W

Waldenstrom's macroglobulinemia
cladribine indicated for, 107
melphalan indicated for, 178
warfarin
aminoglutethimide interaction with, 227
bicalutamide interaction with, 230